Bioactive Natural Products in Drug Discovery

Bioactive Natural Products in Drug Discovery

Editor: Scarlet Mount

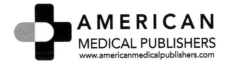

AMERICAN
MEDICAL PUBLISHERS
www.americanmedicalpublishers.com

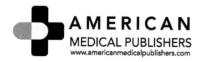

Cataloging-in-Publication Data

Bioactive natural products in drug discovery / edited by Scarlet Mount.
    p. cm.
Includes bibliographical references and index.
ISBN 978-1-63927-917-3
1. Drugs--Design. 2. Drug development. 3. Natural products. 4. Materia medica, Vegetable.
5. Bioactive compounds. 6. Medical microbiology. 7. Pharmaceutical chemistry. I. Mount, Scarlet.
RS420 .B56 2023
615.19--dc23

American Medical Publishers,
41 Flatbush Avenue,
1st Floor, New York,
NY 11217, USA

ISBN 978-1-63927-917-3 (Hardback)

Contents

Preface

A bioactive compound is a type of chemical that can be found in plants and specific foods including nuts, whole grains, fruits, oils and vegetables in small amounts. The actions of bioactive compounds in the body can encourage good health. These compounds are studied in pharmaceutical sciences to treat a variety of medical conditions. Tannins, lycopene, lignan, indoles and resveratrol are few examples of bioactive compounds. Natural products derived from bacteria, marine life, plants, fungi, animals and other organisms are a valuable resource for drug discovery and development. Bioactive natural products have a wide range of biological activities that are beneficial to human health, such as anti-inflammatory, anticancer, antibiotic, biofilm inhibitory effects, antifungal, and immunosuppressive properties. Different natural products from both terrestrial and marine organisms have been identified and characterized, as these products have unique chemical structures and noteworthy biological functions. This book aims to understand the role of bioactive natural products in drug discovery. Researchers and students engaged in drug discovery will be assisted by it.

The researches compiled throughout the book are authentic and of high quality, combining several disciplines and from very diverse regions from around the world. Drawing on the contributions of many researchers from diverse countries, the book's objective is to provide the readers with the latest achievements in the area of research. This book will surely be a source of knowledge to all interested and researching the field.

In the end, I would like to express my deep sense of gratitude to all the authors for meeting the set deadlines in completing and submitting their research chapters. I would also like to thank the publisher for the support offered to us throughout the course of the book. Finally, I extend my sincere thanks to my family for being a constant source of inspiration and encouragement.

Editor

Synthesis of a Novel α-Glucosyl Ginsenoside F1 by Cyclodextrin Glucanotransferase and its In Vitro Cosmetic Applications

Seong Soo Moon [1,†], **Hye Jin Lee** [1,†], **Ramya Mathiyalagan** [2], **Yu Jin Kim** [1], **Dong Uk Yang** [1,3], **Dae Young Lee** [4], **Jin Woo Min** [1], **Zuly Jimenez** [2] and **Deok Chun Yang** [1,2,*]

[1] Department of Oriental Medicinal Biotechnology, College of Life Science, Kyung Hee University, 1 Seocheon-dong, Giheung-gu, Yongin-si, Gyeonggi-do 17104, Korea; ssm8656@hanmail.net (S.S.M.); serendipity27@nate.com (H.J.L.); yujinkim@khu.ac.kr (Y.J.K.); rudckfeo23@naver.com (D.U.Y.); hero304@khu.ac.kr (J.W.M.)

[2] Graduate School of Biotechnology, College of Life Science, Kyung Hee University, 1 Seocheon-dong, Giheung-gu, Yongin-si, Gyeonggi-do 17104, Korea; ramyabinfo@gmail.com (R.M.); zejp78@gmail.com (Z.J.)

[3] K-gen (corp), 218, Gajeong-ro, Yuseong-gu, Daejeon 34129, Korea

[4] Department of Herbal Crop Research, National Institute of Horticultural and Herbal Science, RDA, Eumseong 27709, Korea; dylee0809@gmail.com

* Correspondence: dcyang@khu.ac.kr;

† These authors contributed equally to this work.

Abstract: Ginsenosides from *Panax ginseng* (Korean ginseng) are unique triterpenoidal saponins that are considered to be responsible for most of the pharmacological activities of *P. ginseng*. However, the various linkage positions cause different pharmacological activities. In this context, we aimed to synthesize new derivatives of ginsenosides with unusual linkages that show enhanced pharmacological activities. Novel α-glycosylated derivatives of ginsenoside F1 were synthesized from transglycosylation reactions of dextrin (sugar donor) and ginsenoside F1 (acceptor) by the successive actions of Toruzyme®3.0L, a cyclodextrin glucanotransferase. One of the resultant products was isolated and identified as (20S)-3β,6α,12β-trihydroxydammar-24ene-(20-O-β-D-glucopyranosyl-(1→2)-α-D-glucopyranoside) by various spectroscopic characterization techniques of fast atom bombardment-mass spectrometry (FAB-MS), infrared spectroscopy (IR), proton-nuclear magnetic resonance (^{1}H-NMR), ^{13}C-NMR, gradient heteronuclear single quantum coherence (gHSQC), and gradient heteronuclear multiple bond coherence (gHMBC). As expected, the novel α-glycosylated ginsenoside F1 (G1-F1) exhibited increased solubility, lower cytotoxicity toward human dermal fibroblast cells (HDF), and higher tyrosinase activity and ultraviolet A (UVA)-induced inhibitory activity against matrix metalloproteinase-1 (MMP-1) than ginsenoside F1. Since F1 has been reported as an antiaging and antioxidant agent, the enhanced efficacies of the novel α-glycosylated ginsenoside F1 suggest that it might be useful in cosmetic applications after screening.

Keywords: cyclodextrin glycosyltransferase; cyclodextrin glycosyltransferase (CGTase); ginsenoside F1; α-glucosyl ginsenoside F1

1. Introduction

Ginseng saponins, referred to as ginsenosides, are one of the major bioactive substances of *Panax ginseng* Meyer, a commonly used traditional herbal medicine in Korea, China, and Japan. Ginsenosides have been reported to have antifatigue and antioxidant activities, improve brain function, enhance stamina, and regulate blood circulation with approval from the Korea Food and Drug Administration (KFDA), in addition to various other pharmacological activities including anticancer [1,2], anti-inflammation [3], and antidiabetes [1,4] functions. These various pharmacological activities of ginsenosides typically depend on the types of sugar moieties and the position and linkage of their attachment [4,5]. More than 289 distinct saponins had been identified from different *Panax* sp. up to 2012 [6], and these compounds show different biological activities based on structural differences [3].

Ginsenosides are mainly classified as protopanaxadiol-type (PPD), protopanaxatriol-type (PPT), and oleanane-type saponins and further grouped into major and minor saponins based on the position and linkages of sugar moieties. The minor saponins, which are ginsenoside metabolites, are responsible for most of the pharmacological activities of ginseng which include ginsenoside F1, Rh1, compound K, and Rh2 [7]. These ginsenosides are mainly absorbed into systemic circulation [8]. Ginsenoside F1 is a minor saponin from the leaf of *P. ginseng* that was reported to have skin whitening activity [9], modulate skin diseases [10], and function as an antiaging and antioxidant agent [11], suggesting that it might be a candidate for cosmetic applications.

Synthesis of novel and diversified compounds is a way to extend the efficacy of natural products. Such diversity can be generated by biosynthetic reactions such as glucosylation [12,13]. Especially, enzymatic glycosylation provides more regioselectiveness than conventional chemical synthesis [14]. A number of reports have suggested that transglycosylation by enzymes can be used to improve physiochemical functions such as taste, solubility in water, and oxidative stability of numerous active substances [15,16]. Among these enzymes, cyclodextrin glycosyltransferase (CGTase, 1,4-α-D-glucan: 1,4-α-D-glycopyranosyltransferase, cyclizing, EC 2.4.1.19) [17] has been reported to accelerate reactions between natural products and starch hydrolysate or β-cyclodextrin to produce glucosylated modifications of natural compounds such as hesperidin, glycosylglycerol [14,16] rutin [18], and steroidal saponins [19].

Although the beta isomer was prominent, the alpha isomer has attracted much attention in recent years. The increased solubility of hesperidin [16,18] and decreased bitterness of glycosylated stevioside [15] by CGTase was reported. Other studies reported the mild sweet taste with no odor, no tongue-pricking, and increased stability of O-α-glucosylthiamin compared with thiamin hydrochloride [20] and the powerful skin whitening activity of alpha arbutin [21] compared with beta arbutin [22] as a result of glycosylation by CGTase.

In this study, we aimed to synthesize the unusual alpha glycosylated ginsenoside F1 by a reaction involving ginsenoside F1, dextrin, and CGTase. One of the resultant novel compounds was purified, and the structure was elucidated by various nuclear magnetic resonance (NMR) spectra and Fourier-transform infrared spectroscopy (FTIR). We also evaluated the cytotoxicity and protective effect of α-glycosylated ginsenoside F1 against ultraviolet (UV) damage by measuring matrix metalloproteinase-1 (MMP-1) expression in human dermal fibroblast cells. In addition, the in vitro antityrosinase activity of α-glycosylated ginsenoside F1 was evaluated against mushroom tyrosinase.

2. Materials and Methods

2.1. Materials

Ginsenosides compound K (CK), Rh2, Rh1, F1, aglycone PPD (aPPD), and aglycone PPT (aPPT) were obtained from the laboratory of Hanbangbio, Kyung Hee University, South Korea. Toruzyme 3.0L (the crude enzyme of CGTase) obtained from Novozymes, China, was extracted from *Thermoanaerobacter* sp. Dextrin was supplied by Fluka Chemie AG (Buchs, Switzerland), and all the other chemicals used were of analytical grade and from commercial sources.

2.2. Biotransformation

The preliminary screening of glycosylation was carried out as the method of Wang et al., 2010 [19]. Different ginsenosides, CK (1.6 mM, 1 eq), Rh2 (1.6 mM, 1 eq), Rh1 (1.56 mM,1 eq), F1 (1.56 mM, 1 eq), aPPD (2.17 mM), and aPPT (2.09 mM) together with the sugar donor dextrin (9.9mM, 6 eq, 10–15 units of glucose) were dissolved in 20 mM sodium phosphate buffer (1 mL, pH 7.0). Next, 25 µL of Toruzyme® 3.0L with initial activity of 3.0 KNU (kilo novo units)/g [17] was added to the reaction mixture and reacted at 50 °C for 2 h. and kept in boiling water for 5 min to inactivate the enzyme. The mixture was extracted three times with an equal volume of *n*-butanol, and the *n*-butanol layer was washed twice with distilled water to remove excess dextrin, dried in a rotary evaporator under vacuum [19], and dissolved in methanol for thin-layer chromatography (TLC).

2.3. Glycosylation of Ginsenoside F1

For further experimental analysis, F1 was used as a substrate. The effects of different concentrations of dextrin (0–7 mg) and Toruzyme® (5–30 μL) and different reaction durations (0.5–3 h) on specificity of F1 glycosylation were examined using the procedure described above. For purification of glycosylated F1, F1 (500 mg, 1.56 mM, 1 eq) and dextrin (2g, 7.92 mM, 5 eq) were dissolved in 500 mL of 20 mM sodium phosphate buffer and then treated with 15 mL of Toruzyme® 3.0 L.

2.4. Identification of Glycosylated Ginsenoside F1

Semiqualitative screening of the glycosylated products was carried out by TLC and high-performance liquid chromatography (HPLC) was carried out by Ramya et al., 2015 and Quan et al., 2012 [13,23] with slight modifications. TLC was performed with silica gel plates (60 F254, Merck, Darmstadt, Germany) using the developing solvent $CHCl_3:CH_3OH:H_2O$ (65:35:10, *v/v*, lower phase). The TLC plates were dried, dipped in 10% H_2SO_4, and air dried with heating at 110 to 120 °C. The HPLC analysis was carried out on an Agilent 1260 series with a C_{18} (250 × 4.6 mm, ID 5 μm) column using distilled water as solvent A and acetonitrile as solvent B mobile phases. The following gradient was used: A:B ratios of 80.5:19.5 for 0–29 min, 70:30 for 29–36 min, 68:32 for 36–45 min, 66:34 for 45–47 min, 64.5:35.5 for 47–49 min, 0:100 for 49–61 min, and 80.5:19.5 for 61–66 min with a flow rate of 1.6 mL/min. The sample was detected at a wavelength of 203 nm.

2.5. Nuclear Magnetic Resonance Analysis

Structural elucidation of the new compound by NMR spectra (^1H NMR, ^{13}C NMR, gHSQC (heteronuclear single quantum correlation) and heteronuclear multiple bond correlation (gHMBC)) were performed using a Varian Unity INOVA AS 400 FT-NMR spectrometer (Varian, Palo Alto, CA, USA), and chemical shifts were expressed in δ (ppm), with tetramethylsilane (TMS) used as an internal standard. The dimethyl sulfoxide-d_6 (DMSO-d_6) was used as a solvent. Melting points were obtained using a Fisher-John's melting point apparatus. Optical rotations were measured on a JASCO P-1010 digital polarimeter. Infrared spectra were obtained on a Perkin Elmer Spectrum One FTIR spectrometer (Perkin-Elmer, Walthanm, MA, USA). High resolution fast-atom bombardment mass spectrometry (HR-FAB/MS) were recorded using a JEOL JMS-700 (JEOL, Tokyo, Japan) mass spectrometer.

2.6. Cell Lines and Cell Culture

Human dermal fibroblasts (HDF) were purchased from the Korean Cell Line Bank (Seoul, Korea). The cells were grown in Dulbecco's modified essential media (DMEM) supplemented with 10% fetal bovine serum (FBS) and 1% penicillin–streptomycin at 37 °C in a humidified atmosphere containing 95% air and 5% CO_2.

2.6.1. Ultraviolet Irradiation and Sample Treatment

A high-pressure metal halide lamp (UVASUN 3000, Mutzhas, Munich, Germany) emitting wavelengths in the range of 340 to 450 nm was used as a UV source. Human dermal fibroblasts cells were seeded at 4 × 10 cell/dish in 60-mm culture dishes for 24 h. Prior to UV irradiation, cells were washed twice with phosphate buffer saline (PBS), and the medium was replaced with 1 mL of PBS. The incident dose at the surface of the cells was 66 mW/s. The spectral distribution of the

UVASUN 3000 source was determined with a Beckman UV 5270 spectrophotometer (Beckman, Munich, Germany, FRG).

2.6.2. Cytotoxicity Assay

Human dermal fibroblasts cells were cultured at a density of 1×10^4 cells/well in 96-well flat-bottomed plates in a 5% CO_2 humidified atmosphere at 37 °C. After 24 h of culture, the medium was exchanged with medium containing different concentrations of ginsenoside F1 (F1) and α-glycosylated ginsenoside F1 (Glycosylated F1), and the cells were incubated for a further 24 h. Cell viability was determined by the 3-(4,5-dimethylthiazol-2-yl)-2,5-diphenyltetrazolium bromide (MTT) assay [24] with slight modification. Briefly, 10 µL of MTT solution (5 mg/mL) was added to each well and incubated for 4 h. After removal of MTT, the cells were lysed with 100 µL DMSO, and absorbance was measured at 570 nm using a microplate reader (Bio-Tek Instruments, Winooski, VT, USA).

2.6.3. In Vitro Tyrosinase Inhibition Activity

Tyrosinase from *Agricus bisporus* (mushroom) was purchased from Sigma Chemicals Co. (St Louis, MO, USA). Inhibition of tyrosinase activity was measured as previously described [22]. L-DOPA (3-(3,4-dihydroxyphenyl)-L-alanine, 0.83 or 3.3 mM) was used as the substrate, and 600 units of tyrosinase was added in the presence or absence of F1, glycosylated F1, or arbutin. The absorbance was measured at 475 nm in a microplate reader (Bio-Tek Instruments, Winooski, VT, USA).

2.6.4. Assay for Inhibition of Matrix Metalloproteinase-1 Expression

Matrix metalloproteinase-1 (MMP-1) level was quantified using a sandwich ELISA Quantikine total human MMP-1 kit (R&D Systems Inc., Minneapolis, MN, USA) After UV irradiation, HDF cells were cultured in DMEM with F1, and glycosylated F1, or ((−)-*cis*-3,3',4',5,5',7-hexahydroxy-flavane-3-gallate) (EGCG) as a positive control. The culture supernatants were harvested, and MMP-1 was measured according to the manufacturer's instructions. Absorbance was measured at 490 nm in a microplate reader microplate reader (Bio-Tek Instruments, Winooski, VT, USA).

3. Results and Discussion

3.1. Biotransformation of Minor Ginsenosides by Cyclodextrin glycosyltransferase (CGTase)

Among the major ginsenosides, Rb1, Rc, Re, and Rg1 have already been used as substrates for the synthesis of series of new α-glycosylginsenosides through transglycosylation [13,25,26]. However, after oral administration, the major ginsenosides were converted into minor ginsenosides by intestinal microflora. Therefore, we used minor ginsenosides CK, Rh2, F1, Rh1, aPPD, and aPPT as acceptors with dextrin as a sugar donor during CGTase enzyme transglycosylation. As a result, CK, Rh2, F1, and Rh1 yielded new transglycosylated compounds with different retention factor (R_f) values compared with known ginsenoside standards (Figure S1). Among these, PPT type ginsenosides Rh1 and F1 showed more glycosylated products, possibly due to the glucose attached to α-OH at C-6 and another –OH at C-20 of the dammerendiol steroidal aglycone. We chose F1 for further studies because of the distinct separation of glycosylated products in addition to its previous reported application in cosmetics and skin care. PPD and PPT aglycone did not generate glycosylated products, indicating that sugar molecules are primarily involved in transglycosylation.

3.2. Specificity of Transglycosylation of Ginsenoside F1

Even though the effects of various factors on transglycosylation by Toruzyme were already reported [19,27], this should be validated for the effective synthesis of new compounds. Therefore, the effects of different concentrations of dextrin and CGTase (Toruzyme) on the degree of glycosylation were investigated by HPLC. As shown in Figure S2a, the 5:1 *w/w* ratio of dextrin: F1 showed the highest yield. There was no significant difference for greater than five volumes, and it was difficult to separate saponin after biotransformation due to the combined extraction of sugar with saponin in the recovery process. In addition, increasing the amount of enzyme rapidly increased the yield up to 20 µL of enzyme with 1 mg of F1 and 5 mg of dextrin, as determined by HPLC (Figure S2b).

3.3. Transglycosylation Analysis of Ginsenoside F1

The glycosylation of F1 with dextrin and CGTase for different time durations yielded several new spots that appeared below F1 on TLC (Figure S3). The reaction products were washed several times with water to remove the unreacted excess sugar molecules. The six new spots (G1–F1, G2–F1, G3–F1, G4–F1, G5–F1, and G6–F1) under ginsenoside F1 on TLC (Figure 1a) and the corresponding peaks (G1–F1, G2–F1, G3–F1, G4–F1, G5–F1, and G6–F1), other than ginsenoside F1 on HPLC analysis (Figure 1b), were considered new glycosylated products from F1. G1–F1 (R_f = 0.53) on TLC was isolated as a pure form by silica gel chromatography and elution with $CHCl_3/CH_3OH$ (9:1). The yield of compound G1–F1 was 12% (74 mg) and the structure was identified by ^{1}H-NMR, ^{13}C-NMR, and two-dimensional (2D) NMR and by correlations with the HSQC and HMBC spectra. The low percentage of yield is due to the formation of other products (G2–F1, G3F1, G4–F1, G5–F1, and G6–F1).

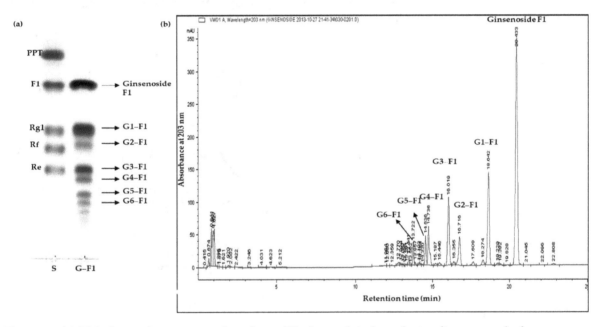

Figure 1. (a) Thin layer chromatography of new F1 glycosylated products after removal of excess sugar. (b) High-performance liquid chromatography (HPLC) analysis of F1 and various glycosylated products after reaction. G1–F1, compound **1**; G2–F1, compound **2**; G3–F1, compound **3**; G4–F1, compound **4**; G5–F1, compound **5**; G6–F1, compound **6**.

Compound **1** (G1–F1) was obtained as a white powder. The molecular formula of G1–F1 was determined to be $C_{42}H_{72}O_{14}$ from the pseudomolecule ion peak m/z 799.4843 [M-H]$^-$ in negative high-resolution fast atom bombardment-mass spectrometry (FAB-MS). The infrared spectrum showed strong absorbance from hydroxyl groups (3366 cm^{-1}) and a double bond (1650 cm^{-1}) in G1–F1 (Figure S4). In the ^{1}H NMR spectrum, proton signals of one olefin methine (δ_H 5.30, dd, J = 6.0, 6.4 Hz, H-24), three oxygenated methines (δ_H 3.48, H-3; 4.10, H-12; 4.38, H-6), and eight singlet methyls (δ_H 1.98 (H-28), 1.58 (H-26), 1.56 (H-27), 1.55 (H-21), 1.45 (H-29), 1.08 (H-18), 1.01 (H-19), 0.98 (H-30)) were observed, indicating that G1–F1 has a protopanaxatriol-type triterpene moiety. Proton signals due to the sugar moiety, two anomeric proton signals at δ_H 5.81 (d, J = 3.6 Hz, H-1″) and 5.04 (d, J = 8.0 Hz, H-1′), and several oxygenated methines and methylene proton signals at δ_H 3.72~4.56 were observed (Figure S5a). The ^{13}C NMR spectrum of G1–F1 (Figure S5b) exhibited 42 carbon signals due to a triterpene with two hexoses. An olefin quaternary carbon signal at δ_C 131.0 (C-25), one olefin methine carbon signal at δ_C 125.9 (C-24), one oxygenated quaternary carbon signal at 83.5 (C-20), three oxygenated methine carbon signals (δ_C 78.6 (C-3), 67.8 (C-6), 70.2 (C-12)), and eight methyl carbon signals (δ_C 32.0 (C-28), 25.7 (C-26), 22.3 (C-21), 17.8 (C-18), 17.6 (C-19), 17.5 (C-27, 30), 16.3 (C-29)) were observed for the protopanaxatriol-type aglycone moiety. The chemical shifts of the sugar moieties signal (δ_C 98.1 (C-1'), 81.2 (C-2'), 78.5 (C-3'), 76.6 (C-5'), 75.5 (C-4'), 62.1 (C-6')) suggested the presence of a glucopyranoside. The coupling constant of the anomeric proton signal (δ_H 5.04, H-1') was 8.0 Hz, confirming β-D-glucopyranoside. Another sugar moiety (δ_C 103.0 (C-1''), 75.2 (C-3''), 74.6 (C-2''), 74.4 (C-5''), 71.9 (C-4''), 62.8 (C-6'')) suggested the presence of glucopyranoside; the coupling constant of the anomeric proton signal (δ_H 5.81, H-1'') was 3.6 Hz, confirming that the glucopyranose had a α-glucosidic linkage. The connection between the β-D-glucopyranosyl unit (C-1') and the C-20 of the aglycone and that of another α-D-glucopyranosyl unit (C-1'') with C-2' of the inner glucose was verified by the cross-peaks observed between the anomer proton signal at δ_H 5.04 (H-1') and the oxygenated quaternary carbon signal at δ_C 83.5 (C-20) and between the anomer proton signal at δ_H 5.81 (H-1'') and the oxygenated methine carbon signal at δ_C 81.2 (C-2') in the HMBC spectrum, respectively (Figure S5c,d). This was confirmed by the downfield shifts of the carbon (δ_C 78.5 (C-3')) and proton signals (δ_H 4.53 (H-3')) due to the glycosylation effect. Ultimately, the structure of G1-F1 was determined to be (20S)-3β,6α,12β -trihydroxydammar-24-ene-(20-O-β-D-glucopyranosyl-(1→2)-α-D-glucopyranoside), which has not been reported previously (Figure 2).

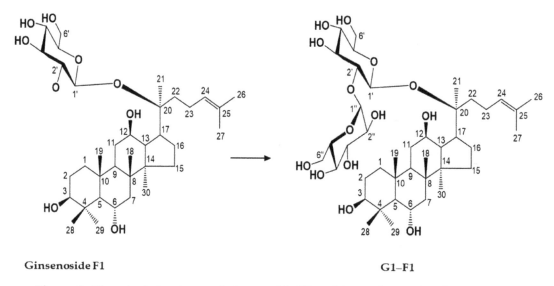

Ginsenoside F1   G1–F1

Figure 2. Chemical structures of ginsenoside F1 and its α-glycosylated F1 (G1–F1).

3.4. Characterization of Novel α-Glycosylated Ginsenoside F1

Water Solubility of Ginsenoside F1 and Novel α-Glycosylated Ginsenoside F1

Transglycosylation reactions catalyzed by CGTase are an efficient method to enhance the water solubility of various compounds [16,18,28]. Accordingly, the water solubility of α-glycosylated ginsenoside F1 was higher than that of F1 alone (data not shown). The soluble α-glycosylated ginsenoside F1 should not only facilitate investigation of the pharmacological activities of ginsenoside F1, but also may be useful as a cosmetics ingredient.

3.5. Cell Cytotoxicity

3.5.1. Comparison of Cell Viability of Ginsenoside F1 and Novel α-Glycosylated Ginsenoside F1 in Human Dermal Fibroblast Cells

To evaluate the effects of α-glycosylated ginsenoside F1 and ginsenoside F1 on the cell viability of HDFs, the cells were treated with different concentrations. Ginsenoside F1 reduced the cell viability of HDFs to a greater extent than α-glycosylated ginsenoside F1 (G1–F1) in a dose-dependent manner

(Figure 3). The α-glycosylated ginsenoside F1 showed lower toxicity toward HDFs than ginsenoside F1 up to a concentration of 5 mg/mL. The cell viability was greater than 90% of that of the control cells up to 2 mg/mL. These results showed that ginsenoside F1 and α-glycosylated ginsenoside F1 have no significant cytotoxicity against skin cells. Thus, the inhibitory effect of these compounds on collagenase expression was not due to cytotoxicity of these compounds at concentrations up to 2 mg/mL.

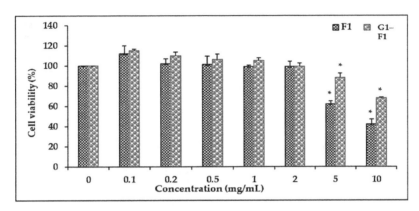

Figure 3. Cytotoxicity of ginsenoside F1 and α-glycosylated ginsenoside F1 in human dermal fibroblast cells. Cells were preincubated with or without compounds for 24 h, and cell viability was evaluated by 3-(4,5-dimethylthiazol-2-yl)-2,5-diphenyltetrazolium bromide (MTT) assay. Data represent the mean ± SD (standard deviation) of triplicate experiments. * $p < 0.05$ compared with the control. F1: ginsenoside F1; G1–F1: α-glycosylated ginsenoside F1.

3.5.2. Inhibition of Tyrosinase Activity by Ginsenoside F1 and G1–F1

To investigate the tyrosinase inhibitory activity of G1–F1, the half maximal inhibitory concentration (IC50) values against mushroom tyrosinase were measured. The tyrosinase inhibitory activity of α-glycosylated ginsenoside F1 was higher than that of ginsenoside F1 but weaker than that of arbutin (Figure 4).

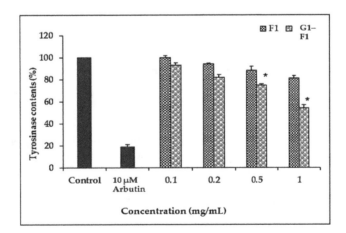

Figure 4. Inhibitory effects of ginsenoside F1 and α-glycosylated ginsenoside F1 on Mushroon tyrosinase activity. Tyrosinase activity was measured using 3.3 mM L-DOPA as a substrate. Results are expressed as the percentage of inhibition by ginsenoside F1 and α-glycosylated compound. Arbutin was used as a positive control. Data represent the mean ± SD of triplicate experiments. * $p < 0.05$ compared with the control. F1: ginsenoside F1; G1–F1: α-glycosylated ginsenoside F1.

It was previously reported that F1 can function as an anti-aging and antioxidant agent [11] and as a drug against skin cancer with antiproliferation and whitening functions [10]. Comparison of the inhibition of tyrosinase activity showed that α-glycosylated ginsenoside F1 had a greater inhibitory effect on tyrosinase activity than ginsenoside F1, indicating that α-glycosylated ginsenoside F1 might be an efficacious anti-tyrosinase agent for use in cosmetics.

3.5.3. Inhibition of Ultraviolet A (UVA)-Induced Matrix Metalloproteinase- (MMP-1) Expression of Ginsenoside F1 and G1–F1

Skin aging occurs as a result of collagen degradation through induction of MMPs by UV irradiation [29]. The α-glycosylated ginsenoside F1 exhibited a greater inhibitory effect against collagenase (MMP-1) than the ginsenoside F1 after UVA irradiation of HDF cell lines (Figure 5), indicating that the C-3-hydroxyl group in the compounds is important for inhibitory activity. (−)-*cis*-3,3′,4′,5,5′,7-Hexahydroxy-flavane-3-gallate (EGCG) was used as a positive control.

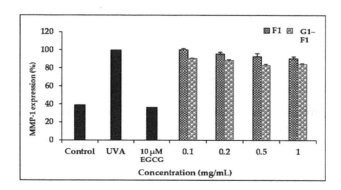

Figure 5. Inhibitory effects of ginsenoside F1 and α-glycosylated ginsenoside F1 on the expression of MMP-1 in UVA-irradiated human dermal fibroblasts. The cells were cultured in the presence of ginsenoside F1 and α-glycosylated ginsenoside F1 (0–1 mg/mL) for 24 h and subjected to ELISA. The results were expressed as the average ± SD of triplicate determinations. * $p < 0.05$ compared with UVA irradiation. F1: ginsenoside F1; G1–F1: α-glycosylated ginsenoside F1.

In addition to the number of sugars, their linkage positions and alpha vs. beta linkages affect pharmacological activities. For example, ginsenoside F1 and Rh1 have the same number of sugar moieties and the same molecular weight but different glucose attachment positions at C-20 and C-6, respectively. F1 showed significantly greater inhibition of viability than Rh1 in prostate cancer cell lines [30]. The glycosylation and nano formulations of ginseng saponins [13,25,26,31–33] and other steroidal saponins [19,27] has recently attracted increased interest.

The alpha isomers of glucose also exhibited significant activity, especially stronger inhibitory activity of α-arbutin on tyrosinase compared with β-arbutin [22]. Similarly, in comparison with the common beta isomers of glucose in ginsenosides, α-glycosyl ginsenoside was reported to have a reduced bitter taste [26], suggesting its potential as an additive in food products.

4. Conclusions

This study describes for the first time the glycosylation of ginsenoside F1 by CGTase and identification of a novel α-glucosylated F1 with an unusual α-D-glcp-(1→2)-β-D-glcp sugar chain (G1–F1). The novel compound G1–F1 showed lower cytotoxicity and stronger inhibitory activity against tyrosinase and collagenase (MMP-1) than ginsenoside F1. This novel G1–F1 may be a potential pharmacological active compound. A single α-glucosylated F1 was purified in this study, and other new glycosylated spots remain to be characterized.

Supplementary Materials:
Figure S1: TLC analysis of transglycosylation of minor ginsenosides (Rh2, CK, PPD, Rh1, F1, PPT). S, standard; (i) Each ginsenoside with CGTase only and (ii) Each ginsenoside with CGTase and dextrin, Figure S2. (a). Effect of dextrin on transglycosylation of ginsenoside F1. Toruzyme® (20 μL) was incubated with ginsenoside F1 (1 mg) in 1 mL of 20 mM sodium phosphate buffer at 60 ± 1 °C for 2 h, (b). Effect of Toruzyme® on transglycosylation of ginsenoside F1. Toruzyme® (5–30 μL) was incubated with ginsenoside F1 (1 mg) and dextrin (5 mg) in 1 mL of 20 mM sodium phosphate buffer at 60 ± 1°C for 2 h. The yield was calculated as the increase in product by HPLC, Figure S3: TLC analysis of transglycosylation of ginsenoside F1 with Toruzyme® and dextrin at different times (min). S, standard of higher molecular weight ginsenosides than F1 in the same protopanaxatriol type ginsenosides; F1+toru (Control 1): Ginsenoside F1 and CGTase Toruzyme enzyme alone; Dextrin+toru (Control 2): Dextrin (sugar donor) and CGTase Toruzyme enzyme alone, Figure S4. (a). Infrared spectrum (FTIR) of novel α-glycosylated ginsenoside F1 (G1–F1), Figure S5. (a). ^{1}H-NMR spectrum of novel α-glycosylated ginsenoside F1 (G1–F1). (b). ^{13}C-NMR spectrum of novel α-glycosylated ginsenoside F1 (G1–F1). (c). gHSQC spectrum of novel α-glycosylated ginsenoside F1 (G1–F1). (d). Key gHMBC spectrum of novel α-glycosylated ginsenoside F1 (G1–F1).

Author Contributions: Conceptualization—H.J.L. and R.M.; Methodology—S.S.M., H.J.L., and J.W.M.; Validation—D.Y.L., Resources—Y.J.K.; Writing—original draft preparation—S.S.M., and H.J.L.; Writing—review, and editing—R.M. and Z.J.; Funding Acquisition—D.U.Y. and D.C.Y.; Project Administration and Supervision—D.C.Y.

Acknowledgments: This research was supported by a grant from the Korea Institute of Planning & Evaluation for Technology in Food, Agriculture, Forestry, & Fisheries (KIPET NO: 317007-3), Republic of Korea.

References

1. Wong, A.S.; Che, C.M.; Leung, K.W. Recent advances in ginseng as cancer therapeutics: A functional and mechanistic overview. *Nat. Prod. Rep.* **2015**, *32*, 256–272. [CrossRef] [PubMed]

2. Mathiyalagan, R.; Subramaniyam, S.; Kim, Y.J.; Kim, Y.C.; Yang, D.C. Ginsenoside compound K-bearing glycol chitosan conjugates: Synthesis, physicochemical characterization, and in vitro biological studies. *Carbohydr. Polym.* **2014**, *112*, 359–366. [CrossRef] [PubMed]

3. Ahn, S.; Siddiqi, M.H.; Noh, H.-Y.; Kim, Y.-J.; Kim, Y.-J.; Jin, C.-G.; Yang, D.-C. Anti-inflammatory activity of ginsenosides in LPS-stimulated RAW 264.7 cells. *Sci. Bull.* **2015**, *60*, 773–784. [CrossRef]

4. Wee, J.J.; Mee Park, K.; Chung, A.S. Biological activities of ginseng and its application to human health. In *Herbal Medicine: Biomolecular and Clinical Aspects*, 2nd ed.; Benzie, I.F.F., Wachtel-Galor, S., Eds.; CRC Press: Boca Raton, FL, USA, 2011.

5. Sathishkumar, N.; Sathiyamoorthy, S.; Ramya, M.; Yang, D.U.; Lee, H.N.; Yang, D.C. Molecular docking studies of anti-apoptotic BCL-2, BCL-XL, and MCL-1 proteins with ginsenosides from *Panax ginseng*. *J. Enzyme Inhib. Med. Chem.* **2012**, *27*, 685–692. [CrossRef] [PubMed]

6. Yang, W.Z.; Hu, Y.; Wu, W.Y.; Ye, M.; Guo, D.A. Saponins in the genus *Panax* L. (Araliaceae): A systematic review of their chemical diversity. *Phytochemistry* **2014**, *106*, 7–24. [CrossRef] [PubMed]

7. Wakabayashi, C.; Murakami, K.; Hasegawa, H.; Murata, J.; Saiki, I. An intestinal bacterial metabolite of ginseng protopanaxadiol saponins has the ability to induce apoptosis in tumor cells. *Biochem. Biophys. Res. Commun.* **1998**, *246*, 725–730. [CrossRef] [PubMed]

8. Tawab, M.A.; Bahr, U.; Karas, M.; Wurglics, M.; Schubert-Zsilavecz, M. Degradation of ginsenosides in humans after oral administration. *Drug Metab. Dispos.* **2003**, *31*, 1065–1071. [CrossRef] [PubMed]

9. Han, J.; Lee, E.; Kim, E.; Yeom, M.H.; Kwon, O.; Yoon, T.H.; Lee, T.R.; Kim, K. Role of epidermal γδ T-cell-derived interleukin 13 in the skin-whitening effect of Ginsenoside F1. *Exp. Dermatol.* **2014**, *23*, 860–862. [CrossRef] [PubMed]

10. Yoo, D.S.; Rho, H.S.; Lee, Y.G.; Yeom, M.H.; Kim, D.H.; Lee, S.-J.; Hong, S.; Lee, J.; Cho, J.Y. Ginsenoside F1 modulates cellular responses of skin melanoma cells. *J. Ginseng Res.* **2011**, *35*, 86–91. [CrossRef]

11. Lee, E.H.; Cho, S.Y.; Kim, S.J.; Shin, E.S.; Chang, H.K.; Kim, D.H.; Yeom, M.H.; Woe, K.S.; Lee, J.; Sim, Y.C.; et al. Ginsenoside F1 protects human HaCaT keratinocytes from ultraviolet-B-induced apoptosis by maintaining constant levels of Bcl-2. *J. Investig. Dermatol.* **2003**, *121*, 607–613. [CrossRef] [PubMed]

12. Shibuya, M.; Nishimura, K.; Yasuyama, N.; Ebizuka, Y. Identification and characterization of glycosyltransferases involved in the biosynthesis of soyasaponin I in *Glycine max*. *FEBS Lett.* **2010**, *584*, 2258–2264. [CrossRef] [PubMed]

13. Mathiyalagan, R.; Kim, Y.-H.; Kim, Y.; Kim, M.-K.; Kim, M.-J.; Yang, D. Enzymatic Formation of Novel Ginsenoside Rg1-α-Glucosides by Rat Intestinal Homogenates. *Appl. Biochem. Biotechnol.* **2015**, *177*, 1701–1715. [CrossRef] [PubMed]

14. Nakano, H.; Kiso, T.; Okamoto, K.; Tomita, T.; Manan, M.B.; Kitahata, S. Synthesis of glycosyl glycerol by cyclodextrin glucanotransferases. *J. Biosci. Bioeng.* **2003**, *95*, 583–588. [CrossRef]

15. Li, S.; Li, W.; Xiao, Q.Y.; Xia, Y. Transglycosylation of stevioside to improve the edulcorant quality by lower substitution using cornstarch hydrolyzate and CGTase. *Food Chem.* **2013**, *138*, 2064–2069. [CrossRef] [PubMed]

16. Kometani, T.; Terada, Y.; Nishimura, T.; Takii, H.; Okada, S. Transglycosylation to hesperidin by cyclodextrin glucanotransferase from an alkalophilic *Bacillus* species in alkaline pH and properties of hesperidin glycosides. *Biosci. Biotechnol. Biochem.* **1994**, *58*, 1990–1994. [CrossRef]

17. Kamaruddin, K.; Illias, R.M.; Aziz, S.A.; Said, M.; Hassan, O. Effects of buffer properties on cyclodextrin glucanotransferase reactions and cyclodextrin production from raw sago (*Cycas revoluta*) starch. *Biotechnol. Appl. Biochem.* **2005**, *41*, 117–125. [PubMed]

18. Suzuki, Y.; Suzuki, K. Enzymatic formation of 4G-α-D-glucopyranosyl-rutin. *Agric. Biol. Chem.* **1991**, *55*, 181–187. [CrossRef] [PubMed]

19. Wang, Y.Z.; Feng, B.; Huang, H.Z.; Kang, L.P.; Cong, Y.; Zhou, W.B.; Zou, P.; Cong, Y.W.; Song, X.B.; Ma, B.P. Glucosylation of steroidal saponins by cyclodextrin glucanotransferase. *Planta Med.* **2010**, *76*, 1724–1731. [CrossRef] [PubMed]

20. Uchida, K.; Suzuki, Y. Enzymatic synthesis of a new derivative of thiamin, O-α-glucosylthiamin. *Biosci. Biotechnol. Biochem.* **1998**, *62*, 221–224. [CrossRef] [PubMed]

21. Seo, D.H.; Jung, J.H.; Ha, S.J.; Cho, H.K.; Jung, D.H.; Kim, T.J.; Baek, N.I.; Yoo, S.H.; Park, C.S. High-yield enzymatic bioconversion of hydroquinone to α-arbutin, a powerful skin lightening agent, by amylosucrase. *Appl. Microbiol. Biotechnol.* **2012**, *94*, 1189–1197. [CrossRef] [PubMed]

22. Sugimoto, K.; Nishimura, T.; Nomura, K.; Sugimoto, K.; Kuriki, T. Syntheses of arbutin-α-glycosides and a comparison of their inhibitory effects with those of α-arbutin and arbutin on human tyrosinase. *Chem. Pharm. Bull.* **2003**, *51*, 798–801. [CrossRef] [PubMed]

23. Quan, L.H.; Min, J.W.; Sathiyamoorthy, S.; Yang, D.U.; Kim, Y.J.; Yang, D.C. Biotransformation of ginsenosides Re and Rg1 into ginsenosides Rg2 and Rh1 by recombinant β-glucosidase. *Biotechnol. Lett.* **2012**, *34*, 913–917. [CrossRef] [PubMed]

24. Sim, G.-S.; Lee, B.-C.; Cho, H.; Lee, J.; Kim, J.-H.; Lee, D.-H.; Kim, J.-H.; Pyo, H.-B.; Moon, D.; Oh, K.-W.; et al. Structure activity relationship of antioxidative property of flavonoids and inhibitory effect on matrix metalloproteinase activity in UVA-irradiated human dermal fibroblast. *Arch. Pharm. Res.* **2007**, *30*, 290–298. [CrossRef] [PubMed]

25. Kim, M.J.; Kim, Y.H.; Song, G.S.; Suzuki, Y.; Kim, M.K. Enzymatic transglycosylation of ginsenoside Rg1 by rice seed α-glucosidase. *Biosci. Biotechnol. Biochem.* **2016**, *80*, 318–328. [CrossRef] [PubMed]

26. Kim, Y.H.; Lee, Y.G.; Choi, K.J.; Uchida, K.; Suzuki, Y. Transglycosylation to ginseng saponins by cyclomaltodextrin glucanotransferases. *Biosci. Biotechnol. Biochem.* **2001**, *65*, 875–883. [CrossRef] [PubMed]

27. Zhou, W.B.; Feng, B.; Huang, H.Z.; Qin, Y.J.; Wang, Y.Z.; Kang, L.P.; Zhao, Y.; Wang, X.N.; Cai, Y.; Tan, D.W.; et al. Enzymatic synthesis of α-glucosyl-timosaponin BII catalyzed by the extremely thermophilic enzyme: *Toruzyme* 3.0L. *Carbohydr. Res.* **2010**, *345*, 1752–1759. [CrossRef] [PubMed]

28. Sato, T.; Nakagawa, H.; Kurosu, J.; Yoshida, K.; Tsugane, T.; Shimura, S.; Kirimura, K.; Kino, K.; Usami, S. α-anomer-selective glucosylation of (+)-catechin by the crude enzyme, showing glucosyl transfer activity, of *Xanthomonas campestris* WU-9701. *J. Biosci. Bioeng.* **2000**, *90*, 625–630. [CrossRef]

29. Kligman, A.M. Early destructive effect of sunlight on human skin. *JAMA* **1969**, *210*, 2377–2380. [CrossRef] [PubMed]

30. Li, W.; Liu, Y.; Zhang, J.W.; Ai, C.Z.; Xiang, N.; Liu, H.X.; Yang, L. Anti-androgen-independent prostate cancer effects of ginsenoside metabolites in vitro: Mechanism and possible structure-activity relationship investigation. *Arch. Pharm. Res.* **2009**, *32*, 49–57. [CrossRef] [PubMed]

31. Luo, S.L.; Dang, L.Z.; Zhang, K.Q.; Liang, L.M.; Li, G.H. Cloning and heterologous expression of UDP-glycosyltransferase genes from *Bacillus subtilis* and its application in the glycosylation of ginsenoside Rh1. *Lett. Appl. Microbiol.* **2015**, *60*, 72–78. [CrossRef] [PubMed]

32. Wang, D.D.; Jin, Y.; Wang, C.; Kim, Y.J.; Perez, Z.E.J.; Baek, N.I.; Mathiyalagan, R.; Markus, J.; Yang, D.C. Rare ginsenoside Ia synthesized from F1 by cloning and overexpression of the UDP-glycosyltransferase gene from *Bacillus subtilis*: Synthesis, characterization, and in vitro melanogenesis inhibition activity in BL6B16 cells. *J. Ginseng Res.* **2018**, *42*, 42–49. [CrossRef] [PubMed]

33. Mathiyalagan, R.; Yang, D.C. Ginseng nanoparticles: A budding tool for cancer treatment. *Nanomedicine* **2017**, *12*, 1091–1094. [CrossRef] [PubMed]

2

Early Celastrol Administration Prevents Ketamine-Induced Psychotic-Like Behavioral Dysfunctions, Oxidative Stress and IL-10 Reduction in The Cerebellum of Adult Mice

Stefania Schiavone, Paolo Tucci, Luigia Trabace * and Maria Grazia Morgese

Department of Clinical and Experimental Medicine, University of Foggia, Viale Pinto, 1 71122 Foggia, Italy; stefania.schiavone@unifg.it (S.S.); paolo.tucci@unifg.it (P.T.); mariagrazia.morgese@unifg.it (M.G.M.)
* Correspondence: luigia.trabace@unifg.it;

Academic Editor: Pinarosa Avato

Abstract: Administration of subanesthetic doses of ketamine during brain maturation represents a tool to mimic an early insult to the central nervous system (CNS). The cerebellum is a key player in psychosis pathogenesis, to which oxidative stress also contributes. Here, we investigated the impact of early celastrol administration on behavioral dysfunctions in adult mice that had received ketamine (30 mg/kg i.p.) at postnatal days (PNDs) 7, 9, and 11. Cerebellar levels of 8-hydroxydeoxyguanosine (8-OHdG), NADPH oxidase (NOX) 1 and NOX2, as well as of the calcium-binding protein parvalbumin (PV), were also assessed. Furthermore, celastrol effects on ketamine-induced alterations of proinflammatory (TNF-α, IL-6 and IL-1β) and anti-inflammatory (IL-10) cytokines in this brain region were evaluated. Early celastrol administration prevented ketamine-induced discrimination index decrease at adulthood. The same was found for locomotor activity elevations and increased close following and allogrooming, whereas no beneficial effects on sniffing impairment were detected. Ketamine increased 8-OHdG in the cerebellum of adult mice, which was also prevented by early celastrol injection. Cerebellar NOX1 levels were enhanced at adulthood following postnatal ketamine exposure. Celastrol *per se* induced NOX1 decrease in the cerebellum. This effect was more significant in animals that were early administered with ketamine. NOX2 levels did not change. Ketamine administration did not affect PV amount in the cerebellum. TNF-α levels were enhanced in ketamine-treated animals; however, this was not prevented by early celastrol administration. While no changes were observed for IL-6 and IL-1β levels, ketamine determined a reduction of cerebellar IL-10 expression, which was prevented by early celastrol treatment. Our results suggest that NOX inhibition during brain maturation prevents the development of psychotic-like behavioral dysfunctions, as well as the increased cerebellar oxidative stress and the reduction of IL-10 in the same brain region following ketamine exposure in postnatal life. This opens novel neuroprotective opportunities against early detrimental insults occurring during brain development.

Keywords: ketamine; psychosis; cerebellum; celastrol; oxidative stress; NADPH oxidases

1. Introduction

The recreational use of the N-methyl-D-aspartate receptor (NMDA-R) antagonist ketamine, at subanesthetic doses, has been widely reported to cause psychedelic effects in humans [1]. Moreover, the development of a psychotic-like state has also been described following prolonged assumption of this psychoactive compound [2,3]. Despite an increasing scientific interest in ketamine's psychotogenic effects, the mechanisms underlying the pathological contribution of this NMDA-R antagonist in psychosis development need to be further elucidated. In this context, the administration of subanesthetic doses of ketamine to rodents represents a reliable tool to mimic neuropathological alterations reminiscent of those observed in psychotic patients, in terms of biomolecular alterations, neurochemical dysfunctions and behavioral impairment [4]. Indeed, in rodents, increased locomotor activity and decreased discrimination abilities have been respectively associated with the agitation and disorganized behavior, as well as with the cognitive impairment observed in subjects suffering from psychosis [5–7]. Moreover, abnormalities in social behavior, such as withdrawal and decreased interactions, have been related to negative symptoms observed in psychotic patients [8].

Numerous lines of evidence have considered the psychotic disease to be the final result of a series of events occurring during the early stages of brain development [9]. Hence, animal models obtained by administering ketamine during a crucial period of central nervous system (CNS) maturation, such as the second postnatal week of life [10], might provide information on the possible pathogenetic contribution of an early insult to an enduring psychotic state in adulthood.

Together with the widely known role of the prefrontal cortex in the pathogenesis of psychosis, in recent years, an emerging interest has been directed towards a possible implication of cerebellum in the development of this mental disorder [11,12]. Indeed, preclinical, clinical, neuroanatomical and neuroimaging reports began to highlight its important role not only in motor function regulation but also in the modulation of emotional and cognitive processes [13–16]. Structural cerebellar abnormalities, such as deficits in its gray matter volume, have also been described in antipsychotic-naive schizophrenic patients [17]. Moreover, vascular insults occurring in this brain region resulted in the onset of unremitting psychosis [18].

Administration of subanesthetic doses of ketamine in both early life stages and adult life has been widely reported to reduce the amount of the calcium-binding protein parvalbumin (PV) in different brain regions, such as prefrontal cortex and hippocampus [19–22]. However, poor evidence is available on the effects of early ketamine administration on cerebellar amount of PV, which has been shown to play a key role in regulating several physiological processes in this brain region [23], such as cell firing, synaptic transmission, as well as the resistance to neuronal degeneration following a variety of acute or chronic insults [24,25].

Oxidative stress, defined as an imbalance between reactive oxygen species (ROS) production and the antioxidant defenses of the cells, has been described as a key player in the pathogenesis of several CNS diseases, going from neurodegenerative to neuropsychiatric disorders [26], including psychosis [27]. The family of the Nicotinamide Adenine Dinucleotide Phosphate (NADPH) oxidase (NOX) enzymes represents one of the major ROS sources in the CNS, where it is involved in several physiological functions [28]. In particular, enhanced levels of NOX1 enzyme have been reported in neuropsychiatric diseases characterized by psychotic symptoms [29,30], and increased NOX2 expression was observed in specific brain regions, such as the prefrontal cortex and nucleus accumbens of environmental [19,31,32] and pharmacologic rodent models of psychosis, including the one obtained by ketamine administration in adult mice [33–35]. NOX1 and NOX2 mRNA and proteins have been detected in rodent cerebellum starting from postnatal day (PND) 4, meaning that the developing cerebellum is able to actively produce ROS. Moreover, administration of antioxidant/NOX inhibitor compounds, such as apocynin, has been demonstrated to decrease ROS levels in Purkinje cells [36]. However, so far, little is known about possible changes of NOX1 and NOX2 enzymes in this brain area following an early CNS insult leading to a later psychotic disease. Together with oxidative stress, increased inflammatory states and/or reduced anti-inflammatory pathways have been reported following ketamine administration [37–39]. Furthermore, the developing CNS has been described as being particularly vulnerable to enhanced peripheral and central inflammation following an external insult [40].

Together with its anti-inflammatory actions [41], celastrol, extracted from the medicinal plant *Tripterygium wilfordii*, has been described to have significant benefits in preventing neuropathological alterations observed in animal models of neurodegenerative diseases [42–44], through numerous mechanisms, including ROS level decrease [45]. In particular, celastrol has been characterized as an effective NOX enzyme inhibitor, with an increased potency against NOX1 and NOX2, acting via the suppression of the association between the enzymatic subunits, located in the cytosol, and the membrane flavocytochrome [46]. Importantly, no available reports investigate the effects of celastrol administration in animal models of psychosis. Moreover, no evidence has been previously published on the possible impact of celastrol administration during a crucial period of brain maturation, or on the development of a psychotic state following an early CNS insult.

A major challenge in the field of oxidative stress in the CNS is represented by the possibility to directly measure ROS production and release in this body district. Therefore, different indirect approaches have been used to quantify free radical amount in the CNS, including the analysis of 8-hydroxydeoxyguanosine (8-OHdG), a reliable marker of DNA oxidation levels [47,48].

Here, we investigated the impact of early celastrol administration on behavioral dysfunctions observed in adult mice exposed to subanesthetic doses of ketamine at PNDs 7, 9 and 11. The effects of this compound on ketamine-induced oxidative stress, as well as on NADPH oxidase expression alterations and PV levels in the cerebellum, were also assessed. Moreover, we also evaluated early celastrol effects on possible ketamine-induced changes of proinflammatory (Tumor Necrosis Factor alpha (TNF-α), interleukin-6 (IL-6) and interleukin-1 beta (IL-1β)), as well as anti-inflammatory [interleukin-10 (IL-10)] cytokines in the same brain region.

2. Results

2.1. Early Celastrol Administration Prevented Cognitive Dysfunctions in Adult Mice Exposed to Ketamine in Postnatal Life

To evaluate the possible effects of early celastrol administration on cognitive dysfunctions induced by ketamine exposure in postnatal life, we performed the Novel Object Recognition (NOR) test in 10 weeks mice. While no differences were detected in the discrimination index among saline, dimethyl sulfoxide (DMSO) and celastrol-treated mice, a significant decrease of this parameter was observed in adult mice who had received ketamine in postnatal life. Early celastrol administration to ketamine-treated mice was able to prevent this cognitive dysfunction (Figure 1, One Way Analysis of variance-ANOVA, followed by Tukey's post hoc test F = 7.387, $p < 0.01$ ketamine vs. saline; $p < 0.05$ ketamine vs. DMSO and vs. ketamine + celastrol; $p < 0.001$ ketamine vs. celastrol; $p > 0.05$ saline vs. DMSO, celastrol and ketamine + celastrol; $p > 0.05$ DMSO vs. celastrol and ketamine + celastrol; $p > 0.05$ celastrol vs. ketamine + celastrol).

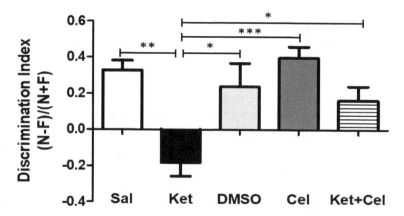

Figure 1. Celastrol administration in postnatal life prevented ketamine-induced cognitive dysfunctions, evaluated at adulthood. Discrimination index (N − F)/(N + F) (N = time spent in exploration of the novel object during the T2; F = time spent in exploration of the familiar object in the T2) in adult mice receiving saline (Sal, $n = 6$) or ketamine (Ket, $n = 13$) or a 50% DMSO in phosphate-buffered saline (PBS) (DMSO, $n = 7$) or celastrol (Cel, $n = 6$) or ketamine + celastrol (Ket + Cel, $n = 14$) at PNDs 7, 9 and 11. One Way ANOVA, followed by Tukey's post hoc test F = 7.387, *** $p < 0.001$; ** $p < 0.01$; * $p < 0.05$.

2.2. Early Celastrol Administration Prevented Locomotor Dysfunctions in Adult Mice Exposed to Ketamine in Postnatal Life

To assess the possible impact of early celastrol administration on ketamine-induced locomotor alterations, we performed the Open Field (OF) test in adult mice. Ketamine administration in postnatal life significantly enhanced locomotor activity at 10 weeks of age, with respect to the saline, DMSO and celastrol-treated groups, within which no differences were observed. Celastrol co-administered with ketamine at PNDs 7, 9 and 11 was able to prevent the observed hyperlocomotion (Figure 2, One Way ANOVA, followed by Tukey's post hoc test, F = 10.34, $p < 0.001$ ketamine vs. saline, DMSO, celastrol and ketamine + celastrol; $p > 0.05$ saline vs. DMSO, celastrol and ketamine + celastrol; $p > 0.05$ DMSO vs. celastrol and ketamine + celastrol; $p > 0.05$ celastrol vs. ketamine + celastrol).

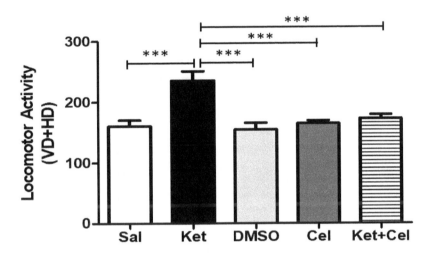

Figure 2. Celastrol administration in postnatal life prevented ketamine-induced increased in locomotor activity in later adulthood. Locomotor activity (VD = vertical displacements; HD = horizontal displacements) in adult mice receiving saline (Sal, $n = 7$) or ketamine (Ket, $n = 13$) or a 50% DMSO in PBS (DMSO, $n = 7$) or celastrol (Cel, $n = 8$) or ketamine + celastrol (Ket + Cel, $n = 14$) at PNDs 7, 9 and 11. One Way ANOVA, followed by Tukey's post hoc test F = 10.34, *** $p < 0.001$.

2.3. Early Celastrol Administration Prevented Social Behavior Dysfunctions in Adult Mice Exposed to Ketamine in Postnatal Life

To investigate the effects of early celastrol administration on ketamine-induced social behavior impairments, we performed the Social Interaction (SI) test in adult mice. Animals receiving ketamine at PNDs 7, 9 and 11 showed a decrease in the sniffing time with respect to saline, DMSO- and celastrol-treated mice. A significant difference in this parameter was also observed in ketamine-treated mice who had also received celastrol in postnatal life compared to the saline group (Figure 3A, One Way ANOVA, followed by Tukey's post hoc test, F = 6.856, $p < 0.01$ ketamine vs. saline; $p < 0.05$ ketamine vs. DMSO and celastrol; $p < 0.05$ ketamine + celastrol vs. saline; $p > 0.05$ saline vs. DMSO and celastrol; $p > 0.05$ DMSO vs. celastrol; $p > 0.05$ ketamine vs. ketamine + celastrol). Postnatal ketamine exposure caused a significant increase in the close following time, which was prevented by the concomitant treatment with celastrol (Figure 3B, One Way ANOVA, followed by Tukey's post hoc test, F = 13.10, $p < 0.05$ ketamine vs. saline; $p < 0.001$ ketamine vs. DMSO, celastrol and ketamine + celastrol; $p > 0.05$ saline vs. DMSO, celastrol and ketamine + celastrol; $p > 0.05$ DMSO vs. celastrol and ketamine + celastrol; $p > 0.05$ celastrol vs. ketamine + celastrol). The same pattern was observed for the celastrol effects on ketamine-induced elevation of time spent in allogroming (Figure 3C, One Way ANOVA, followed by Tukey's post hoc test, F = 12.50, $p < 0.001$ ketamine vs. saline and DMSO; $p < 0.01$ ketamine vs. celastrol and ketamine + celastrol; $p > 0.05$ saline vs. DMSO, celastrol and ketamine + celastrol; $p > 0.05$ DMSO vs. celastrol and ketamine + celastrol; $p > 0.05$ celastrol vs. ketamine + celastrol).

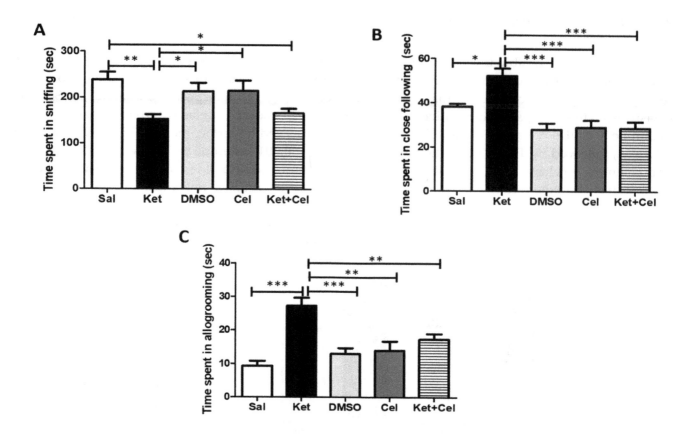

Figure 3. Celastrol administration in postnatal life prevented ketamine-induced social behavior dysfunctions in later adulthood. (**A**). Time spent in sniffing (seconds, sec) in adult mice receiving saline (Sal, $n = 4$) or ketamine (Ket, $n = 8$) or a 50% DMSO in PBS (DMSO, $n = 4$) or celastrol (Cel, $n = 4$) or ketamine + celastrol (Ket + Cel, $n = 7$) at PNDs 7, 9 and 11. One Way ANOVA, followed by Tukey's post hoc test F = 6.856, ** $p < 0.01$; * $p < 0.05$. (**B**). Time spent in close following (seconds, sec) in adult mice receiving saline (Sal, $n = 4$) or ketamine (Ket, $n = 7$) or a 50% DMSO in PBS (DMSO, $n = 4$) or celastrol (Cel, $n = 4$) or ketamine + celastrol (Ket + Cel, $n = 7$) at PNDs 7, 9 and 11. One Way ANOVA, followed by Tukey's post hoc test F = 13.10, *** $p < 0.001$; * $p < 0.05$. (**C**). Time spent in allogroming (seconds, sec) in adult mice receiving saline (Sal, $n = 5$) or ketamine (Ket, $n = 6$) or a 50% DMSO in PBS (DMSO, $n = 4$) or celastrol (Cel, $n = 4$) or ketamine + celastrol (Ket + Cel, $n = 6$) at PNDs 7, 9 and 11. One Way ANOVA, followed by Tukey's post hoc test F = 12.50, *** $p < 0.001$; ** $p < 0.01$.

2.4. Early Celastrol Administration Prevented Oxidative Stress Increase in the Cerebellum of Adult Mice Exposed to Ketamine in Postnatal Life

To assess the effects of early celastrol administration on ketamine-induced oxidative stress in the cerebellum of adult mice, we quantified 8-OHdG levels in this brain region. Mice receiving ketamine at PNDs 7, 9 and 11 showed a significant elevation of this biomarker of oxidative stress with respect to saline-treated animals whose 8-OHdG amount was comparable to the one of the DMSO and celastrol-treated animals. Early celastrol administration was able to prevent ketamine-induced enhancement of this biomarker (Figure 4, One Way ANOVA, followed by Tukey's post hoc test, F = 6.361, $p < 0.05$ ketamine vs. saline; $p < 0.01$ ketamine vs. ketamine + celastrol; $p > 0.05$ saline vs. DMSO, celastrol and ketamine + celastrol; $p > 0.05$ DMSO vs. celastrol and ketamine + celastrol; $p > 0.05$ celastrol vs. ketamine + celastrol).

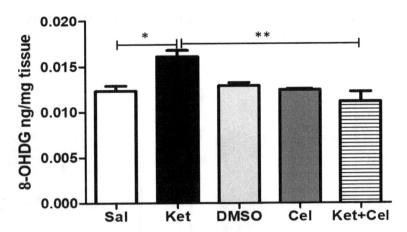

Figure 4. Celastrol administration in postnatal life prevented ketamine-induced oxidative stress in the cerebellum in later adulthood. 8-OHdG levels (ng/mg tissue) in the cerebellum of adult mice receiving saline (Sal, $n = 3$) or ketamine (Ket, $n = 5$) or a 50% DMSO in PBS (DMSO, $n = 3$) or celastrol (Cel, $n = 3$) or ketamine + celastrol (Ket + Cel, $n = 5$) at PNDs 7, 9 and 11. One Way ANOVA, followed by Tukey's post hoc test F = 6.361 * $p < 0.05$; ** $p < 0.01$.

2.5. Early Celastrol Administration Decreased NOX1 Levels in the Cerebellum of Adult Mice Per Se and Following Ketamine Exposure

To evaluate the effects of early celastrol administration on ketamine-induced NADPH oxidase alterations in the cerebellum, we measured NOX1 and NOX2 levels in this area. NOX1 amount was significantly increased by ketamine administration in postnatal life. Celastrol, injected as single treatment at the same time point, reduced NOX1 levels compared to both saline or ketamine-treated mice. The amount of this NADPH oxidase isoform was further reduced when celastrol was administered early to ketamine-treated animals (Figure 5, One Way ANOVA, followed by Tukey's post hoc test F = 50.30, $p < 0.05$ ketamine vs. saline and ketamine + celastrol vs. celastrol; $p < 0.01$ celastrol vs. saline; $p < 0.001$ ketamine + celastrol vs. saline and vs. DMSO and ketamine vs. DMSO, celastrol and ketamine + celastrol; $p > 0.05$ saline vs. DMSO).

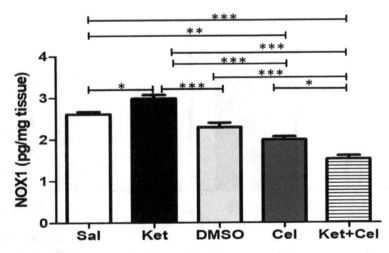

Figure 5. Celastrol administration in postnatal life decreased NOX1 levels in the cerebellum of adult mice. NOX1 levels (pg/mg tissue) in the cerebellum of adult mice receiving saline (Sal, $n = 3$) or ketamine (Ket, $n = 5$) or a 50% DMSO in PBS (DMSO, $n = 3$) or celastrol (Cel, $n = 3$) or ketamine + celastrol (Ket + Cel, $n = 5$) at PNDs 7, 9 and 11. One Way ANOVA, followed by Tukey's post hoc test F = 50.30, * $p < 0.05$; ** $p < 0.01$; *** $p < 0.001$.

Ketamine administration at PNDs 7, 9 and 11 did not significantly alter NOX2 amount in the cerebellum of adult mice, and no differences in the levels of this NADPH oxidase isoform were detected among all the other experimental groups (Figure 6, One Way ANOVA, followed by Tukey's post hoc test F = 1.158, $p > 0.05$ for all comparisons).

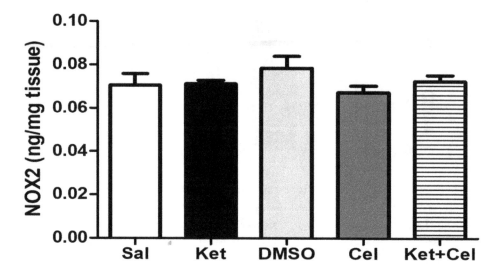

Figure 6. NOX2 levels were not altered in the cerebellum of adult mice exposed to ketamine in postnatal life. NOX2 levels (ng/mg tissue) in the cerebellum of adult mice receiving saline (Sal, $n = 3$) or ketamine (Ket, $n = 5$) or a 50% DMSO in PBS (DMSO, $n = 3$) or celastrol (Cel, $n = 3$) or ketamine + celastrol (Ket + Cel, $n = 5$) at PNDs 7, 9 and 11. One Way ANOVA, followed by Tukey's post hoc test F = 1.158 $p > 0.05$ for all comparisons.

The same was observed for cerebellar PV levels (Figure 7, One Way ANOVA, followed by Tukey's post hoc test, F = 2.632, $p > 0.05$ for all comparisons).

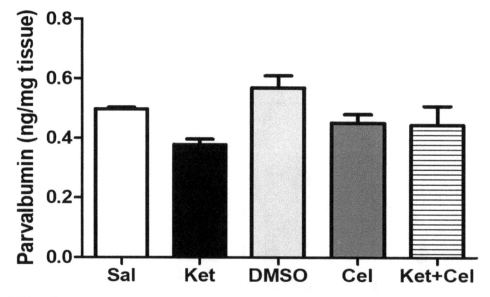

Figure 7. PV levels were not altered in the cerebellum of adult mice exposed to ketamine in postnatal life. PV levels (ng/mg tissue) in the cerebellum of adult mice receiving saline (Sal, $n = 3$) or ketamine (Ket, $n = 5$) or a 50% DMSO in PBS (DMSO, $n = 3$) or celastrol (Cel, $n = 3$) or ketamine + celastrol (Ket + Cel, $n = 5$) at PNDs 7, 9 and 11. One Way ANOVA, followed by Tukey's post hoc test F = 2.632, $p > 0.05$ for all comparisons.

2.6. Early Celastrol Administration Did not Prevent TNF-α Increase in the Cerebellum of Adult Mice Exposed to Ketamine in Postnatal Life

To investigate the effects of early celastrol administration on ketamine-induced inflammation in the cerebellum, we measured levels of TNF-α, IL-6 and IL-1β in this brain area. Ketamine administration in postnatal life determined an enhancement of cerebellar TNF-α in later adulthood compared to controls which showed comparable TNF-α amount with respect to the DMSO and celastrol-treated groups. Increased TNF-α were also detectable in adult mice receiving both ketamine and celastrol at PNDs 7, 9 and 11 (Figure 8A, One Way ANOVA, followed by Tukey's post hoc test F = 7.382, $p < 0.05$ ketamine vs. saline, saline vs. ketamine + celastrol and celastrol vs. ketamine + celastrol), whereas no significant alterations in the amount of IL-6 (Figure 8B, One Way ANOVA, followed by Tukey's post hoc test F = 1.444 $p > 0.05$ for all comparisons) and IL-1β (Figure 8C, One Way ANOVA, followed by Tukey's post hoc test F = 2.103 $p > 0.05$ for all comparisons) in the same brain region were found.

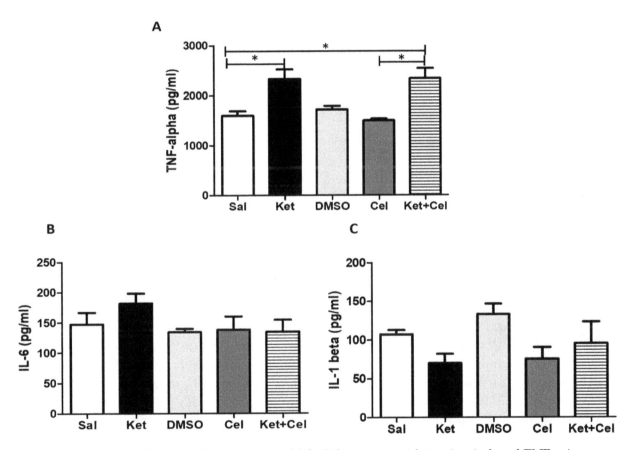

Figure 8. Celastrol administration in postnatal life did not prevent ketamine-induced TNF-α increase in the cerebellum in later adulthood. (**A**). TNF-α levels (pg/mg tissue) in the cerebellum of adult mice receiving saline (Sal, $n = 3$) or ketamine (Ket, $n = 5$) or a 50% DMSO in PBS (DMSO, $n = 3$) or celastrol (Cel, $n = 3$) or ketamine + celastrol (Ket + Cel, $n = 5$) at PNDs 7, 9 and 11. One Way ANOVA, followed by Tukey's post hoc test F = 7.382, * $p < 0.05$. (**B**). IL-6 levels (pg/mg tissue) in the cerebellum of adult mice receiving saline (Sal, $n = 3$) or ketamine (Ket, $n = 5$) or a 50% DMSO in PBS (DMSO, $n = 3$) or celastrol (Cel, $n = 3$) or ketamine + celastrol (Ket + Cel, $n = 5$) at PNDs 7, 9 and 11. One Way ANOVA, followed by Tukey's post hoc test F = 1.444, $p > 0.05$. (**C**). IL-1β levels (pg/mg tissue) in the cerebellum of adult mice receiving saline (Sal, $n = 3$) or ketamine (Ket, $n = 5$) or a 50% DMSO in PBS (DMSO, $n = 3$) or celastrol (Cel, $n = 3$) or ketamine + celastrol (Ket + Cel, $n = 5$) at PNDs 7, 9 and 11. One Way ANOVA, followed by Tukey's post hoc test F = 2.103 $p > 0.05$.

2.7. Early Celastrol Administration Prevented IL-10 Decrease in the Cerebellum of Adult Mice Exposed to Ketamine in Postnatal Life

To assess the effects of early celastrol administration on ketamine-induced decrease of anti-inflammatory cytokines in the cerebellum, we quantified IL-10 levels in this brain region. Mice administered with ketamine at PNDs 7, 9 and 11 showed reduced IL-10 amounts in later adulthood compared to saline-treated animals, whose levels of this cytokine were comparable to the ones detected in mice receiving DMSO or celastrol. Early celastrol administration in ketamine-treated animals was able to prevent IL-10 reduction in the cerebellum (Figure 9, One Way ANOVA, followed by Tukey's post hoc test F = 15.19, $p < 0.001$ ketamine vs. saline, ketamine vs. celastrol and ketamine vs. ketamine + celastrol; $p < 0.01$ ketamine vs. DMSO).

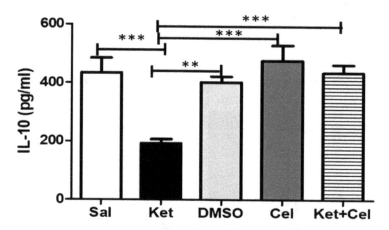

Figure 9. Celastrol administration in postnatal life prevented ketamine-induced IL-10 decrease in the cerebellum in later adulthood. IL-10 levels (pg/mL) in the cerebellum of adult mice receiving saline (Sal, $n = 3$) or ketamine (Ket, $n = 5$) or a 50% DMSO in PBS (DMSO, $n = 3$) or celastrol (Cel, $n = 3$) or ketamine + celastrol (Ket + Cel, $n = 5$) at PNDs 7, 9 and 11. One Way ANOVA, followed by Tukey's post hoc test F = 15.19, *** $p < 0.001$, ** $p < 0.01$.

3. Discussion

In this work, we demonstrated that early celastrol administration prevented discrimination ability dysfunctions, locomotor activity alterations and social behavior impairment in adult mice that had received ketamine at PNDs 7, 9 and 11. Previously published in vivo studies investigating possible beneficial effects of celastrol on CNS disorders have mainly regarded neurodegenerative disorders, including Alzheimer's disease [43–45], Parkinson's diseases [49–51], amyotrophic lateral sclerosis [42,52] and multiple sclerosis [53,54], epilepsy [55,56], cerebral ischemia and ischemic stroke [57–59] as well as traumatic brain injury [60,61]. One in vitro report indirectly investigated the impact of celastrol on the expression of specific genes, such as Fragile X Mental Retardation 1 (FMR1), linked to different psychiatric diseases, including schizophrenia [62]. Therefore, a novelty of our study with respect to the existing literature in the field is related to the evaluation of the effects of celastrol in psychotic disease by using a mouse model of the disorder. Importantly, this was obtained by negatively impacting the process of brain maturation with an early detrimental insult, represented by ketamine administration. Indeed, it has been reported that the developing brain is more vulnerable to the neurotoxicity induced by this psychoactive compound compared to the mature brain, in terms of enhanced neuronal cell death, neurogenesis alterations, disruptions of γ-aminobutyric acid (GABA)ergic interneuron development, altered NMDA-R expression, impaired synaptogenesis and increased oxidative stress production [63]. These disturbances during a critical period of brain maturation, i.e., the first 2–3 weeks of life in rodents, when brain growth spurt occurs, have been reported to trigger brain dysfunctions later in life, resulting finally in psychotic-like neuropathological and behavioral alterations [64]. Thus, our observations suggest that early administration of celastrol concomitantly to a brain insult might block the detrimental effects of ketamine with respect to the development of CNS and stop the progression of cerebral damage.

Decreased discrimination ability in rodents has been considered a behavioral feature mimicking the cognitive dysfunctions observed in psychotic patients [6]. Our findings regarding the preventive effects of early celastrol administration on ketamine-induced decrease in cognitive functions are in line with previous observations reporting a beneficial impact of this compound on learning and memory dysfunctions induced by metabolic alterations [65] or by neurodegenerative processes, induced by aggregation of specific proteins [45,66]. However, these studies were mainly focused on the behavioral effects of celastrol administration in adult life or even later, when the CNS insults leading to brain damage might have already been consolidated.

Elevations in locomotor activity in rodents are known to mimic the psychomotor agitation observed in subjects suffering from psychosis [5]. In our experimental conditions, early celastrol-treated mice, also exposed to ketamine in postnatal life, did not show an increase in locomotor activity with respect to the other experimental groups. Accordingly, the beneficial effects of celastrol on locomotor activity dysfunctions have been previously described in animal models of epilepsy, where motor function alterations were rapidly reduced by celastrol administration [67].

In this work, we also showed that ketamine administration at PNDs 7,9 and 11 induced dysfunctions in social behavior at adulthood. In particular, we reported decreased sniffing time in ketamine-treated mice with respect to controls. Together with its relation to social hierarchy in rodents, the sniffing behavior has been shown to be related to the establishment of normal social interactions [68]. Importantly, decreased social interactions in rodents have been paralleled to a negative symptom observed in psychotic patients, i.e., the social withdrawal [5]. Our findings are in line with previous work reporting a decreased sniffing time in rats treated with another NMDA-R antagonist, phencyclidine [69], together with a positive effects of antipsychotic treatment in reverting this social deficit [70]. Moreover, decreased duration of sniffing was observed in animal models of neuropsychiatric diseases also characterized by psychotic symptoms, such as autism [71]. In our experimental conditions, mice receiving ketamine in postnatal life also showed increased time spent in close-following and allogrooming. Close following is generally considered a mutual investigation behavior, while allogroming has been described as a standard behavior of altruism and reciprocal cooperation [72]. However, despite their general classification as non-aggressive behaviors, elevations in these social outcomes have been associated with subordination of the partner and abnormal dominance establishment [73], which could be seen as aggressive-like behaviors [74]. Accordingly, Becker et al. described a decrease in non-aggressive behavior in ketamine-treated rats [72]. Our findings might appear to be in contradiction with a previous work reporting that ketamine ameliorates aggressive-like behavior induced by neonatal maternal separation in mice [75]. However, in this study, lower doses of ketamine (15 mg/kg) were used and the administration time (post-natal days 35–49) was not comparable to those followed in our research procedure. In our experimental conditions, celastrol did not show beneficial effects on the ketamine-induced social withdrawal at adulthood but was able to prevent the observed increase in aggressive-like behavior. This is in line with previous findings reporting beneficial effects of antioxidant therapies in attenuating aggressive behavior induced by different stimuli [76] and describing aggressivity enhancement in mice with a genetic reduction of antioxidant functions [77]. In apparent contrast with our findings, Phensy and co-workers demonstrated that antioxidant treatment with N-acetyl cysteine was able to prevent social interaction dysfunctions induced by ketamine administration during postnatal life. However, in this work, administration of this antioxidant compound was performed throughout the entire period of brain development. Thus, we cannot exclude that prolonged administration of celastrol during brain maturation might also have an impact on social withdrawal observed at adulthood.

In our study, we found that early celastrol administration prevented elevations in cerebellar oxidative stress observed in mice treated with ketamine in postnatal life. The cerebellum has been gaining increasing importance in the pathogenic mechanisms underlying the development of psychosis [11,78–80] and of other psychiatric diseases, clinically characterized by psychotic symptoms [81]. In addition to the ketamine-induced detrimental effects on the prefrontal cortex [22,82,83], the negative impact of this NMDA-R antagonist also on the developing cerebellum has been shown in non-human primates [84]. In good agreement with our observations, previous works have reported increased direct and indirect biomarkers of oxidative stress in the cerebellum of animal models of neuropsychiatric disorders [85,86]. In particular, Filiou and co-workers described cerebellar oxidative stress-induced structural alterations in the G72/G30 transgenic schizophrenia mouse model [87]. Moreover, antipsychotic medication has been demonstrated to inhibit the activity of specific enzymes, which can also produce free radicals in rodent cerebellum [88,89]. The increased oxidative stress observed in this brain region may also be considered a possible trigger of the cerebello-thalamo-cortical network dysfunctions which have been described as predictors of disease progression in individuals at ultra-high risk for psychosis [12,90]. In support of this concept, interesting lines of evidence describe a positive effects of antioxidant treatments in preventing cerebellar dysfunctions observed in neuropsychiatric diseases also characterized by psychotic symptoms, such as autism spectrum disorder [91].

An important finding of our study consists in the observed increased cerebellar NOX1 levels in adult mice who had received ketamine in postnatal life, whereas NOX2 amount was not affected by this early detrimental insult. A physiological role of the NADPH oxidase enzymatic family in different stages of cerebellum development has been previously described [36]. Moreover, Olguín-Albuerne and Morán reported a key role of NADPH oxidase-derived ROS in controlling the development of cerebellar granule neurons during brain maturation [92]. However, in vitro and in vivo evidence highlighted a crucial role of NOX enzymes in the development of structural and functional alterations in cerebellum following different insults [93–95]. Increased NOX1 enzyme expression and activity has been implicated not only in the pathogenesis of neurodegenerative disorders [96–98], but also in neurotoxic processes mediated by sustained microglia activation [99]. Thus, the observed NOX1 increase following postnatal ketamine administration should also be considered in the context of the effects that this NMDA-R antagonist has on the inflammatory states of the brain. Supporting this perspective, it has been reported that exposure to subanesthetic doses of ketamine is able to activate neuroinflammatory pathways [83] and to induce microglia activation in rodent brains [100]. In our experimental conditions, early celastrol administration was able per se to decrease NOX1 levels in the cerebellum of adult mice which did not receive ketamine in postnatal life. Although speculative, a possible explanation for this result could be related to possible celastrol effects on other ketamine-independent events occurring in mature brain and implicating a role of the NADPH oxidase system, such as protein aggregation [101] or specific heat shock proteins expression and/or activation [102,103]. Hence, in the presence of a neurodetrimental insult, i.e., ketamine, early celastrol administration was able to further lower cerebellar NOX1 levels. With respect to these findings, additional investigations are needed to further unravel molecular mechanisms of actions of celastrol and its possible impact on NOX1 enzyme expression. Indeed, in this context, a limitation of this study is represented by the absence of the evaluation of the enzyme activation in the cerebellum. The lack of NOX2 increase following postnatal ketamine exposure observed in our experimental conditions could be explained by a region-specific effect of this NMDA-receptor antagonist in inducing an enhancement of this NADPH oxidase isoform. In line with this hypothesis, Zhang and co-workers previously described that cortical NOX2 was upregulated in adult rats treated with ketamine from PND6 to PND8 [20]. Moreover, in further support, an interesting study of Boczek et al. analyzed the effects of repeated ketamine administration on different brain areas, i.e., cortex, cerebellum, hippocampus and striatum, revealing region-specific effects of this NMDA-R antagonist [104]. However, we cannot totally exclude that the observed celastrol effects might be related to other pathways, other than the inhibition of NOX enzymes, finally resulting in decreased ROS levels, such as the enhancement of antioxidant capacity [105], the increase of antioxidant enzyme activity [106] and the targeting of mitochondria respiratory chain [107].

Decreased PV levels and loss of phenotype of PV-positive interneurons have been described in brain regions other than cerebellum, such as prefrontal cortex and hippocampus, in pharmacologic and non-pharmacologic animal models of psychosis [22,108]. With respect to this issue, a novelty of the present study is the absence, at least in our experimental conditions, of the reduction of PV amount in the cerebellum of adult mice administered with ketamine in the early stages of life, suggesting a region-specific effect of this NMDA-R antagonist. Moreover, our findings should also be considered in the light of the link existing between NADPH oxidases and PV. Indeed, NOX2 enzyme alterations have been reported to mediate cortical PV changes induced by different neurodetrimental insults, such as ketamine administration [34] or traumatic brain injury [109]. Thus, the lack of PV alterations observed in our experimental conditions might be related to the absence of NOX2 changes in the same brain region, suggesting a different mechanism of action underlying ketamine effects in the cerebellum with respect to what observed in the prefrontal cortex.

Here, we also showed that ketamine administration in early life stages caused increased levels of a specific proinflammatory cytokine, the TNF-α, in the cerebellum, without affecting cerebellar levels of IL-6 and IL-1β. Behavioral manifestations in psychiatric disorders such as schizophrenia and autism have been reported to be sustained by early neuroinflammatory processes which involve specific brain regions, including the cerebellum [110]. Moreover, patients with first psychotic episode, drug-naive schizophrenia, and subjects at ultra-high risk of psychosis have been described to share altered cerebellar-default mode network connectivity which appears to be modulate by inflammation in this brain region [111]. Moreover, in good agreement with our findings, previous evidence has reported a crucial role of TNF-α in regulating ketamine-induced neurotoxicity in the hippocampus [112,113], which is known to be functionally connected with the cerebellum [114,115]. In our experimental conditions, early celastrol administration was not able to prevent the ketamine-induced TNF-α increase in the cerebellum. This finding might appear in apparent contradiction with previous lines of evidence showing an effect of this compound in lowering TNF-α in monocytes and macrophages [45], as well as in the brain of animal models of neurodegenerative disorders, such as Alzheimer's disease [116,117], amyotrophic lateral sclerosis [42] and Parkinson's disease [50]. However, in most of the animal models on which celastrol has previously been tested for the evaluation of its effects on TNF-α, the pathological and/or neurotoxic insult leading to the neurodegenerative condition mainly occurred at adulthood. Moreover, other routes of administration (such as the oral one), as well as different doses and considered brain regions might also explain our findings. Further research is certainly needed to highlight possible different effects of celastrol on pro-inflammatory cytokines based on the time of the insult occurring in the brain. The lack of ketamine-induced cerebellar IL-6 increase that we observed might also be considered in the light of the unaltered NOX2 and PV expression we found in the same brain region. Indeed, a molecular association between IL-6, NOX2 and PV has been previously reported in the ketamine model of psychosis [35].

In this study, we also reported that early celastrol administration prevented ketamine-induced decrease of IL-10, an anti-inflammatory cytokine, in the cerebellum. Accordingly, an imbalance between pro-inflammatory and anti-inflammatory cytokines has been described in both schizophrenia [118] and other psychiatric disorders characterized by psychotic symptoms, such as bipolar disorders [119]. Intriguingly, IL-10 has been described as the most important player both in the resolution of the inflammatory cascade [120] and in the protection against possible detrimental effects following a neurotoxic insults [121,122]. Moreover, a key role of this anti-inflammatory cytokine in preventing glutamate-mediated cerebellar granule cell death has been reported [123], together with the regulation of synapses formation and functioning in the developing brain [124]. Thus, we could hypothesize that, at least in our experimental conditions, early celastrol administration might exert a protective effect against a neurotoxic insult, represented by ketamine, on the developing cerebellum, acting also on the anti-inflammatory pathways related to IL-10.

In conclusion, our study suggests that early NOX inhibition by celastrol during a crucial period of CNS maturation can prevent the development of psychotic-like behavioral dysfunctions, the increased oxidative stress and the IL-10 reduction in the cerebellum of adult mice exposed to an early neurodetrimental insult, i.e., ketamine. This might open new pharmacological insights into the possible use of this compound for neuroprotective purposes during brain development.

4. Materials and Methods

4.1. Animals

Mice were housed at constant room temperature (22 ± 1 °C) and relative humidity (55 ± 5%) under a 12 h light/dark cycle (lights on from 7:00 AM to 7:00 PM), with free access to food and water. Experimental procedures involving animals and their care were performed in conformity with the institutional guidelines of the Italian Ministry of Health (D.Lgs. n.26/2014), the Guide for the Care and Use of Laboratory Animals: Eight Edition, the Guide for the Care and Use of Mammals in Neuroscience and Behavioral Research (National Research Council, 2004), the Directive 2010/63/EU of the European Parliament and of the Council of 22 September 2010 on the protection of animals used for scientific purposes, as well as the ARRIVE guidelines. We daily monitored animal welfare during the entire period of experimental procedures. All efforts were made to minimize the number of animals used and their suffering. The experimental protocol was approved by the Italian Ministry of Health (approval number 679/2017-PR, protocol n. B2EF8.17).

4.2. Experimental Design

Five C57/Bl6 adult male mice and 10 adult females (Envigo, San Pietro al Natisone, Italy) weighing 25–30 g (8–10 weeks of age) were mated (one male and two females per cage).

Male pups were divided into the following five experimental groups:

1. pups administered with saline (10 mL/kg i.p.);
2. pups administered with ketamine (Sigma-Aldrich Corporation, Saint Louis, MO, US; 30 mg/kg i.p., dissolved in saline) [10,33];
3. pups administered with celastrol (Sigma Aldrich, Milano, Italy; 1 mg/kg i.p., dissolved in 50% DMSO/PBS) [43];
4. pups administered with a 50% DMSO/PBS solution (5 mL/kg i.p.)—we have referred to this treatment throughout the text as "DMSO";
5. pups administered with ketamine (30 mg/kg i.p., dissolved in saline, injected in the right side of the peritoneum) and celastrol (1 mg/kg i.p., dissolved in 50% DMSO/PBS, injected in the left side of the peritoneum)—we have referred to this treatment throughout the text as "ketamine + celastrol".

The above-mentioned treatments were repeated at PNDs 7, 9 and 11.

All pups were grown until adulthood, i.e., 10 weeks of age, when behavioral tests were performed. Immediately after, mice were euthanized by cervical dislocation for the collection of cerebella on which neurochemical and biomolecular analysis were conducted. The tissue was frozen in isopentane and stored at −80 °C until analysis was performed.

Body weight gain during the experimental protocol was calculated as the difference between body weight at PND 7 (the time of the first ketamine and/or celastrol injection) and body weight at 10 weeks of age (the time at which the behavioral tests were performed). No statistical differences were detected among the experimental groups (Supplementary Material A). Moreover, body weight at the time of the behavioral tests (10 weeks of age) was comparable among experimental groups (Supplementary Material B). No evident signs of hair loss and/or alopecia were observed during the experimental protocol for all the animals included in this study.

4.3. Behavioral Tests

4.3.1. NOR Test

The NOR test was performed as previously described [19,125] in a squared plastic-made arena (40 cm × 40 cm × 40 cm). For the habituation, mice were allowed to freely explore the arena for 10 min over five days. Mice were acclimatized to the testing room for one hour prior the beginning of the test. The test included two trials (training trial, T1 and testing trial, T2) of 3 min with an intertrial time of 1 min [126,127]. In T1, mice were put in the center of the arena and left free to explore two identical objects (two white light bulbs, fixed on the floor of the arena by velcro) for 3 min. In the testing trial (T2), one of the light bulbs was substituted with a novel object (a light blue plastic-made brick). At the beginning of the experimental procedure and between T1 and T2, the objects were cleaned with 20% *v/v* ethanol to remove any olfactory cues. Moreover, the arena was cleaned each time to remove mouse feces. Both T1 and T2 were videorecorded using a fixed camera. Then, an investigator, blind to the identity of the tested mouse, analyzed the animal behavior, including in the scoring of object sniffing and touching, as well as having moved the vibrissae while directing the nose toward the object at a distance of 1 cm. The following behaviors were not considered: sitting on, leaning against, and chewing the objects. The discrimination index was calculated using the following formula: $(N - F)/(N + F)$ (N = times spent in exploration of the novel object during the T2; F = times spent in exploration of the familiar object in the T2) [19].

4.3.2. OF Test

The OF test was performed as previously described [128], in a square plastic arena (40 cm × 40 cm × 40 cm), virtually divided into nine equal squares with black horizontal and vertical lines [129]. Mice were acclimatized to the testing room for one hour prior the beginning of the test. For the habituation, mice were allowed to freely move into the arena for 10 min over five days. The day of the test, mice were initially placed in the same corner and then left to move freely in the arena for 5 min. The experimental procedures were videorecorded using a fixed camera and then analyzed by a blind investigator who manually scored as spontaneous locomotor activity the total of horizontal and vertical displacements performed during the test (squares crossed with the four paws).

4.3.3. SI Test

The SI test was performed, as previously described [130–132], in a plexiglass rectangular cage (45cm × 30cm × 25cm), located under a fixed camera. Briefly, 24 h before, as well as on the morning of the test, the cages were cleaned, the testing mouse was weighed in order to choose an appropriate intruder, which was labelled with a white, sticking tape on the tail. Mice were acclimatized to the testing room for one hour prior the beginning of the test. The testing mouse was left undisturbed in the cage for 15 min. Then, the intruder was introduced, and the social behavior was videorecorded for 10 min. Analysis of behavior was conducted by a blind researcher and the following parameters were considered for the scoring: time (seconds) spent by the testing mouse in sniffing the intruder, time (seconds) spent by the testing mouse in close following the intruder and time (seconds) spent by the testing mouse in the allogrooming to the intruder.

4.4. Enzyme-Linked Immunosorbent Assays (ELISAs)

Samples were homogenized in 10 volumes of PBS with protease inhibitors, as previously described [133,134]. Commercially available ELISA kits were used for measurement of 8-OHdG (JaICA, Shizuoka, Japan), NOX2 (MyBiosource, San Diego, CA, USA), NOX1 (MyBiosource, San Diego, CA, USA), PV (MyBiosource, San Diego, CA, USA), TNF-α (MyBiosource, San Diego, CA, USA), IL-6 (MyBiosource, San Diego, CA, USA), IL-1β (MyBiosource, San Diego, CA, USA) and IL-10 (MyBiosource, San Diego, CA, USA) in the cerebellum, according to the manufacturer's instructions. Each sample analysis was performed in duplicate to avoid intra-assay variations.

4.5. Blindness of the Study

Researchers performing data analysis were blind with respect to the treatment conditions. The blindness was maintained until the end of the analysis process.

4.6. Statistical Analysis

GraphPad 5.0 software for Windows was used to perform statistical analyses. Data were analyzed by One Way ANOVA, followed by Tukey's post hoc test. For all tests, a p value < 0.05 was considered statistically significant. Results are expressed as means ± mean standard error (SEM).

Author Contributions: Conceptualization, S.S., P.T., L.T. and M.G.M.; Data curation, S.S., P.T., L.T. and M.G.M.; Formal analysis, S.S. and M.G.M.; Funding acquisition, S.S., P.T. and L.T.; Investigation, S.S., P.T. and M.G.M.; Methodology, S.S., P.T. and M.G.M.; Project administration, L.T.; Resources, S.S., P.T. and L.T.; Software, S.S. and M.G.M.; Supervision, L.T.; Validation, S.S., P.T., L.T. and M.G.M.; Visualization, S.S., P.T., L.T. and M.G.M.; Writing—original draft, S.S.; Writing—review & editing, S.S., P.T., L.T. and M.G.M.

Acknowledgments: The authors thank Stefania Di Monte for technical support.

References

1. Curran, H.V.; Nutt, D.; de Wit, H. Psychedelics and related drugs: Therapeutic possibilities, mechanisms and regulation. *Psychopharmacology* **2018**, *235*, 373–375. [CrossRef] [PubMed]
2. Vlisides, P.E.; Bel-Bahar, T.; Nelson, A.; Chilton, K.; Smith, E.; Janke, E.; Tarnal, V.; Picton, P.; Harris, R.E.; Mashour, G.A. Subanaesthetic ketamine and altered states of consciousness in humans. *Br. J. Anaesth.* **2018**, *121*, 249–259. [CrossRef] [PubMed]
3. Pomarol-Clotet, E.; Honey, G.D.; Murray, G.K.; Corlett, P.R.; Absalom, A.R.; Lee, M.; McKenna, P.J.; Bullmore, E.T.; Fletcher, P.C. Psychological effects of ketamine in healthy volunteers. Phenomenological study. *Br. J. Psychiatry J. Ment. Sci.* **2006**, *189*, 173–179. [CrossRef]
4. Frohlich, J.; Van Horn, J.D. Reviewing the ketamine model for schizophrenia. *J. Psychopharmacol.* **2014**, *28*, 287–302. [CrossRef]
5. Powell, S.B.; Zhou, X.; Geyer, M.A. Prepulse inhibition and genetic mouse models of schizophrenia. *Behav. Brain Res.* **2009**, *204*, 282–294. [CrossRef]
6. Watson, D.J.; Marsden, C.A.; Millan, M.J.; Fone, K.C. Blockade of dopamine D(3) but not D(2) receptors reverses the novel object discrimination impairment produced by post-weaning social isolation: Implications for schizophrenia and its treatment. *Int. J. Neuropsychopharmacol. Off. Sci. J. Coll. Int. Neuropsychopharmacol.* **2012**, *15*, 471–484. [CrossRef]
7. Forrest, A.D.; Coto, C.A.; Siegel, S.J. Animal models of psychosis: Current state and future directions. *Curr. Behav. Neurosci. Rep.* **2014**, *1*, 100–116. [CrossRef]
8. Mattei, D.; Schweibold, R.; Wolf, S.A. Brain in flames—Animal models of psychosis: Utility and limitations. *Neuropsychiatr. Dis. Treat.* **2015**, *11*, 1313–1329.
9. Owen, M.J.; O'Donovan, M.C.; Thapar, A.; Craddock, N. Neurodevelopmental hypothesis of schizophrenia. *Br. J. Psychiatry J. Ment. Sci.* **2011**, *198*, 173–175. [CrossRef] [PubMed]
10. Jeevakumar, V.; Driskill, C.; Paine, A.; Sobhanian, M.; Vakil, H.; Morris, B.; Ramos, J.; Kroener, S. Ketamine administration during the second postnatal week induces enduring schizophrenia-like behavioral symptoms and reduces parvalbumin expression in the medial prefrontal cortex of adult mice. *Behav. Brain Res.* **2015**, *282*, 165–175. [CrossRef]
11. Yeganeh-Doost, P.; Gruber, O.; Falkai, P.; Schmitt, A. The role of the cerebellum in schizophrenia: From cognition to molecular pathways. *Clinics* **2011**, *66* (Suppl. S1), 71–77. [CrossRef] [PubMed]

12. Bernard, J.A.; Orr, J.M.; Mittal, V.A. Cerebello-thalamo-cortical networks predict positive symptom progression in individuals at ultra-high risk for psychosis. *Neuroimage. Clin.* **2017**, *14*, 622–628. [CrossRef] [PubMed]

13. Villanueva, R. The cerebellum and neuropsychiatric disorders. *Psychiatry Res.* **2012**, *198*, 527–532. [CrossRef] [PubMed]

14. Bernard, J.A.; Orr, J.M.; Dean, D.J.; Mittal, V.A. The cerebellum and learning of non-motor associations in individuals at clinical-high risk for psychosis. *Neuroimage Clin.* **2018**, *19*, 137–146. [CrossRef] [PubMed]

15. Schmahmann, J.D. The cerebellum and cognition. *Neurosci. Lett.* **2019**, *688*, 62–75. [CrossRef] [PubMed]

16. Andreasen, N.C.; Pierson, R. The role of the cerebellum in schizophrenia. *Biol. Psychiatry* **2008**, *64*, 81–88. [CrossRef]

17. Arasappa, R.; Rao, N.; Venkatasubramanian, G.; Jayakumar, P.; Gangadhar, B. Structural cerebellar abnormalities in antipsychotic-naive schizophrenia: Evidence for cognitive dysmetria. *Indian J. Psychol. Med.* **2008**, *30*, 83–89. [CrossRef]

18. Bielawski, M.; Bondurant, H. Psychosis following a stroke to the cerebellum and midbrain: A case report. *Cerebellum Ataxias* **2015**, *2*, 17. [CrossRef]

19. Schiavone, S.; Sorce, S.; Dubois-Dauphin, M.; Jaquet, V.; Colaianna, M.; Zotti, M.; Cuomo, V.; Trabace, L.; Krause, K.H. Involvement of NOX2 in the development of behavioral and pathologic alterations in isolated rats. *Biol. Psychiatry* **2009**, *66*, 384–392. [CrossRef]

20. Zhang, H.; Sun, X.R.; Wang, J.; Zhang, Z.Z.; Zhao, H.T.; Li, H.H.; Ji, M.H.; Li, K.Y.; Yang, J.J. Reactive oxygen species-mediated loss of phenotype of parvalbumin interneurons contributes to long-term cognitive impairments after repeated neonatal ketamine exposures. *Neurotox. Res.* **2016**, *30*, 593–605. [CrossRef]

21. Sabbagh, J.J.; Murtishaw, A.S.; Bolton, M.M.; Heaney, C.F.; Langhardt, M.; Kinney, J.W. Chronic ketamine produces altered distribution of parvalbumin-positive cells in the hippocampus of adult rats. *Neurosci. Lett.* **2013**, *550*, 69–74. [CrossRef] [PubMed]

22. Schiavone, S.; Morgese, M.G.; Bove, M.; Colia, A.L.; Maffione, A.B.; Tucci, P.; Trabace, L.; Cuomo, V. Ketamine administration induces early and persistent neurochemical imbalance and altered NADPH oxidase in mice. *Prog. Neuro-Psychopharmacol. Biol. Psychiatry* **2019**, *96*, 109750. [CrossRef] [PubMed]

23. Schwaller, B.; Meyer, M.; Schiffmann, S. 'New' functions for 'old' proteins: The role of the calcium-binding proteins calbindin D-28k, calretinin and parvalbumin, in cerebellar physiology. Studies with knockout mice. *Cerebellum* **2002**, *1*, 241–258. [CrossRef] [PubMed]

24. Bastianelli, E. Distribution of calcium-binding proteins in the cerebellum. *Cerebellum* **2003**, *2*, 242–262. [CrossRef] [PubMed]

25. Liu, F.F.; Yang, L.D.; Sun, X.R.; Zhang, H.; Pan, W.; Wang, X.M.; Yang, J.J.; Ji, M.H.; Yuan, H.M. NOX2 mediated-parvalbumin interneuron loss might contribute to anxiety-like and enhanced fear learning behavior in a rat model of post-traumatic stress disorder. *Mol. Neurobiol.* **2016**, *53*, 6680–6689. [CrossRef]

26. Schiavone, S.; Trabace, L. Pharmacological targeting of redox regulation systems as new therapeutic approach for psychiatric disorders: A literature overview. *Pharmacol. Res.* **2016**, *107*, 195–204. [CrossRef]

27. Barron, H.; Hafizi, S.; Andreazza, A.C.; Mizrahi, R. Neuroinflammation and oxidative stress in psychosis and psychosis risk. *Int. J. Mol. Sci.* **2017**, *18*, 651. [CrossRef]

28. Sorce, S.; Krause, K.H. NOX enzymes in the central nervous system: From signaling to disease. *Antioxid. Redox Signal.* **2009**, *11*, 2481–2504. [CrossRef]

29. Ibi, M.; Liu, J.; Arakawa, N.; Kitaoka, S.; Kawaji, A.; Matsuda, K.I.; Iwata, K.; Matsumoto, M.; Katsuyama, M.; Zhu, K.; et al. Depressive-like behaviors are regulated by NOX1/NADPH oxidase by redox modification of NMDA receptor 1. *J. Neurosci. Off. J. Soc. Neurosci.* **2017**, *37*, 4200–4212. [CrossRef]

30. Ma, M.W.; Wang, J.; Zhang, Q.; Wang, R.; Dhandapani, K.M.; Vadlamudi, R.K.; Brann, D.W. NADPH oxidase in brain injury and neurodegenerative disorders. *Mol. Neurodegener.* **2017**, *12*, 7. [CrossRef]

31. Schiavone, S.; Jaquet, V.; Sorce, S.; Dubois-Dauphin, M.; Hultqvist, M.; Backdahl, L.; Holmdahl, R.; Colaianna, M.; Cuomo, V.; Trabace, L.; et al. NADPH oxidase elevations in pyramidal neurons drive psychosocial stress-induced neuropathology. *Transl. Psychiatry* **2012**, *2*, e111. [CrossRef] [PubMed]

32. Schiavone, S.; Mhillaj, E.; Neri, M.; Morgese, M.G.; Tucci, P.; Bove, M.; Valentino, M.; Di Giovanni, G.; Pomara, C.; Turillazzi, E.; et al. Early loss of blood-brain barrier integrity precedes NOX2 elevation in the prefrontal cortex of an animal model of psychosis. *Mol. Neurobiol.* **2017**, *54*, 2031–2044. [CrossRef] [PubMed]

33. Sorce, S.; Schiavone, S.; Tucci, P.; Colaianna, M.; Jaquet, V.; Cuomo, V.; Dubois-Dauphin, M.; Trabace, L.; Krause, K.H. The NADPH oxidase NOX2 controls glutamate release: A novel mechanism involved in psychosis-like ketamine responses. *J. Neurosci. Off. J. Soc. Neurosci.* **2010**, *30*, 11317–11325. [CrossRef] [PubMed]

34. Behrens, M.M.; Ali, S.S.; Dao, D.N.; Lucero, J.; Shekhtman, G.; Quick, K.L.; Dugan, L.L. Ketamine-induced loss of phenotype of fast-spiking interneurons is mediated by NADPH-oxidase. *Science* **2007**, *318*, 1645–1647. [CrossRef] [PubMed]

35. Behrens, M.M.; Ali, S.S.; Dugan, L.L. Interleukin-6 mediates the increase in NADPH-oxidase in the ketamine model of schizophrenia. *J. Neurosci. Off. J. Soc. Neurosci.* **2008**, *28*, 13957–13966. [CrossRef]

36. Coyoy, A.; Olguin-Albuerne, M.; Martinez-Briseno, P.; Moran, J. Role of reactive oxygen species and NADPH-oxidase in the development of rat cerebellum. *Neurochem. Int.* **2013**, *62*, 998–1011. [CrossRef]

37. Fraguas, D.; Diaz-Caneja, C.M.; Rodriguez-Quiroga, A.; Arango, C. Oxidative stress and inflammation in early onset first episode psychosis: A systematic review and meta-Analysis. *Int. J. Neuropsychopharmacol. Off. Sci. J. Coll. Int. Neuropsychopharmacol.* **2017**, *20*, 435–444. [CrossRef]

38. Khandaker, G.M.; Cousins, L.; Deakin, J.; Lennox, B.R.; Yolken, R.; Jones, P.B. Inflammation and immunity in schizophrenia: Implications for pathophysiology and treatment. *Lancet. Psychiatry* **2015**, *2*, 258–270. [CrossRef]

39. Kirkpatrick, B.; Miller, B.J. Inflammation and schizophrenia. *Schizophr. Bull.* **2013**, *39*, 1174–1179. [CrossRef]

40. Hagberg, H.; Mallard, C. Effect of inflammation on central nervous system development and vulnerability. *Curr. Opin. Neurol.* **2005**, *18*, 117–123. [CrossRef]

41. Ng, S.W.; Chan, Y.; Chellappan, D.K.; Madheswaran, T.; Zeeshan, F.; Chan, Y.L.; Collet, T.; Gupta, G.; Oliver, B.G.; Wark, P.; et al. Molecular modulators of celastrol as the keystones for its diverse pharmacological activities. *Biomed. Pharmacother. Biomed. Pharmacother.* **2019**, *109*, 1785–1792. [CrossRef] [PubMed]

42. Kiaei, M.; Kipiani, K.; Petri, S.; Chen, J.; Calingasan, N.Y.; Beal, M.F. Celastrol blocks neuronal cell death and extends life in transgenic mouse model of amyotrophic lateral sclerosis. *Neuro-Degener. Dis.* **2005**, *2*, 246–254. [CrossRef] [PubMed]

43. Paris, D.; Ganey, N.J.; Laporte, V.; Patel, N.S.; Beaulieu-Abdelahad, D.; Bachmeier, C.; March, A.; Ait-Ghezala, G.; Mullan, M.J. Reduction of beta-amyloid pathology by celastrol in a transgenic mouse model of Alzheimer's disease. *J. Neuroinflamm.* **2010**, *7*, 17. [CrossRef] [PubMed]

44. Choi, B.S.; Kim, H.; Lee, H.J.; Sapkota, K.; Park, S.E.; Kim, S.; Kim, S.J. Celastrol from 'Thunder God Vine' protects SH-SY5Y cells through the preservation of mitochondrial function and inhibition of p38 MAPK in a rotenone model of Parkinson's disease. *Neurochem. Res.* **2014**, *39*, 84–96. [CrossRef] [PubMed]

45. Tarafdar, A.; Pula, G. The Role of NADPH Oxidases and Oxidative Stress in Neurodegenerative Disorders. *Int. J. Mol. Sci.* **2018**, *19*, E3824. [CrossRef]

46. Jaquet, V.; Marcoux, J.; Forest, E.; Leidal, K.G.; McCormick, S.; Westermaier, Y.; Perozzo, R.; Plastre, O.; Fioraso-Cartier, L.; Diebold, B.; et al. NADPH oxidase (NOX) isoforms are inhibited by celastrol with a dual mode of action. *Br. J. Pharmacol.* **2011**, *164*, 507–520. [CrossRef]

47. Schiavone, S.; Jaquet, V.; Trabace, L.; Krause, K.H. Severe life stress and oxidative stress in the brain: From animal models to human pathology. *Antioxid. Redox Signal.* **2013**, *18*, 1475–1490. [CrossRef]

48. Kawanishi, S.; Oikawa, S. Mechanism of telomere shortening by oxidative stress. *Ann. N. Y. Acad. Sci.* **2004**, *1019*, 278–284. [CrossRef]

49. Konieczny, J.; Jantas, D.; Lenda, T.; Domin, H.; Czarnecka, A.; Kuter, K.; Smialowska, M.; Lason, W.; Lorenc-Koci, E. Lack of neuroprotective effect of celastrol under conditions of proteasome inhibition by lactacystin in in vitro and in vivo studies: Implications for Parkinson's disease. *Neurotox. Res.* **2014**, *26*, 255–273. [CrossRef]

50. Cleren, C.; Calingasan, N.Y.; Chen, J.; Beal, M.F. Celastrol protects against MPTP- and 3-nitropropionic acid-induced neurotoxicity. *J. Neurochem.* **2005**, *94*, 995–1004. [CrossRef]

51. Faust, K.; Gehrke, S.; Yang, Y.; Yang, L.; Beal, M.F.; Lu, B. Neuroprotective effects of compounds with antioxidant and anti-inflammatory properties in a Drosophila model of Parkinson's disease. *BMC Neurosci.* **2009**, *10*, 109. [CrossRef] [PubMed]

52. Brown, I.R. Heat shock proteins and protection of the nervous system. *Ann. N. Y. Acad. Sci.* **2007**, *1113*, 147–158. [CrossRef] [PubMed]

53. Abdin, A.A.; Hasby, E.A. Modulatory effect of celastrol on Th1/Th2 cytokines profile, TLR2 and CD3 + T-lymphocyte expression in a relapsing-remitting model of multiple sclerosis in rats. *Eur. J. Pharmacol.* **2014**, *742*, 102–112. [CrossRef] [PubMed]

54. Wang, Y.; Cao, L.; Xu, L.M.; Cao, F.F.; Peng, B.; Zhang, X.; Shen, Y.F.; Uzan, G.; Zhang, D.H. Celastrol Ameliorates EAE Induction by Suppressing Pathogenic T Cell Responses in the Peripheral and Central Nervous Systems. *J. Neuroimmune Pharmacol. Off. J. Soc. Neuroimmune Pharmacol.* **2015**, *10*, 506–516. [CrossRef]

55. Malkov, A.; Ivanov, A.I.; Latyshkova, A.; Bregestovski, P.; Zilberter, M.; Zilberter, Y. Activation of nicotinamide adenine dinucleotide phosphate oxidase is the primary trigger of epileptic seizures in rodent models. *Ann. Neurol.* **2019**, *85*, 907–920. [CrossRef]

56. Von Ruden, E.L.; Wolf, F.; Gualtieri, F.; Keck, M.; Hunt, C.R.; Pandita, T.K.; Potschka, H. Genetic and pharmacological targeting of heat shock protein 70 in the mouse amygdala-kindling model. *ACS Chem. Neurosci.* **2019**, *10*, 1434–1444. [CrossRef]

57. Jiang, M.; Liu, X.; Zhang, D.; Wang, Y.; Hu, X.; Xu, F.; Jin, M.; Cao, F.; Xu, L. Celastrol treatment protects against acute ischemic stroke-induced brain injury by promoting an IL-33/ST2 axis-mediated microglia/macrophage M2 polarization. *J. Neuroinflamm.* **2018**, *15*, 78. [CrossRef]

58. Li, Y.; He, D.; Zhang, X.; Liu, Z.; Zhang, X.; Dong, L.; Xing, Y.; Wang, C.; Qiao, H.; Zhu, C.; et al. Protective effect of celastrol in rat cerebral ischemia model: Down-regulating p-JNK, p-c-Jun and NF-kappaB. *Brain Res.* **2012**, *1464*, 8–13. [CrossRef]

59. Zhu, F.; Li, C.; Jin, X.P.; Weng, S.X.; Fan, L.L.; Zheng, Z.; Li, W.L.; Wang, F.; Wang, W.F.; Hu, X.F.; et al. Celastrol may have an anti-atherosclerosis effect in a rabbit experimental carotid atherosclerosis model. *Int. J. Clin. Exp. Med.* **2014**, *7*, 1684–1691.

60. Kim, J.Y.; Kim, N.; Zheng, Z.; Lee, J.E.; Yenari, M.A. The 70 kDa heat shock protein protects against experimental traumatic brain injury. *Neurobiol. Dis.* **2013**, *58*, 289–295. [CrossRef]

61. Eroglu, B.; Kimbler, D.E.; Pang, J.; Choi, J.; Moskophidis, D.; Yanasak, N.; Dhandapani, K.M.; Mivechi, N.F. Therapeutic inducers of the HSP70/HSP110 protect mice against traumatic brain injury. *J. Neurochem.* **2014**, *130*, 626–641. [CrossRef] [PubMed]

62. Readhead, B.; Hartley, B.J.; Eastwood, B.J.; Collier, D.A.; Evans, D.; Farias, R.; He, C.; Hoffman, G.; Sklar, P.; Dudley, J.T.; et al. Expression-based drug screening of neural progenitor cells from individuals with schizophrenia. *Nat. Commun.* **2018**, *9*, 4412. [CrossRef] [PubMed]

63. Cheung, H.M.; Yew, D.T.W. Effects of perinatal exposure to ketamine on the developing brain. *Front. Neurosci.* **2019**, *13*, 138. [CrossRef] [PubMed]

64. Coronel-Oliveros, C.M.; Pacheco-Calderon, R. Prenatal exposure to ketamine in rats: Implications on animal models of schizophrenia. *Dev. Psychobiol.* **2018**, *60*, 30–42. [CrossRef]

65. Liao, W.T.; Xiao, X.Y.; Zhu, Y.; Zhou, S.P. The effect of celastrol on learning and memory in diabetic rats after sevoflurane inhalation. *Arch. Med. Sci. AMS* **2018**, *14*, 370–380. [CrossRef]

66. Hooper, P.L.; Durham, H.D.; Torok, Z.; Hooper, P.L.; Crul, T.; Vigh, L. The central role of heat shock factor 1 in synaptic fidelity and memory consolidation. *Cell Stress Chaperones* **2016**, *21*, 745–753. [CrossRef]

67. Barker-Haliski, M.L.; Loscher, W.; White, H.S.; Galanopoulou, A.S. Neuroinflammation in epileptogenesis: Insights and translational perspectives from new models of epilepsy. *Epilepsia* **2017**, *58* (Suppl. S3), 39–47. [CrossRef]

68. Wesson, D.W. Sniffing behavior communicates social hierarchy. *Curr. Biol.* **2013**, *23*, 575–580. [CrossRef]

69. Lee, P.R.; Brady, D.L.; Shapiro, R.A.; Dorsa, D.M.; Koenig, J.I. Social interaction deficits caused by chronic phencyclidine administration are reversed by oxytocin. *Neuropsychopharmacol. Off. Publ. Am. Coll. Neuropsychopharmacol.* **2005**, *30*, 1883–1894. [CrossRef]

70. Snigdha, S.; Neill, J.C. Efficacy of antipsychotics to reverse phencyclidine-induced social interaction deficits in female rats–a preliminary investigation. *Behav. Brain Res.* **2008**, *187*, 489–494. [CrossRef]

71. Bozdagi, O.; Sakurai, T.; Papapetrou, D.; Wang, X.; Dickstein, D.L.; Takahashi, N.; Kajiwara, Y.; Yang, M.; Katz, A.M.; Scattoni, M.L.; et al. Haploinsufficiency of the autism-associated Shank3 gene leads to deficits in synaptic function, social interaction, and social communication. *Mol. Autism* **2010**, *1*, 15. [CrossRef] [PubMed]

72. Becker, A.; Peters, B.; Schroeder, H.; Mann, T.; Huether, G.; Grecksch, G. Ketamine-induced changes in rat behaviour: A possible animal model of schizophrenia. *Prog. Neuro Psychopharmacol. Biol. Psychiatry* **2003**, *27*, 687–700. [CrossRef]

73. Schweinfurth, M.K.; Stieger, B.; Taborsky, M. Experimental evidence for reciprocity in allogrooming among wild-type Norway rats. *Sci. Rep.* **2017**, *7*, 4010. [CrossRef] [PubMed]

74. Alleva, E. 7—Assessment of Aggressive Behavior in Rodents. In *Methods in Neurosciences*; Conn, P.M., Ed.; Academic Press: Cambridge, MA, USA, 1993; Volume 14, pp. 111–137.

75. Shin, S.Y.; Baek, N.J.; Han, S.H.; Min, S.S. Chronic administration of ketamine ameliorates the anxiety- and aggressive-like behavior in adolescent mice induced by neonatal maternal separation. *Korean J. Physiol. Pharmacol. Off. J. Korean Physiol. Soc. Korean Soc. Pharmacol.* **2019**, *23*, 81–87. [CrossRef] [PubMed]

76. Hira, S.; Saleem, U.; Anwar, F.; Ahmad, B. Antioxidants Attenuate Isolation- and L-DOPA-Induced Aggression in Mice. *Front. Pharmacol.* **2017**, *8*, 945. [CrossRef] [PubMed]

77. Garratt, M.; Brooks, R.C. A genetic reduction in antioxidant function causes elevated aggression in mice. *J. Exp. Biol.* **2015**, *218 Pt 2*, 223–227. [CrossRef]

78. Kim, T.; Lee, K.H.; Oh, H.; Lee, T.Y.; Cho, K.I.K.; Lee, J.; Kwon, J.S. Cerebellar structural abnormalities associated with cognitive function in patients with first-episode psychosis. *Front. Psychiatry* **2018**, *9*, 286. [CrossRef]

79. Moberget, T.; Ivry, R.B. Prediction, Psychosis, and the Cerebellum. *Biol. Psychiatry Cogn. Neurosci. Neuroimaging* **2019**, *4*, 820–831. [CrossRef]

80. Jones, C.A.; Watson, D.J.; Fone, K.C. Animal models of schizophrenia. *Br. J. Pharmacol.* **2011**, *164*, 1162–1194. [CrossRef]

81. Shinn, A.K.; Roh, Y.S.; Ravichandran, C.T.; Baker, J.T.; Ongur, D.; Cohen, B.M. Aberrant cerebellar connectivity in bipolar disorder with psychosis. *Biol. Psychiatry. Cogn. Neurosci. Neuroimaging* **2017**, *2*, 438–448. [CrossRef]

82. Yadav, M.; Parle, M.; Jindal, D.K.; Dhingra, S. Protective effects of stigmasterol against ketamine-induced psychotic symptoms: Possible behavioral, biochemical and histopathological changes in mice. *Pharmacol. Rep. Pr* **2018**, *70*, 591–599. [CrossRef] [PubMed]

83. Yadav, M.; Jindal, D.K.; Dhingra, M.S.; Kumar, A.; Parle, M.; Dhingra, S. Protective effect of gallic acid in experimental model of ketamine-induced psychosis: Possible behaviour, biochemical, neurochemical and cellular alterations. *Inflammopharmacology* **2018**, *26*, 413–424. [CrossRef] [PubMed]

84. Brambrink, A.M.; Evers, A.S.; Avidan, M.S.; Farber, N.B.; Smith, D.J.; Martin, L.D.; Dissen, G.A.; Creeley, C.E.; Olney, J.W. Ketamine-induced neuroapoptosis in the fetal and neonatal rhesus macaque brain. *Anesthesiology* **2012**, *116*, 372–384. [CrossRef] [PubMed]

85. Tobe, E.H. Mitochondrial dysfunction, oxidative stress, and major depressive disorder. *Neuropsychiatr. Dis. Treat.* **2013**, *9*, 567–573. [CrossRef] [PubMed]

86. Zhang, D.; Cheng, L.; Craig, D.W.; Redman, M.; Liu, C. Cerebellar telomere length and psychiatric disorders. *Behav. Genet.* **2010**, *40*, 250–254. [CrossRef]

87. Filiou, M.D.; Teplytska, L.; Otte, D.M.; Zimmer, A.; Turck, C.W. Myelination and oxidative stress alterations in the cerebellum of the G72/G30 transgenic schizophrenia mouse model. *J. Psychiatr. Res.* **2012**, *46*, 1359–1365. [CrossRef]

88. Streck, E.L.; Rezin, G.T.; Barbosa, L.M.; Assis, L.C.; Grandi, E.; Quevedo, J. Effect of antipsychotics on succinate dehydrogenase and cytochrome oxidase activities in rat brain. *Naunyn-Schmiedeberg's Arch. Pharmacol.* **2007**, *376*, 127–133. [CrossRef]

89. Assis, L.C.; Scaini, G.; Di-Pietro, P.B.; Castro, A.A.; Comim, C.M.; Streck, E.L.; Quevedo, J. Effect of antipsychotics on creatine kinase activity in rat brain. *Basic Clin. Pharmacol. Toxicol.* **2007**, *101*, 315–319. [CrossRef]

90. Cao, H.; Chen, O.Y.; Chung, Y.; Forsyth, J.K.; McEwen, S.C.; Gee, D.G.; Bearden, C.E.; Addington, J.; Goodyear, B.; Cadenhead, K.S.; et al. Cerebello-thalamo-cortical hyperconnectivity as a state-independent functional neural signature for psychosis prediction and characterization. *Nat. Commun.* **2018**, *9*, 3836. [CrossRef]

91. Gu, F.; Chauhan, V.; Chauhan, A. Impaired synthesis and antioxidant defense of glutathione in the cerebellum of autistic subjects: Alterations in the activities and protein expression of glutathione-related enzymes. *Free Radic. Biol. Med.* **2013**, *65*, 488–496. [CrossRef]

92. Olguin-Albuerne, M.; Moran, J. ROS produced by NOX2 control in vitro development of cerebellar granule neurons development. *ASN Neuro* **2015**, *7*. [CrossRef] [PubMed]

93. Coyoy, A.; Valencia, A.; Guemez-Gamboa, A.; Moran, J. Role of NADPH oxidase in the apoptotic death of cultured cerebellar granule neurons. *Free Radic. Biol. Med.* **2008**, *45*, 1056–1064. [CrossRef] [PubMed]

94. Sorce, S.; Nuvolone, M.; Keller, A.; Falsig, J.; Varol, A.; Schwarz, P.; Bieri, M.; Budka, H.; Aguzzi, A. The role of the NADPH oxidase NOX2 in prion pathogenesis. *PLoS Pathog.* **2014**, *10*, e1004531. [CrossRef] [PubMed]

95. Nadeem, A.; Ahmad, S.F.; Al-Harbi, N.O.; Attia, S.M.; Alshammari, M.A.; Alzahrani, K.S.; Bakheet, S.A. Increased oxidative stress in the cerebellum and peripheral immune cells leads to exaggerated autism-like repetitive behavior due to deficiency of antioxidant response in BTBR T + tf/J mice. *Prog. Neuro-Psychopharmacol. Biol. Psychiatry* **2019**, *89*, 245–253. [CrossRef] [PubMed]

96. Cristovao, A.C.; Guhathakurta, S.; Bok, E.; Je, G.; Yoo, S.D.; Choi, D.H.; Kim, Y.S. NADPH oxidase 1 mediates alpha-synucleinopathy in Parkinson's disease. *J. Neurosci. Off. J. Soc. Neurosci.* **2012**, *32*, 14465–14477. [CrossRef] [PubMed]

97. Jiang, T.; Sun, Q.; Chen, S. Oxidative stress: A major pathogenesis and potential therapeutic target of antioxidative agents in Parkinson's disease and Alzheimer's disease. *Prog. Neurobiol.* **2016**, *147*, 1–19. [CrossRef] [PubMed]

98. Belarbi, K.; Cuvelier, E.; Destée, A.; Gressier, B.; Chartier-Harlin, M.C. NADPH oxidases in Parkinson's disease: A systematic review. *Mol. Neurodegener.* **2017**, *12*, 84. [CrossRef]

99. Cheret, C.; Gervais, A.; Lelli, A.; Colin, C.; Amar, L.; Ravassard, P.; Mallet, J.; Cumano, A.; Krause, K.H.; Mallat, M. Neurotoxic activation of microglia is promoted by a nox1-dependent NADPH oxidase. *J. Neurosci. Off. J. Soc. Neurosci.* **2008**, *28*, 12039–12051. [CrossRef]

100. Nakki, R.; Nickolenko, J.; Chang, J.; Sagar, S.M.; Sharp, F.R. Haloperidol prevents ketamine- and phencyclidine-induced HSP70 protein expression but not microglial activation. *Exp. Neurol.* **1996**, *137*, 234–241. [CrossRef]

101. Vasconcellos, L.R.; Dutra, F.F.; Siqueira, M.S.; Paula-Neto, H.A.; Dahan, J.; Kiarely, E.; Carneiro, L.A.; Bozza, M.T.; Travassos, L.H. Protein aggregation as a cellular response to oxidative stress induced by heme and iron. *Proc. Natl. Acad. Sci. USA* **2016**, *113*, E7474–E7482. [CrossRef]

102. Chen, F.; Pandey, D.; Chadli, A.; Catravas, J.D.; Chen, T.; Fulton, D.J. Hsp90 regulates NADPH oxidase activity and is necessary for superoxide but not hydrogen peroxide production. *Antioxid. Redox Signal.* **2011**, *14*, 2107–2119. [CrossRef] [PubMed]

103. Troyanova, N.I.; Shevchenko, M.A.; Boyko, A.A.; Mirzoyev, R.R.; Pertseva, M.A.; Kovalenko, E.I.; Sapozhnikov, A.M. Modulating effect of extracellular HSP70 on generation of reactive oxigen species in populations of phagocytes. *Bioorganicheskaia Khimiia* **2015**, *41*, 305–315. [CrossRef] [PubMed]

104. Boczek, T.; Lisek, M.; Ferenc, B.; Wiktorska, M.; Ivchevska, I.; Zylinska, L. Region-specific effects of repeated ketamine administration on the presynaptic GABAergic neurochemistry in rat brain. *Neurochem. Int.* **2015**, *91*, 13–25. [CrossRef] [PubMed]

105. Wang, C.; Shi, C.; Yang, X.; Yang, M.; Sun, H.; Wang, C. Celastrol suppresses obesity process via increasing antioxidant capacity and improving lipid metabolism. *Eur. J. Pharmacol.* **2014**, *744*, 52–58. [CrossRef]

106. Divya, T.; Dineshbabu, V.; Soumyakrishnan, S.; Sureshkumar, A.; Sudhandiran, G. Celastrol enhances Nrf2 mediated antioxidant enzymes and exhibits anti-fibrotic effect through regulation of collagen production against bleomycin-induced pulmonary fibrosis. *Chem. Biol. Interact.* **2016**, *246*, 52–62. [CrossRef]

107. Chen, G.; Zhang, X.; Zhao, M.; Wang, Y.; Cheng, X.; Wang, D.; Xu, Y.; Du, Z.; Yu, X. Celastrol targets mitochondrial respiratory chain complex I to induce reactive oxygen species-dependent cytotoxicity in tumor cells. *BMC Cancer* **2011**, *11*, 170. [CrossRef]

108. Braun, I.; Genius, J.; Grunze, H.; Bender, A.; Möller, H.J.; Rujescu, D. Alterations of hippocampal and prefrontal GABAergic interneurons in an animal model of psychosis induced by NMDA receptor antagonism. *Schizophr. Res.* **2007**, *97*, 254–263. [CrossRef]

109. Schiavone, S.; Neri, M.; Trabace, L.; Turillazzi, E. The NADPH oxidase NOX2 mediates loss of parvalbumin interneurons in traumatic brain injury: Human autoptic immunohistochemical evidence. *Sci. Rep.* **2017**, *7*, 8752. [CrossRef]

110. Meyer, U.; Feldon, J.; Dammann, O. Schizophrenia and autism: Both shared and disorder-specific pathogenesis via perinatal inflammation? *Pediatric Res.* **2011**, *69*, 26–33. [CrossRef]

111. Wang, H.; Guo, W.; Liu, F.; Wang, G.; Lyu, H.; Wu, R.; Chen, J.; Wang, S.; Li, L.; Zhao, J. Patients with first-episode, drug-naive schizophrenia and subjects at ultra-high risk of psychosis shared increased cerebellar-default mode network connectivity at rest. *Sci. Rep.* **2016**, *6*, 26124. [CrossRef]

112. Zheng, X.; Zhou, J.; Xia, Y. The role of TNF-α in regulating ketamine-induced hippocampal neurotoxicity. *Arch. Med. Sci. AMS* **2015**, *11*, 1296–1302. [CrossRef] [PubMed]

113. Li, Y.; Shen, R.; Wen, G.; Ding, R.; Du, A.; Zhou, J.; Dong, Z.; Ren, X.; Yao, H.; Zhao, R.; et al. Effects of ketamine on levels of inflammatory cytokines IL-6, IL-1beta, and TNF-alpha in the hippocampus of mice following acute or chronic administration. *Front. Pharmacol.* **2017**, *8*, 139. [PubMed]

114. Onuki, Y.; Van Someren, E.J.W.; De Zeeuw, C.I.; Van der Werf, Y.D. Hippocampal–cerebellar interaction during spatio-temporal prediction. *Cereb. Cortex* **2013**, *25*, 313–321. [CrossRef] [PubMed]

115. Babayan, B.M.; Watilliaux, A.; Viejo, G.; Paradis, A.-L.; Girard, B.; Rondi-Reig, L. A hippocampo-cerebellar centred network for the learning and execution of sequence-based navigation. *Sci. Rep.* **2017**, *7*, 17812. [CrossRef] [PubMed]

116. Decourt, B.; Lahiri, D.K.; Sabbagh, M.N. Targeting tumor necrosis factor alpha for Alzheimer's disease. *Curr. Alzheimer Res.* **2017**, *14*, 412–425. [CrossRef]

117. Allison, A.; Cacabelos, R.; Lombardi, V.; Alvarez, X.; Vigo, C. Celastrol, a potent antioxidant and anti-inflammatory drug, as a possible treatment for Alzheimer's disease. *Prog. Neuro-Psychopharmacol. Biol. Psychiatry* **2001**, *25*, 1341–1357. [CrossRef]

118. Müller, N. Inflammation in Schizophrenia: Pathogenetic Aspects and Therapeutic Considerations. *Schizophr. Bull.* **2018**, *44*, 973–982. [CrossRef]

119. Kim, Y.-K.; Jung, H.-G.; Myint, A.-M.; Kim, H.; Park, S.-H. Imbalance between pro-inflammatory and anti-inflammatory cytokines in bipolar disorder. *J. Affect. Disord.* **2007**, *104*, 91–95. [CrossRef]

120. Garcia, J.M.; Stillings, S.A.; Leclerc, J.L.; Phillips, H.; Edwards, N.J.; Robicsek, S.A.; Hoh, B.L.; Blackburn, S.; Dore, S. Role of Interleukin-10 in Acute Brain Injuries. *Front. Neurol.* **2017**, *8*, 244. [CrossRef]

121. Stoll, G.; Jander, S.; Schroeter, M. *Cytokines in CNS Disorders: Neurotoxicity versus Neuroprotection*; Advances in Dementia Research, Vienna, 2000//; Jellinger, K., Schmidt, R., Windisch, M., Eds.; Springer Vienna: Vienna, Austria, 2000; pp. 81–89.

122. Zhu, Y.; Chen, X.; Liu, Z.; Peng, Y.P.; Qiu, Y.H. Interleukin-10 Protection against lipopolysaccharide-induced neuro-inflammation and neurotoxicity in ventral mesencephalic cultures. *Int. J. Mol. Sci.* **2015**, *17*, 25. [CrossRef]

123. Bachis, A.; Colangelo, A.M.; Vicini, S.; Doe, P.P.; De Bernardi, M.A.; Brooker, G.; Mocchetti, I. Interleukin-10 prevents glutamate-mediated cerebellar granule cell death by blocking caspase-3-like activity. *J. Neurosci.* **2001**, *21*, 3104–3112. [CrossRef] [PubMed]

124. Lim, S.H.; Park, E.; You, B.; Jung, Y.; Park, A.R.; Park, S.G.; Lee, J.R. Neuronal synapse formation induced by microglia and interleukin 10. *PLoS ONE* **2013**, *8*, e81218. [CrossRef] [PubMed]

125. Lueptow, L.M. Novel object recognition test for the investigation of learning and memory in mice. *J. Vis. Exp. Jove* **2017**, *126*, e55718. [CrossRef] [PubMed]

126. Trabace, L.; Cassano, T.; Colaianna, M.; Castrignano, S.; Giustino, A.; Amoroso, S.; Steardo, L.; Cuomo, V. Neurochemical and neurobehavioral effects of ganstigmine (CHF2819), a novel acetylcholinesterase inhibitor, in rat prefrontal cortex: An in vivo study. *Pharmacol. Res.* **2007**, *56*, 288–294. [CrossRef]

127. Carratu, M.R.; Borracci, P.; Coluccia, A.; Giustino, A.; Renna, G.; Tomasini, M.C.; Raisi, E.; Antonelli, T.; Cuomo, V.; Mazzoni, E.; et al. Acute exposure to methylmercury at two developmental windows: Focus on neurobehavioral and neurochemical effects in rat offspring. *Neuroscience* **2006**, *141*, 1619–1629. [CrossRef]

128. Nogueira Neto, J.D.; de Almeida, A.A.; da Silva Oliveira, J.; Dos Santos, P.S.; de Sousa, D.P.; de Freitas, R.M. Antioxidant effects of nerolidol in mice hippocampus after open field test. *Neurochem. Res.* **2013**, *38*, 1861–1870. [CrossRef]

129. Fortes, A.C.; Almeida, A.A.; Mendonca-Junior, F.J.; Freitas, R.M.; Soares-Sobrinho, J.L.; de La Roca Soares, M.F. Anxiolytic properties of new chemical entity, 5TIO1. *Neurochem. Res.* **2013**, *38*, 726–731. [CrossRef]

130. Crawley, J.N.; Chen, T.; Puri, A.; Washburn, R.; Sullivan, T.L.; Hill, J.M.; Young, N.B.; Nadler, J.J.; Moy, S.S.; Young, L.J.; et al. Social approach behaviors in oxytocin knockout mice: Comparison of two independent lines tested in different laboratory environments. *Neuropeptides* **2007**, *41*, 145–163. [CrossRef]

131. Silverman, J.L.; Turner, S.M.; Barkan, C.L.; Tolu, S.S.; Saxena, R.; Hung, A.Y.; Sheng, M.; Crawley, J.N. Sociability and motor functions in Shank1 mutant mice. *Brain Res.* **2011**, *1380*, 120–137. [CrossRef]

132. Kaidanovich-Beilin, O.; Lipina, T.; Vukobradovic, I.; Roder, J.; Woodgett, J.R. Assessment of social interaction behaviors. *J. Vis. Exp. Jove* **2011**, *25*, e2473. [CrossRef]

133. Schiavone, S.; Tucci, P.; Mhillaj, E.; Bove, M.; Trabace, L.; Morgese, M.G. Antidepressant drugs for beta amyloid-induced depression: A new standpoint? *Prog. Neuro-Psychopharmacol. Biol. Psychiatry* **2017**, *78*, 114–122. [CrossRef] [PubMed]

134. Morgese, M.G.; Tucci, P.; Mhillaj, E.; Bove, M.; Schiavone, S.; Trabace, L.; Cuomo, V. Lifelong nutritional omega-3 deficiency evokes depressive-like state through soluble beta amyloid. *Mol. Neurobiol.* **2017**, *54*, 2079–2089. [CrossRef] [PubMed]

3

The Effects of 2′,4′-Dihydroxy-6′-methoxy-3′,5′-dimethylchalcone from *Cleistocalyx operculatus* Buds on Human Pancreatic Cancer Cell Lines

Huynh Nhu Tuan [1,†], Bui Hoang Minh [2,†], Phuong Thao Tran [3], Jeong Hyung Lee [3], Ha Van Oanh [1], Quynh Mai Thi Ngo [4], Yen Nhi Nguyen [5], Pham Thi Kim Lien [6] and Manh Hung Tran [6,*]

[1] Hanoi University of Pharmacy, 13 Le Thanh Tong Street, Hoan Kiem District, Hanoi 100100, Vietnam
[2] Faculty of Pharmacy, Nguyen Tat Thanh University, 300C Nguyen Tat Thanh Street, District 4, Hochiminh City 72820, Vietnam
[3] Department of Biochemistry, College of Natural Sciences, Kangwon National University, Chuncheon, Gangwon-Do 24414, Korea
[4] College of Pharmacy, Hai Phong University of Medicine and Pharmacy, 72A Nguyen Binh Khiem, Hai Phong 180000, Vietnam
[5] Faculty of Biology and Biotechnology, University of Science, Vietnam National University Hochiminh City, 227 Nguyen Van Cu, District 5, Hochiminh City 748000, Vietnam
[6] Biomedical Sciences Department, Institute for Research & Executive Education (VNUK), The University of Danang, 158A Le Loi, Hai Chau District, Danang City 551000, Vietnam
* Correspondence: tmhung801018@gmail.com
† These authors contributed equally to this research.

Academic Editor: Pinarosa Avato

Abstract: 2′,4′-Dihydroxy-6′-methoxy-3′,5′-dimethylchalcone (DMC), a principal natural chalcone of *Cleistocalyx operculatus* buds, suppresses the growth of many types of cancer cells. However, the effects of this compound on pancreatic cancer cells have not been evaluated. In our experiments, we explored the effects of this chalcone on two human pancreatic cancer cell lines. A cell proliferation assay revealed that DMC exhibited concentration-dependent cytotoxicity against PANC-1 and MIA PACA2 cells, with IC$_{50}$ values of 10.5 ± 0.8 and 12.2 ± 0.9 μM, respectively. Treatment of DMC led to the apoptosis of PANC-1 by caspase-3 activation as revealed by annexin-V/propidium iodide double-staining. Western blotting indicated that DMC induced proteolytic activation of caspase-3 and -9, degradation of caspase-3 substrate proteins (including poly[ADP-ribose] polymerase [PARP]), augmented bak protein level, while attenuating the expression of bcl-2 in PANC-1 cells. Taken together, our results provide experimental evidence to support that DMC may serve as a useful chemotherapeutic agent for control of human pancreatic cancer cells.

Keywords: *Cleistocalyx operculatus*; 2′,4′-dihydroxy-6′-methoxy-3′,5′-dimethylchalcone (DMC); pPancreatic cancer; PANC-1

1. Introduction

Pancreatic cancer (PC) causes significant mortality in the USA and other countries [1]. The GLOBOCAN 2012 summit reported that PC is responsible for over 331,000 deaths annually, and is the seventh leading cause of cancer deaths in both males and females [2,3]. PC includes adenocarcinomas, accounting for approximately 85% of cases, with an overall 5-year survival rate of 5–10%, and endocrine tumors constituting less than 5% of all cases [2,3]. The causes remain insufficiently known; however, previous studies have established that the risk factors include obesity, a genetic predisposition, diabetes, a poor diet, and physical inactivity. In addition, smoking was recognized to be a risk factor of PC. [4,5]. Over the past 10 years, PC mortality has increased in both genders in the USA, Europe, Japan, and China [4,5]. Currently, there are no effective screening recommendations for PC; therefore a better understanding of the cause and identification of risk factors is essential to prevent this disease [6]. Several therapies for PC such as radiotherapy, chemotherapy, and immunotherapy have been developed; however, drug development for this cancer remains challenging. In the search for new anti-PC drugs, natural products have been identified as potential sources for the development of new drugs [7,8].

Cleistocalyx operculatus, a member of Myrtaceae family, had been used as a beverage since ancient times in Vietnam for the treatment of cold, fever, inflammation, and gastrointestinal disorders [9]. A bud water extract increased contractility and decreased the frequency of contraction in an isolated rat heart perfusion system. Moreover, data from several studies also suggested that this extract protected lipid peroxidation in rat liver microsomes and the trauma of PC12 cells; and inhibited α-glucosidase, rat-intestinal maltase, and sucrase activities [10–13]. The plant contains chalcones, flavanones, flavones, and triterpenoids exhibiting many pharmaceutical activities, including anti-tumor effects; inhibition of cancer cell growth; and anti-cholinesterase, anti-oxidation, anti-hyperglycemia, anti-influenza, and anti-inflammation activities [14–18]. Of the active compounds, the chalcone 2',4'-dihydroxy-6'-methoxy-3',5'-dimethylchalcone (DMC) exhibited both cytotoxic and anti-tumor effects in vivo and was cytotoxic to several cancer cell lines in vitro. DMC could reverse multi-drug resistance in HCC cell lines. Moreover, this compound displayed hepatoprotection and neuroprotection, promoted glucose uptake, affected the differentiation of 3T3-L1 cells into adipocytes; and reduced drug efflux by suppressing Nrf2/ARE signaling in human HCC BEL-7402/5-FU cells [19–22]. DMC triggers SMMC-7721 cell apoptosis via the mitochondrion-dependent pathway, inhibiting Bcl-2 expression and thus causing outer mitochondrial membrane disintegration [23]. DMC is the most cytotoxic agent isolated from the plant to date. Here, we isolated DMC (Figure 1A) from buds of C. operculatus using several chromatographic steps, and explored the effects thereof on some human cancer cell lines. We also provide the first evidence that DMC induces apoptosis of the human pancreatic cancer cell lines PANC-1.

2. Results

2.1. Cell Proliferation Activity

To investigate the effects of DMC on the human pancreatic cancer cell lines PANC-1 and MIA PACA2 growth, cells were treated with DMC (3–30 μM) for 48 h, and after that, cell numbers and viability were measured using a Dojindo kit. DMC significantly inhibited PANC-1 (Figure 1B) and MIA PACA2 cell proliferation (Figure 1C) in concentration-dependent manners, with IC_{50} values of 10.5 ± 0.8 and 12.2 ± 0.9 μM, respectively. Inverted microscopy revealed that exposure to DMC for 24 h greatly affected the number of cell death of PANC-1 cells (Figure 1D). Considering that DMC showed stronger toxicity against PANC-1 than MIA PACA2 our subsequent studies focused on the mechanism of action of DMC in PANC-1.

2.2. Caspase-3 activity

Caspase-3 is a member of the cysteine-aspartic acid protease family and usually exists as an inactive precursor of 32 kDa in size. When it is in activation mode, this causes the death of cell by an apoptosis pathway via cleavage of proteins into heterozygous substances. DMC (3–30 μM) was added to PANC-1 cells (1×10^6/well) followed by incubation for 12, 24, and 48 h; this enhanced caspase-3 activation was measured by assaying the levels of Ac-Asp-Glu-Val-Asp-8- amino-4-trifluoromethylcoumarin (Av-DEVD-AFC).

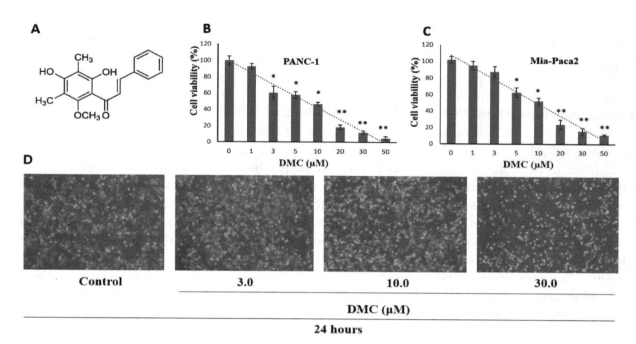

Figure 1. (**A**) Chemical structure of DMC; Effect of DMC on PANC-1 (**B**), and MIA-PACA2 (**C**) cell viability; and (**D**) PANC-1 cell morphology visualized by light microscopy (scale bar 500 μm), cells were seeded into 6-well plates at 1×10^5 cells/well and treated with the indicated concentration of DMC for 24 h. Data are presented as the mean ± standard deviation of three independent experiments performed in duplicate (*$p < 0.01$; **$p < 0.05$).

Figure 2 shows that caspase-3 activity increased 3–9-fold in a dose-dependent manner, when DMC-induced activities were compared to those of the vehicle.

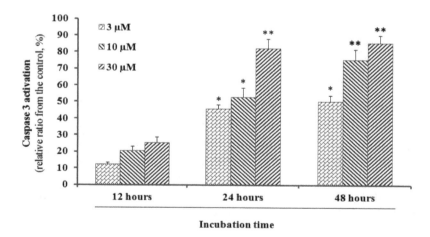

Figure 2. The increment of caspase-3 activity in PANC-1 cells treated by DMC in vitro. After 12 h, 24 h and 48 h incubation with DMC (3–30 μM), the cell lysates were incubated at 37 °C with caspase-3 substrate (Ac-DEVD-AFC) for 1 h. The fluorescence intensity of the cell lysates was measured to determine the caspase-3 activity. The blank group was used as 0.1% DMSO-treated cells. Data are presented as the mean ± SD of results from three independent experiments (* $p < 0.01$; ** $p < 0.05$).

2.3. Induction of Apoptosis by DMC

Next, PANC-1 cells (5×10^5) were treated with DMC (3–30 μM) for 48 h, stained with annexin V/PI, and subjected to flow cytometry using a BD Biosciences platform. Early and late apoptotic cells, and necrotic cells, were counted; and total and early apoptosis quantified (Figure 3). Apoptotic cell numbers increased in a DMC dose-dependent manner.

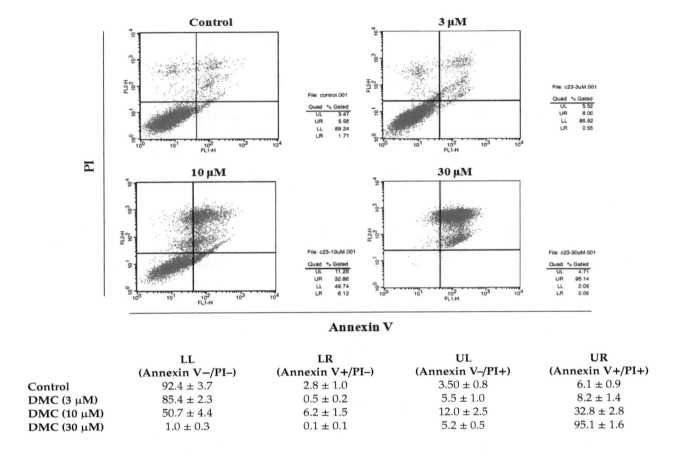

	LL (Annexin V−/PI−)	LR (Annexin V+/PI−)	UL (Annexin V−/PI+)	UR (Annexin V+/PI+)
Control	92.4 ± 3.7	2.8 ± 1.0	3.50 ± 0.8	6.1 ± 0.9
DMC (3 μM)	85.4 ± 2.3	0.5 ± 0.2	5.5 ± 1.0	8.2 ± 1.4
DMC (10 μM)	50.7 ± 4.4	6.2 ± 1.5	12.0 ± 2.5	32.8 ± 2.8
DMC (30 μM)	1.0 ± 0.3	0.1 ± 0.1	5.2 ± 0.5	95.1 ± 1.6

Figure 3. Effect of DMC on apoptosis of PANC-1 cells. Apoptosis quantification using annexin V/PI double staining assay after treatment with DMC (3–30 μM) for 48 h. PANC-1 cells were harvested and stained with PI and annexin V-FITC in darkness for 15 min. Data are presented as the mean ± SD of results from three independent experiments.

2.4. Effect of DMC on the Expression of Apoptosis-Related Protein

As the apoptotic cell population thus increased dramatically, we next measured the levels of apoptotic proteins. We used western blotting to detect death receptors and pro-apoptotic ligands that might be involved in DMC (3–30 μM)-induced PANC-1 apoptosis. As shown in Figure 4, DMC significantly inhibited expression of the anti-apoptotic Bcl-2 protein in a dose-dependent manner. Notably, the levels of the pro-apoptotic Bax protein were also changed by DMC. Recent evidences have suggested that the mitochondrial mutilation expedited cytochrome c (Cyt-c) which was discharged from mitochondria into the cytoplasm, triggering apoptotic progression. This process caused the stimulation of the caspase signaling and mitochondria-facilitated apoptosis so we assessed whether DMC triggers apoptosis via this mechanism in PANC-1 cells. We used western blotting to measure Cyt-c protein levels. DMC upregulated cytosolic Cyt-c expression and downregulated Bcl-2 synthesis compared to untreated cells (Figure 5). One of the other substrates for caspase during apoptosis is PARP, an enzyme that appears to be involved in DNA repair and genome surveillance and integrity in response to environmental stress. The beginning of caspase signaling activation might cause PARP cleavage which was considered as the main pathway in triggering apoptosis. As shown in Figure 4, exposure to DMC (3–30 μM) for 48 h triggered progressive PARP proteolytic cleavage and/or downregulation. We used western blotting to quantitate the levels of cleaved caspase-3 and -9; DMC upregulated cleavage of both proteins (Figure 4), explaining the Bcl-2 downregulation evident in Figure 5.

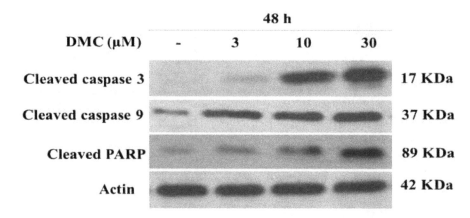

Figure 4. Effect of DMC on caspase activation and PARP degradation protein expression in PANC-1 cells. Cells were treated with DMC (3–30 µM) for 48 h. Protein 50 µg/lane from cells lysates were electrophoresed on SDS-PAGE gels, then transferred to total blot PVDF membranes. β-Actin was used as a control, (–), 0.1% DMSO-treated cells. The experiments were carried out in three replicates.

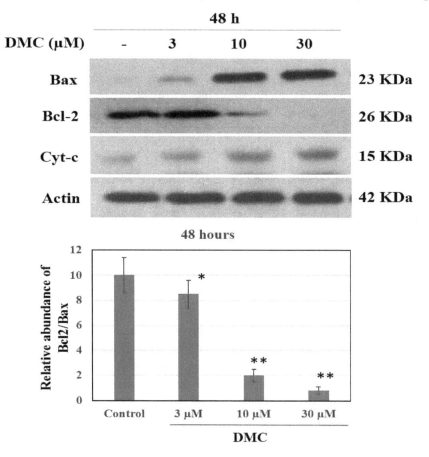

Figure 5. Effect of DMC on Bcl-2, Bax and Cyt-c protein expression in PANC-1 cells. Cells were treated with DMC (3–30 µM) for 48 h. Protein 50 µg/lane from cells lysates were electrophoresed on SDS-PAGE gels, then transferred to total blot PVDF membranes. β-Actin was used as a control, (–) 0.1% DMSO-treated cells. The experiments were carried out in three replicates. * $P < 0.05$ and $P < 0.01$ compared with control group.

3. Discussion

The pear-shaped pancreas—an abdominal organ located horizontally behind the lower part of the stomach—is an important component of the digestive system, secreting hormones, including insulin, that regulate sugar metabolism and digestive enzymes. Pancreatic cancer begins in the tissues of the pancreas. This cancer usually has a poor prognosis, even when the patient is diagnosed at the early stage because its signs and symptoms are hard to identify. The symptoms of pancreatic cancer generally mostly appear at the advanced stages of the disease. Some of the signs and symptoms of pancreatic cancer patients that might be identified include upper abdominal pain that spreads to the back, jaundice, yellow eyes, loss of appetite, weight loss, and depression. At present, the causes of the cancer remain unclear. There are two types of pancreatic cancer, including cancer formed in the pancreas (adenocarcinoma) and cancer formed in hormone-producing cells which is called endocrine. Pancreatic cancer is one of the most prevalent malignant tumors in the world and the treatment regimens for pancreatic cancer primarily depend on the cancer stages [7,8]. Nowadays, about 15–20% of patients undergo surgery and only 5% of them survive to 5 years [8]. The recent increase in cancer incidence, the absence of a cure, and severe side effects of existing drugs render it essential to find new effective therapeutics. In Vietnam, both Western and Oriental (natural plant) medicines are used to treat pancreatic cancer. Oriental medicines have fewer side effects and are less expensive than Western drugs. The herbal remedies used also target cancer-related impacts on the spleen, and sputum production. The recommended medicines include Radix Astragali membranacei, *Scutellaria barbata*, *Plumbago zeylanica*, *Poria cocos*, *Angelica sinensis*, and Rhizoma atrclylodis macrocephalae [9]. However, one of the limitations in the treatment of this disease by traditional oriental medicine method is due to the lack of scientific research perspectives in using of medicinal herbs with different ingredients and amounts.

In the last 10 years, many natural medicinal products have been used to treat pancreatic cancer. Fucoidan from a seaweed collected in Okinawa destroyed pancreatic tumor cells, and tumors regressed after 4–5 years of treatment [24]. α-Bisabolol (a sesquiterpene essential oil ingredient) reduced proliferation and survival of the pancreatic cancer cell lines KLM1, KP4, Panc1, and MIA Paca2; but not a pancreatic epithelial cell line (ACBRI515) [25]. Daily intake of plants rich in flavonoids and proanthocyanidins reduces the risk of pancreatic cancer by 25% [26–28]. Ethyl acetate extracts of *Coreopsis tinctoria* rich in flavonoids such as marein and flavanomarein kill pancreatic tumor cells by inducing apoptosis [29]. *Scutellaria baicalensis* extracts containing baicalein, wogonin, oroxylin A, and a glucuronide effectively countered pancreatic cancer in a mouse xenograft model [30,31]. The natural flavonoids and chalcons have many pharmaceutical applications, including antioxidant and anticancer ones. 2',4'-Dihydroxy-6'-methoxy-3',5'-dimethylchalcone (DMC) is also an important natural chalcone that has been shown to exhibit tremendous pharmacological activities which include anticancer activity against the wide range of cancer types. However, the anti-pancreatic cancer activity of DMC has not been previously investigated. In this study, DMC was selected to investigate the capability against PANC-1 cell lines. To clarify mechanism responsible for its anticancer activity, DMC at the concentration of 3–30 μM enhanced annexin-V uptake in PANC-1 cells signifying traslocation of the cell membrane phospholpids, phosphatidylsenin, from inner face to the outer surface of plasma membrane of PANC-1 cells then led to the cell apoptosis (Figure 3). Apoptosis, however, is known to be triggered by different routes, and the mitochondrials enhancement is a popularly crucial signalling pathway in the induction of apoptosis progress. Among these mitochindrials, the Bcl-2 family proteins are frequently main factors in apoptotic pathway due to their natural functional property. Bcl-2 family proteins play major roles in apoptosis and it has been suggested that such proteins exert either pro- or anti-apoptotic effects. The proteins either activate or inactivate transport through inner mitochondrial membrane pores, thus regulating the matrix Ca^{2+} level, the pH, and the cell membrane potential. Some pro-apoptotic Bcl-2 proteins may induce cytochrome c (Cyt-c) release to the cytosol; anti-apoptotic Bcl-2 proteins may inhibit such release. Cytosolic Bcl-2 proteins activated caspase-9 and -3, triggering apoptosis, meanwhile Bax was once termed Bcl-2-like protein 4, and is a pro-apoptotic protein; Bcl-2 is a major anti-apoptotic protein. Bax in the outer mitochondrial membrane enables the release of Cyt-c and activates caspase-9, a cysteine-aspartic protease involved in apoptosis and cytokine signaling. Caspase-3 is activated by proteolytic cleavage of caspase 9 to play a key role in apoptosis, further stimulating Cyt-c release by mitochondria and activating apaf-1 (the apoptosome), which then cleaves the caspase-9 pro-enzyme to the active dimer. In human cancer cells, this enzyme is regulated via phosphorylation mediated by an allosteric inhibitor, inhibiting dimerization and inducing a conformational change. Stimulation of caspase signaling and the accompanying cleavage of PARP are the principal features of the apoptotic cascade. We found that DMC activated enzymes and the PARP pathway to induce PANC-1 cell death, augmented by changes in Bcl-2 and Bax expression levels. DMC triggered the dose-dependent release of Cyt-c from mitochondria into the cytoplasm of PANC-1 cells.

DMC induces apoptosis in several human cancer cell lines including SMMC-7721 (human hepatocarcinoma cancer cells), 8898 (pancreas cancer cells), HeLa (cervical cancer cells), SPC-A-1 (lung cancer cells), 95-D (metastatic lung carcinoma cells), and GBC-SD (gall bladder carcinoma cells). When SMMC-7721 cells were treated with DMC for 48 h, the DNA became fragmented and the chromatin condensed. Also, the proportion of hypodiploid SMMC-7721 cells increased after DMC treatment [32]. At a low concentration, DMC inhibited proliferation of the human leukemia cell line K562. Notably, DMC downregulated Bcl-2 protein expression but did not affect Bax protein expression, thus reducing the Bcl-2:Bax ratio [33]. DMC was not toxic to normal human liver L-02 or normal human fetal lung fibroblast HFL-1 cell lines. In SMMC-7721 cells, DMC induced apoptosis by increasing intracellular ROS generation via inhibition of N-acetylcysteine activity [23]. Our data partly explained why DMC triggers PANC-1 cell apoptosis. We conclude that DMC exhibits significant anti-PANC-1 cancer cell activity; however, further in vivo evaluation in a mouse model of pancreatic cancer is essential.

4. Material and Methods

4.1. General Experimental Procedures

NMR experiments were conducted on a Unity INOVA 400 spectrometer (Varian, IL, USA). ^{1}H- and ^{13}C-NMR spectra were recorded at 400 and 100 MHz, respectively, and tetramethylsilane was used as the internal standard. ESI MS analyses were performed on a Micromass QTQF2 mass spectrometer (Water, Milford, MA, USA). The untraviloet (UV) was measured with a Shimadzu UV-1800 UV-Vis spectrophotometer (Shimadzu, Japan). IR spectrum was measured with a Shimadzu IR-408 spectrophotometer in $CHCl_3$ solution (Shimadzu, Japan). TLC was carried out on silica gel F_{254}-precoated glass plates and RP-18 F_{254S} plates (Merck, Germany). Dulbecco's modified Eagle medium (DMEM), fetal bovine serum (FBS), trypsin-EDTA 0.25%, streptomycin and penicillin were obtained from Hyclone (Logan, UT, USA). Dimethyl sulfoxide (DMSO), and a Dojindo Kit was purchased from Dojindo Molecular Technology INC (Maryland, USA). Annexin V-FITC/PI double staining detection kit, mitochondrial membrane potential assay kit with caspase-3 activity assay kit, propidium iodide (PI) were purchased from Beyotime (Beyotime Institute of Biotechnology, Shanghai, China). All used chemicals and reagents were of analytical grade.

4.2. Plant Material

The buds of *Cleistocalyx operculatus* were collected at Quang Nam province, Vietnam, in July 2017 and identified by Dr Pham Cong Tuan, Danang Traditional Medicine Hospital (Danang city, Vietnam). A voucher specimen (TMH-22-2017) was deposited in the Pharmaceutical Biology Laboratory of the University of Danang (Danang city, Vietnam).

4.3. Isolation of DCM

The air-dried buds (2.0 kg) were extracted with 70% ethanol (2 liters × 3 times). The 70% EtOH extract was combined and concentrated in vacuo to yield a residue which was suspended in water and then successively partitioned with *n*-hexane, EtOAc, and *n*-BuOH. After removal of solvent *in vacuo*, the *n*-hexane fraction was obtained (16.8 g). The *n*-hexane soluble fraction (HEX) was separated by silica gel column chromatography using a gradient of *n*-hexane−EtOAc (from 40:1 to 1:1) to yield 20 fractions (HEX.1 ~ HEX.20) according to their TLC profiles. Fraction HEX-5 (5.62 g) was further fractionated on a Sephadex LH-20 column eluting with MeOH to divide to six sub-fractions

(HEX.5.1-HEX.5.6). 2',4'-Dihydroxy-6'-methoxy-3',5'-dimethylchalcone (DMC, 1.6 g) was obtained from HEX.5.2 by crystallization from MeOH.

2',4'-Dihydroxy-6'-methoxy-3',5'-dimethylchalcone (DMC): Orange yellow needles (MeOH), mp 124–125 °C, UV λ_{max} (MeOH) nm (log ε): 284 (4.15), 320 (4.13); IR (KBr) cm^{-1}: 3460, 2875, 2750, 1630, 1550, 1450; ESI-MS *m/z* 312.1 [M]$^+$ (calcd for $C_{18}H_{16}O_5$), for ^{1}H and ^{13}C-NMR spectral data please see Supplementary Materials and in the comparison with previous reference [10].

4.4. Cell Lines and Culture

The human pancreatic cancer cell lines PANC-1 (human pancreas) and MIA-PACA2 (human pancreatic carcinoma) were obtained from the American Type Culture Collection (ATCC, Manassas, VA, USA). The cells were maintained in DMEM (GibcoBRL, NY, USA) with 10% fetal bovine serum (FBS) supplemented with 2% penicillin and 100 µg/mL of streptomycin at 37 °C in a 95% humidified atmosphere containing 5% CO_2.

4.5. Cell Proliferation Activity Assay

Cell proliferation activity of DMC was determined against PANC-1 and MIA-PACA2 cancer cell lines using a Dojindo kit with a slight modification. Viable cells were seeded in the growth medium into 96-well microtiter plates (95 µL, concentration 1×10^4 cells/well) and incubated at 37 °C in a 5% CO_2 incubator. The test sample DCM was dissolved in DMSO and adjusted to final sample concentrations ranging from 3 to 30 µM by diluting with the growth medium. Each sample was prepared in triplicate. The final DMSO concentration was adjusted to <0.1%. After standing for 4 h, the test sample was added to each well. The same volume of medium with 0.1% DMSO was added to the control wells. After 48 h incubation, Dojindo reagent was added to the each well (10 µL). 4 h later, the plate was removed from incubator and the optical density (O.D) was measured at 450 nm using a Molecular Devices microplate reader (Molecular Devices, Sunnyvale, CA, USA). The IC$_{50}$ value was defined as the concentration of sample which reduced absorbance by 50% relative to the vehicle-treated control.

4.6. Caspase-3 Actyivation Assay

Caspase-3 enzyme activity was measured by proteolytic cleavage of the fluorogenic substrate Ac-DEVD-AFC by counting on a fluorescence plate reader (Twinkle LB970 microplate fluorometer, Berthold Technologies, Bad Wildbad, Germany). PANC-1 cells (1×10^5 cell/well) were treated with DCM (3–30 µM). After incubation for 24 h, cells were harvested and washed with cold PBS. The pellets were lyzed using 15 µL of lysis buffer [10 mM Tris-HCL (pH 8.0), 10 mM EDTA, 0.5% Triton X-100] at room temperature for 10 min, and then placed on ice; 100 µL of assay buffer [100 mM Hepes (pH 7.5), 10 mM dithiothreitol, 10% (*w/v*) sucrose, 0.1% (*v/v*) Chaps, 0.1% (*v/v*) BSA] and 10 µL of substrate solutin (200 µm substrate in assay buffer) were added. After incubation at 37 °C for 1 h, fluorescence was measured with excitation at 370 nm and emission at 505 nm.

4.7. Detection of Apoptosis by Double Stanning

The Annexin V-FITC/PI staining kit was used to detect the phosphatidylserine translocation, an important characteristic at an early stage of cell apoptosis. Briefly, PANC-1 cells were seeded in 6 well plates at a density of 2×10^5 cells/mL and incubated for 24 h. After that, cells were treated with different concentrations of DMC for 48 h. The cells were collected and washed in PBS, then were resuspended in 195 µL binding buffer, and incubated with 10 µL Annexin V-FITC and 5 µL PI in the dark for 20 min. Thereafter, the solutions were immediately measured by FCM (Beckman, Fullerton, CA, USA).

4.8. Preparation of Total Cell Extract and Immuno Blot Analysis

Immunoblot analysis, and immunoreactive proteins were visualized by an enhanced chemiluminescence (ECL) procedure according to the manufacturer's protocol. PANC-1 cells

$(5 \times 10^5$ cells/mL) were treated with DMC (3-30 μM) for 24 h at 37 °C. Cell lysates were prepared in 100 μL of lysis buffer (Sigma, Ronkonkoma, NY, USA) containing a protease inhibitor cocktail (Roche, Mannheim, Germany). Insoluble material was removed by centrifugation at 14,000 rpm for 10 min. And then the protein contents in the supernatant were measured using a Bio-Rad DC protein assay kit. The protein extract (50 μg/well) was separated by SDS-PAGE and then transferred onto PVDF membranes (Bio-Rad, Hercules, CA, USA). The membranes were bloked with 5% (*w/v*) non-fat dry milk in TBS-T [Tris-buffered saline containing 0.1% (*v/v*) Tween-20] at 4 °C overnight and incubated with primary antibodies at room temperature for 1.5 h. The membranes were washed three times with TBS-T, and blotted with secondary antibodies conjugated with horse-radish peroxidase at room temperature for 1.5 h, followed by washing three times in TBST-T. Immunoreactive proteins were visualized by an enhanced chemiluminescence (ECL) procedure according to the manufacturer's protocol (Santa Cruz Biotechnology, Santa Cruz, CA, USA) and exposed to X ray films. Protein contents were normalized by reprobing the same membrane with anti-β-actin detection; previously used membranes were soaked in stripping buffer (Gene Bio-Application Ltd., Yavne, Israel) at room temperature for 20 min.

4.9. Statistical Analysis

All treatments were conducted in triplicate and the results are presented as the mean ± standard deviation (S.D). The statistical significance of all treatment effects was evaluated by Student's *t*-test with a probability limit for significance of $p < 0.05, p < 0.001$.

Author Contributions: M.H.T., P.T.K.L. carried out the conception and designed the experiments. H.N.T., B.H.M., P.T.T., Q.M.T.N. and Y.N.N. performed sampling, extractions, and bioassay activities. H.V.O. performed identification and description of the plant. J.H.L. and M.H.T. performed N.M.R. experiments. J.H.L., P.T.K.L. and M.H.T. contributed to the preparation of the manuscript.

References

1. Howlader, N.; Noone, A.M.; Krapcho, M.; Miller, D.; Bishop, K.; Altekruse, S.F.; Kosary, C.L.; Yu, M.; Ruhl, J.; Tatalovich, Z.; et al. *SEER Cancer Statistics Review, 1975–2013*; National Cancer Institute: Bethesda, MD, USA, 2016.
2. Ferlay, J.; Soerjomataram, I.; Dikshit, R.; Eser, S.; Mathers, C.; Rebelo, M.; Parkin, D.M.; Forman, D.; Bray, F. *GLOBOCAN 2012 v1.0, Cancer Incidence and Mortality Worldwide: IARC CancerBase No. 11*; International Agency for Research on Cancer: Lyon, France, 2013.
3. Ferlay, J.; Soerjomataram, I.; Dikshit, R.; Eser, S.; Mathers, C.; Rebelo, M. Cancer incidence and mortality worldwide: Sources, methods and major patterns in GLOBOCAN 2012. *Int. J. Cancer* **2015**, *136*, E359–E386. [CrossRef] [PubMed]
4. Hidalgo, M.; Cascinu, S.; Kleeff, J.; Labianca, R.; Löhr, J.M.; Neoptolemos, J.; Real, F.X.; Van Laethem, J.L.; Heinemann, V. Addressing the challenges of pancreatic cancer: Future directions for improving outcomes. *Pancreatology* **2013**, *15*, 8–18. [CrossRef] [PubMed]
5. Vincent, A.; Herman, J.; Schulick, R.; Hruban, R.H.; Goggins, M. Pancreatic cancer. *Lancet* **2011**, *378*, 607–620. [CrossRef]
6. Ilic, M.; Ilic, I. Epidemiology of pancreatic cancer. *World J. Gastroenterol.* **2016**, *22*, 9694–9705. [CrossRef] [PubMed]
7. Chhoda, A.; Lu, L.; Clerkin, B.M.; Risch, H.; Farrell, J.J. Current approaches to pancreatic cancer screening. *Am. J. Pathol.* **2019**, *189*, 22–35. [CrossRef] [PubMed]

8. Cheng, X.; Zhao, G.; Zhao, Y. Combination Immunotherapy Approaches for Pancreatic Cancer Treatment. *Can. J. Gastroenterol. Hepatol.* **2018**, *2018*, 6240467. [CrossRef] [PubMed]

9. Loi, D.T. *Vietnamese Medicinal Plants and Ingredients*; Medical Publishing House: Hanoi, Vietnam, 2001; pp. 423–424.

10. Ye, C.L.; Lu, Y.H.; Wei, D.Z. Flavonoids from Cleistocalyx operculatus. *Phytochemistry* **2004**, *65*, 445–447. [CrossRef]

11. Woo, A.Y.; Waye, M.M.; Kwan, H.S.; Chan, M.C.; Chau, C.F.; Cheng, C.H. Inhibition of ATPases by Cleistocalyx operculatus. A possible mechanism for the cardiotonic actions of the herb. *Vasc. Pharmacol.* **2002**, *38*, 163–168. [CrossRef]

12. Mai, T.T.; Chuyen, N.V. Anti-hyperglycemic activity of an aqueous extract from flower buds of Cleistocalyx operculatus (Roxb.) Merr and Perry. *Biosci. Biotechnol. Biochem.* **2007**, *71*, 69–76. [CrossRef]

13. Mai, T.T.; Thu, N.N.; Tien, P.G.; Van Chuyen, N. Alpha-glucosidase inhibitory and antioxidant activities of Vietnamese edible plants and their relationships with polyphenol contents. *J. Nutr. Sci. Vitaminol.* **2007**, *53*, 267–276. [CrossRef]

14. Wang, C.; Wu, P.; Tian, S.; Xue, J.; Xu, L.; Li, H.; Wei, X. Bioactive pentacyclic triterpenoids from the leaves of Cleistocalyx operculatus. *J. Nat. Prod.* **2016**, *79*, 2912–2923. [CrossRef] [PubMed]

15. Su, J.C.; Wang, S.; Cheng, W.; Huang, X.J.; Li, M.M.; Jiang, R.W.; Li, Y.L.; Wang, L.; Ye, W.C.; Wang, Y. Phloroglucinol derivatives with unusual skeletons from Cleistocalyx operculatus and their in vitro antiviral activity. *J. Org. Chem.* **2018**, *83*, 8522–8532. [CrossRef] [PubMed]

16. Ha, T.K.; Dao, T.T.; Nguyen, N.H.; Kim, J.; Kim, E.; Cho, T.O.; Oh, W.K. Antiviral phenolics from the leaves of Cleistocalyx operculatus. *Fitoterapia* **2016**, *110*, 135–141. [CrossRef] [PubMed]

17. Min, B.S.; Cuong, T.D.; Lee, J.S.; Shin, B.S.; Woo, M.H.; Hung, T.M. Cholinesterase inhibitors from Cleistocalyx operculatus buds. *Arch. Pharm. Res.* **2010**, *33*, 1665–1670. [CrossRef] [PubMed]

18. Dung, N.T.; Bajpai, V.K.; Yoon, J.I.; Kang, S.C. Anti-inflammatory effects of essential oil isolated from the buds of Cleistocalyx operculatus (Roxb.) Merr and Perry. *Food Chem. Toxicol.* **2009**, *47*, 449–453. [CrossRef] [PubMed]

19. Huang, H.Y.; Niu, J.L.; Zhao, L.M.; Lu, Y.H. Reversal effect of 2',4'-dihydroxy-6'-methoxy-3',5'-dimethylchalcone on multi-drug resistance in resistant human hepatocellular carcinoma cell line BEL-7402/5-FU. *Phytomedicine* **2011**, *18*, 1086–1092. [CrossRef] [PubMed]

20. Huang, H.Y.; Niu, J.L.; Lu, Y.H. Multidrug resistance reversal effect of DMC derived from buds of Cleistocalyx operculatus in human hepatocellular tumor xenograft model. *J. Sci. Food Agric.* **2012**, *92*, 135–140. [CrossRef]

21. Yu, W.G.; Qian, J.; Lu, Y.H. Hepatoprotective effects of 2', 4'-dihydroxy-6'-methoxy-3', 5'-dimethylchalcone on CCl4-induced acute liver injury in mice. *J. Agric. Food Chem.* **2011**, *59*, 12821–12829. [CrossRef]

22. Su, M.Y.; Huang, H.Y.; Li, L.; Lu, Y.H. Protective effects of 2', 4'-dihydroxy-6'-methoxy-3', 5'-dimethylchalcone to PC12 cells against cytotoxicity induced by hydrogen peroxide. *J. Agric. Food Chem.* **2011**, *59*, 521–527. [CrossRef]

23. Ye, C.L.; Lai, Y.F. 2',4'-Dihydroxy-6'-methoxy-3',5'-dimethylchalcone, from buds of *Cleistocalyxoperculatus*, induces apoptosis in human hepatoma SMMC-7721 cells through a reactive oxygen species-dependent mechanism. *Cytotechnology* **2016**, *68*, 331–341. [CrossRef]

24. Fitton, J.H.; Stringer, D.N.; Karpiniec, S.S. Therapies from Fucoidan: An Update. *Mar. Drugs* **2015**, *13*, 5920–5946. [CrossRef] [PubMed]

25. Seki, T.; Kokuryo, T.; Yokoyama, Y.; Suzuki, H.; Itatsu, K.; Nakagawa, A.; Mizutani, T.; Miyake, T.; Uno, M.; Yamauchi, K.; et al. Antitumor effects of α-bisabolol against pancreatic cancer. *Cancer Sci.* **2011**, *102*, 2199–2205. [CrossRef] [PubMed]

26. Paluszkiewicz, P.; Smolińska, K.; Dębińska, I.; Turski, W.A. Main dietary compounds and pancreatic cancer risk. The quantitative analysis of case-control and cohort studies. *Cancer Epidemiol.* **2012**, *36*, 60–67. [CrossRef] [PubMed]

27. Jansen, R.J.; Robinson, D.P.; Stolzenberg-Solomon, R.Z.; Bamlet, W.R.; de Andrade, M.; Oberg, A.L.; Hammer, T.J.; Rabe, K.G.; Anderson, K.E.; Olson, J.E.; et al. Fruit and vegetable consumption is inversely associated with having pancreatic cancer. *Cancer Causes Control* **2011**, *22*, 1613–1625. [CrossRef] [PubMed]

28. Rossi, M.; Lugo, A.; Lagiou, P.; Zucchetto, A.; Polesel, J.; Serraino, D.; Negri, E.; Trichopoulos, D.; La Vecchia, C. Proanthocyanidins and other flavonoids in relation to pancreatic cancer: A case-control study in Italy. *Ann. Oncol.* **2012**, *23*, 1488–1493. [CrossRef] [PubMed]

29. Dias, T.; Liu, B.; Jones, P.; Houghton, P.J.; Mota-Filipe, H.; Paulo, A. Cytoprotective effect of Coreopsis tinctoria extracts and flavonoids on tBHP and cytokine-induced cell injury in pancreatic MIN6 cells. *J. Ethnopharmacol.* **2012**, *139*, 485–492. [CrossRef] [PubMed]

30. Lu, Q.Y.; Zhang, L.; Moro, A.; Chen, M.C.; Harris, D.M.; Eibl, G.; Go, V.L. Detection of baicalin metabolites baicalein and oroxylin-a in mouse pancreas and pancreatic xenografts. *Pancreas* **2012**, *41*, 571–576. [CrossRef] [PubMed]

31. Wu, X.; Zhang, H.; Salmani, J.M.; Fu, R.; Chen, B. Advances of wogonin, an extract from Scutellaria baicalensis for the treatment of multiple tumors. *Onco Targets Ther.* **2016**, *9*, 2935–2943. [PubMed]

32. Ye, C.L.; Liu, J.W.; Wei, D.Z.; Lu, Y.H.; Qian, F. In vitro anti-tumor activity of 2′, 4′-dihydroxy-6′-methoxy-3′, 5′-dimethylchalcone against six established human cancer cell lines. *Pharmacol. Res.* **2004**, *50*, 505–510. [CrossRef]

33. Ye, C.L.; Qian, F.; Wei, D.Z.; Lu, Y.H.; Liu, J.W. Induction of apoptosis in K562 human leukemia cells by 2′, 4′-dihydroxy-6′-methoxy-3′, 5′-dimethylchalcone. *Leuk. Res.* **2005**, *29*, 887–892. [CrossRef]

4

Spectroscopic Characterization and Cytotoxicity Assessment towards Human Colon Cancer Cell Lines of Acylated Cycloartane Glycosides from *Astragalus boeticus* L.

Vittoria Graziani [1], Assunta Esposito [1], Monica Scognamiglio [2,*], Angela Chambery [1], Rosita Russo [1], Fortunato Ciardiello [3], Teresa Troiani [3], Nicoletta Potenza [1], Antonio Fiorentino [1,4,*] and Brigida D'Abrosca [1,4]

[1] Dipartimento di Scienze e Tecnologie Ambientali Biologiche e Farmaceutiche (DiSTABiF), Università degli Studi della Campania "Luigi Vanvitelli", via Vivaldi 43, I-81100 Caserta, Italy; vittoria.graziani@unicampania.it (V.G.); assunta.esposito@unicampania.it (A.E.); angela.chambery@unicampania.it (A.C.); rosita.russo@unicampania.it (R.R.); nicoletta.potenza@unicampania.it (N.P.); brigida.dabrosca@unicampania.it (B.D.A.)

[2] Department of Biochemistry, Max Planck Institute for Chemical Ecology-Beutenberg Campus, Hans-Knöll-Straße, 8 D-07745 Jena, Germany

[3] Dipartimento di Medicina di Precisione, Università degli Studi della Campania "Luigi Vanvitelli" - Via Pansini, 5, 80131 Napoli, Italy; fortunato.ciardiello@unicampania.it (F.C.); teresa.troiani@unicampania.it (T.T.)

[4] Dipartimento di Biotecnologia Marina, Stazione Zoologica Anton Dohrn, Villa Comunale, 80121 Naples, Italy

* Correspondence: mscognamiglio@ice.mpg.de (M.S.); antonio.fiorentino@unicampania.it (A.F.);

Abstract: In several European countries, especially in Sweden, the seeds of the species *Astragalus boeticus* L. were widely used as coffee substitutes during the 19th century. Nonetheless, data regarding the phytochemistry and the pharmacological properties of this species are currently extremely limited. Conversely, other species belonging to the *Astragalus* genus have already been extensively investigated, as they were used for millennia for treating various diseases, including cancer. The current work was addressed to characterize cycloartane glycosides from *A. boeticus*, and to evaluate their cytotoxicity towards human colorectal cancer (CRC) cell lines. The isolation of the metabolites was performed by using different chromatographic techniques, while their chemical structures were elucidated by nuclear magnetic resonance (NMR) (1D and 2D techniques) and electrospray-ionization quadrupole time-of-flight (ESI-QTOF) mass spectrometry. The cytotoxic assessment was performed in vitro by 3-(4,5-dimethylthiazol-2-yl)-2,5-diphenyltetrazolium bromide (MTT) assays in Caco-2, HT-29 and HCT-116 CRC cells. As a result, the targeted phytochemical study of *A. boeticus* enabled the isolation of three new cycloartane glycosides, 6-*O*-acetyl-3-*O*-(4-*O*-malonyl)-β-D-xylopyranosylcycloastragenol (**1**), 3-*O*-(4-*O*-malonyl)-β-D-xylopyranosylcycloastragenol (**2**), 6-*O*-acetyl-25-*O*-β-D-glucopyranosyl-3-*O*-β-D-xylopyranosylcycloastragenol (**3**) along with two known compounds, 6-*O*-acetyl-3-*O*-β-D-xylopyranosylcycloastragenol (**4**) and 3-*O*-β-D-xylopyranosylcycloastragenol (**5**). Importantly, this work demonstrated that the acetylated cycloartane glycosides **1** and **4** might preferentially inhibit cell growth in the CRC cell model resistant to epidermal growth factor receptor (EGFR) inhibitors.

Keywords: *Astragalus boeticus* L.; spectroscopic analysis; cytotoxic activity; human colon cancer cell lines; acetylated astragalosides; Fabaceae

1. Introduction

Astragalus genus is the largest in the Fabaceae family and it is widely distributed throughout the cool, temperate, semiarid and arid regions of the world [1]. *Astragalus boeticus* L. is a Steno-Mediterranean species, which has represented an important cultivation in several countries of Europe, as its seeds have been widely used as coffee substitutes in times of poverty and coffee prohibition. In Sweden, during the 19th century, the monarchy introduced an extensive cultivation of the aforementioned species to produce the so-called Swedish coffee. After the beginning of the 20th century, its cultivation declined, and it was replaced by other substitutes [2]. In addition to this information, available literature data describing the phytochemistry and the bioactivities of A. boeticus are currently extremely limited.

On the contrary, a plethora of works regarding other species of the same genus exists. The *Astragalus* species were employed as forage for animals, albeit many species were found to be toxic, and responsible for causing locoism in cattle [3,4]. In both folk and modern medicine, several *Astragalus* spp. were considered medicinal plants of great importance, as these have been successfully used to cure a broad range of ailments [5]. In the Traditional Chinese Medicine "Astragali radix" (dried roots of *Astragalus membranaceus* Bunge and other *Astragalus* spp.) was a very well-known drug for its immune stimulant, hepato-protective, anti-diabetic, analgesic, expectorant and sedative properties [6].

Previous works investigated the chemical profile of *Astragalus* spp. in order to identify the active principles responsible for the bioactivity of the plant's crude extracts. Results from these studies described imidazoline alkaloids, nitro toxins and selenium derivatives as toxic compounds, while polysaccharides, phenols and saponins as biologically active constituents [6]. *Astragalus* saponins include both oleanane and cycloartane-type glycosides, yet the former occur far less in nature, thus the *Astragalus* genus was especially employed as an ideal source to find cycloartane saponins [7].

These compounds were the most extensively studied secondary metabolites from *Astragalus*, as they exhibited a wide range of biological and pharmacological properties. Indeed, these molecules were found to exert immunomodulatory, anti-cancer, anti-fungal, hepato-, kidney-, neuro- and vascular-protective activities [7–12]. So far, the most well-characterized biological effects were those related to their immune stimulant properties, which made these compounds ideal vaccine adjuvant candidates [13]. Alongside the capacity to modulate key immunity pathways, recent evidence supported the effectiveness of *Astragalus* saponins as anti-tumor compounds and/or as adjuvants in combination with orthodox chemotherapeutic agents [14,15].

The anti-cancer activities of these compounds have been evaluated towards a wide range of human malignancies, and a large part of these works evidenced the effectiveness of *Astragalus* saponins against gastric and colorectal cancers [16]. Consistent with this, our group recently demonstrated the anti-proliferative effects of A. *boeticus* in human colorectal cancer (CRC) cells [17].

Colorectal cancer is one of the most frequently-diagnosed malignant diseases in Europe, and one of the leading causes of cancer-related deaths worldwide [18]. Even if the outcome of patients with metastatic colorectal cancer (mCRC) has clearly improved during the last years, the current therapies are still not entirely efficient. Nowadays, resistance to both chemotherapy and molecularly-targeted therapies represents a major problem for setting up effective treatment. The EGFR, which was found overexpressed in 60% to 80% of colorectal cancers, is a transmembrane tyrosine kinase receptor that, once activated, triggers two main signaling pathways. These include the RAS-RAF-MAPK axis, which is mainly involved in cell proliferation, and the PI3KPTEN-AKT pathway, which is especially involved in cell survival and motility [19]. Thus, EGFR inhibitors, such as Cetuximab and Panitumumab, have been developed to block specifically the abnormal activation of those pathways in wild-type KRAS CRC patients [20].

In this study, we aimed at providing a detailed chemical characterization of cycloartane glycosides from A. *boeticus*, and at assessing their anti-proliferative activity towards human colorectal cancer cells endowed with diverse mutation profiles and drug sensitiveness. The ultimate goal of this research is to contribute to the search for new effective agents against refractory CRCs. As a result, we isolated and characterized five cycloartane glycosides (**1–5**), identifying compound **4** as a strong inhibitor of proliferation in CRC cell models resistant to anti-EGFR therapies.

2. Results and Discussion

2.1. Structural Elucidation of Cycloartane Glycosides from Astragalus boeticus L.

A crude hydro-alcoholic extract of *A. boeticus* leaves was partitioned between EtOAc and H_2O. The purification process, which was performed by using different chromatographic techniques, enabled the isolation of compounds 1, 2, 4 from the organic phase, while we also obtained 3 and 5 from the aqueous fraction (Figure 1). The structures of these metabolites were elucidated through a combination of NMR spectroscopy (1D and 2D techniques) and ESI-QTOF mass spectrometry.

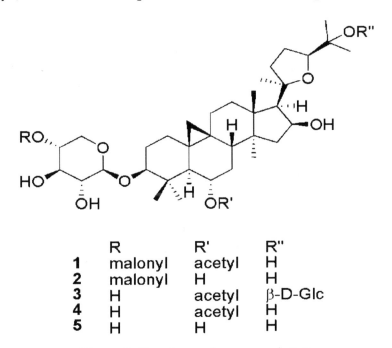

	R	R'	R"
1	malonyl	acetyl	H
2	malonyl	H	H
3	H	acetyl	β-D-Glc
4	H	acetyl	H
5	H	H	H

Figure 1. Structures of compounds **1–5**.

Compound **1** showed a molecular formula $C_{40}H_{62}O_{13}$ on the basis of the NMR data and ESI-QTOF mass spectrum. In fact, the ^{13}C NMR displayed 40 signals, which were identified using the HSQC experiment as eight methyls (—CH_3), eleven methylenes (=CH_2), eleven methines (=CH−), and ten quaternary carbons. The ESI-QTOF spectrum displayed the sodiated adduct of the quasimolecular ion at *m/z* 773.49, and a strong peak at *m/z* 687.46, which indicated the easy loss of an 86 Da fragment. In the ^{1}H NMR spectrum (Table 1), two methylene protons at δ_H 0.40 and δ_H 0.61 (δ_C 30.1), along with six singlet methyls at δ_H 0.98, 1.01, 1.05, 1.13, 1.22, 1.26, and 1.27 allowed compound **1** to be identified as a cycloartane triterpene. The doublet at δ_H 4.32 (δ_C 105.9), as well as other protons that resonated in the range between 3.18 and 4.85 ppm, suggested the presence of a sugar unit. Meanwhile, a methyl singlet at δ_H 1.99 supported the presence of an acetate group in the molecule. The above-mentioned methylene signals (δ_H 0.40 and δ_H 0.61) were assigned to H-19 protons; these, in the CIGAR-HMBC experiment (Figure 2), showed cross peaks with the C-9 (δ_C 21.8), C-10 (δ_C 29.6), C-1 (δ_C 32.8) C-11 (δ_C 26.8), C-5 (δ_C 51.2) and C-8 (δ_C 46.7). In the same experiment, the H-5 proton correlated with the C-1 methylene, the C-4 quaternary carbon at δ_C 42.8, and with two carbinols at δ_C 89.1 and δ_C 72.0. Thanks to the long-range heterocorrelations between the H-6 proton (δ_H 4.75) and the C-4, C-5, and C-8 carbons, it was feasible to assign the first carbinol to the C-3 methine, and then the second to the C-6 carbon. Moreover, the H-6 proton also had cross peaks with the carbonyl at δ_C 171.7, which in turn correlated with the methyl at δ_H 1.99. These data allowed the acetoxy (CH_3-COO-) group to be located at position 6. On the other hand, the H-3 proton correlated with the anomeric carbon at δ_C 105.9, suggesting that the glycosylation site was located on the hydroxyl at the C-3 carbon. Furthermore, the C-4 carbon showed correlations with the methyls at δ_H 0.98 and δ_H 1.05, values that were consequently assigned to the H-29 and H-28 protons, respectively. In addition, the methyls at δ_H 1.27 (δ_C 21.4) and 1.01 (δ_C 20.3) were attributed to the H-18 and H-30 protons, respectively, on the basis of the long range heterocorrelations between the C-18 carbon with the proton at δ_H 2.38 (H-17), which in turn correlated with the H-21 methyl at δH 1.22 (δ_C 28.4).

In the COSY experiment, the H-17 proton had cross peaks with a proton geminal to oxygen at δH 4.65 (H-16), which homocorrelated with the methylene protons at δ_H 1.87 and δ_H 1.45 (H-15), suggesting the presence of another hydroxyl at the C-16 carbon. Consequently, the remaining methyls at δ_H 1.13 and δ_H 1.26 were attributed to the H-26 and H-27 protons, respectively. In the CIGAR-HMBC experiment, these latter protons displayed heterocorrelations with a quaternary carbinol carbon at δ_C 71.2 (C-25), and with a carbinol methine at δ_C 82.6, which was bound to a proton at δ_H 3.76. This latter signal evidenced heterocorrelations with the diasterotopic protons at δ_H 2.02 and δ_H 1.73, while homocorrelations were with the methylene protons at δ_H 2.62 and 1.87 (δ_C 35.5). All these data supported the presence of a tetrahydrofuran moiety formed by an oxygen bridge among the C-20 and C-24 carbons of the side chain. Besides the ester carbonyl of the acetate group, two additional carbonyls at δ_C 170.6 and 171.7 were also evident in the ^{13}C NMR spectrum. In the CIGAR-HMBC experiment, both of them revealed cross peaks with the methylene at δ_H 3.69 (δ_H 51.8), while the carbon at δ_C 170.6 was further correlated with a proton at δ_C 4.72. These data were in agreement with the presence of a malonyl that was bound to the saccharide unit. In the HSQCTOXY experiment, the anomeric carbon at δ_C 105.9 showed cross peaks with the signals at δ_C 75.4, 75.2, 73.6 and δ_C 63.3. These carbons in the HSQC experiment correlated with the methines at δ_H 3.26, 3.57, 4.72 and to the methylene protons at δ_H 3.96 and 3.28, respectively. The H2BC experiment displayed the following correlations: Starting from the anomeric proton at δ_C 4.32 (H-1′)→75.4 (C-2′)→3.57 (H3′)→73.6 (C-4′)→3.96/3.28 (H-5′); starting from the anomeric carbon at δ_C 105.9 (C-1′)→3.26 (H-2′)→75.2 (C-3′)→4.72 (H-4′)→63.3 (C-5′). These data further supported the presence of a pentose that was bound to a malonyl group at the C-4′ carbon.

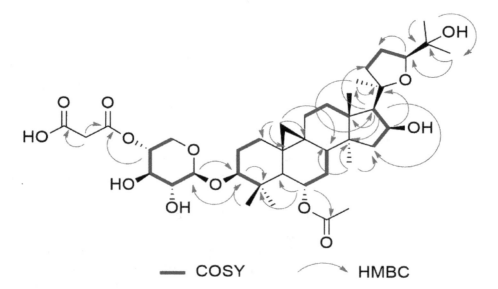

Figure 2. Selected H–H and H–C long range correlations of compound **1** evidenced in COSY and HMBC, respectively.

The stereostructure of the molecule was assigned on the basis of the nOe observed in the NOESY experiment (Figure 3). The sugar was identified as xylose by the GC-MS analysis of the acetylated alditol, which was obtained from the hydrolysis, reduction and acetylation of compound **1**. The coupling constant value of the anomeric proton allowed a β configuration for the anomeric carbon to be determined. The absolute configuration of the sugar was assigned by GC-MS, after a reaction of hydrolyzed saponins with L-cisteine methyl ester and acetylation [21].

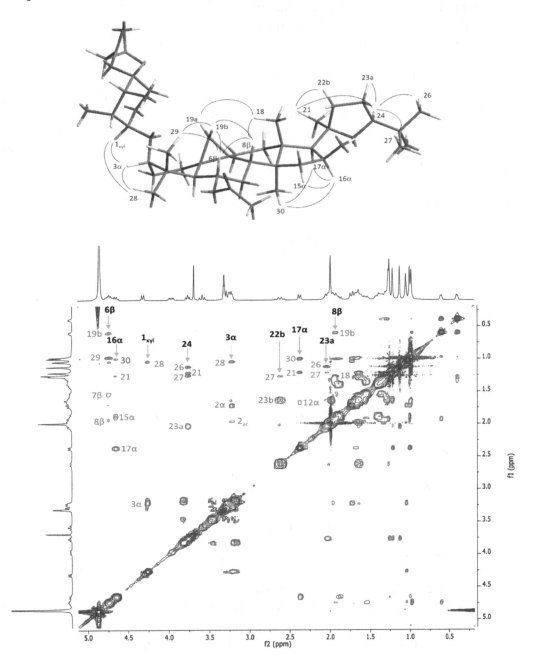

Figure 3. Key nOe correlation of compound **1** (top); NOESY experiment of compound **1** in CD$_3$OD (bottom).

The nOe evidenced in the NOESY experiments (Figure 3) allowed the configuration at the C-6 and C-16 carbons to be assigned. Based on these data, compound **1** was unequivocally identified as 6-*O*-acetyl-3-*O*-(4-*O*-malonyl)-β-D-xylopyranosylcycloastragenol (Figures S1–S9).

Compound **2** showed the molecular formula C$_{38}$H$_{60}$O$_{12}$ on the basis of the NMR data, and the presence of a quasimolecular peak at *m/z* 731.41 in the ESI-QTOF MS spectrum. The loss of an 86 Da fragment was demonstrated by the peak at *m/z* 645.39, indicating the presence of a malonyl moiety also in this molecule.

The ^{1}H NMR spectrum showed the H-19 protons at δ$_H$ 0.37 and 0.53, and seven singlet methyls at δ$_H$ 0.96 (H-30), 0.98 (H-28), 1.15 (H-26), 1.24 (H-27), 1.26 (H-29 and H-21). The absence of the characteristic signal associated with the methyl group of the acetate moiety demonstrated that compound **2** was the deacetylated form of compound **1**, and all the NMR data confirmed this hypothesis. In addition, the C3-sugar was characterized as xylose, and the malonyl was positioned to the C-4' carbon of this saccharide moiety. Based on these data, compound **2** was unequivocally identified as 3-O-β-D-(4-O-malonyl)xylopyranosylcycloastragenol.

Compound **3** showed the molecular formula $C_{43}H_{70}O_{15}$, calculated on the basis of its spectro-scopic features. In the ^{1}H-NMR spectrum, the signals of the aglycone, and those belonging to the C3-xylopyranose, were in good agreement with the previous metabolite. However, a further anomeric doublet at δ_C 4.51 suggested the presence of a second sugar. The heterocorrelation between this anomeric signal and the C-25 carbon at δ_H 79.9 allowed the second site of glycosylation to be located at position 25. The HSQCTOCSY experiment revealed the presence of an additional spin system due to this sugar, in which the anomeric proton (δ_C 4.51) correlated with the carbons at δ_C 99.6, 75.0, 78.2, 71.2, 77.5 and 62.7. These data were in agreement with the presence of a glucopyranose, a hypothesis that was confirmed by GC-MS analysis. Moreover, the coupling constant value indicated a β configuration for the anomeric carbon, while the D-series was established by GC-MS after the reaction of hydrolyzed saponins with L-cisteine methyl ester and acetylation. Based on these data, compound **3** was unequivocally identified as 6-O-acetyl-25-O-β-D-glucopyranosyl-3-O-β-D-xylo-pyranosylcycloastragenol.

Compound **4** showed a molecular formula $C_{37}H_{60}O_{10}$, calculated on the basis of its spectroscopic data. Of interest, this compound was also obtained by the mild acidic hydrolysis of compound **1**. In fact, when this compound was dissolved in water, after one day at room temperature, it was quantitatively converted in **4** by loss of the C4'-malonyl. All the NMR data confirmed this hypothesis, and allowed the identification of compound **4** as 6-O-acetyl-3-O-β-D-xylopyranosylcycloastragenol [22].

Compound **5** showed a molecular formula $C_{35}H_{58}O_9$, calculated on the basis of its spectroscopic data. The ^{1}H-NMR and ^{13}C-NMR signals of the aglycone and those belonging to the C3-xylopyranose were superimposable with the previous metabolites. Conversely, the lack of the singlet peak at δ_H 1.99 proved the absence of the C6-acetyl. All of these data enabled the identification of compound **5** as 3-O-β-D-xylopyranosylcycloastragenol [23].

2.2. Cytotoxicity of Cycloartane Glycosides from Astragalus boeticus Against Human Colorectal Cancer Cells

The cytotoxic activity of the isolated compounds (**1–5**) was assessed on three human colorectal cancer cell lines (Caco-2, HT-29 and HCT-116), using MTT (3-[4,5-dimethylthiazol-2-yl]-2,5-diphenyltetrazolium bromide) tetrazolium salt colorimetric assay (Figure 4). Results from these experiments demonstrated that cell proliferation was reduced by the treatment with compounds **1** and **4** in a dose-dependent manner, while **2**, **3** and **5** did not exert any significant effect. To our knowledge, no mechanistic studies regarding the proliferation reducing-effect of compounds **1** and **4** are available in literature. Yet, several previous works shed the light on the anticancer activity of other cycloartane glycosides (most of them isolated from *A. membranaceus*), which act by inducing apoptosis and modulating crucial cellular signaling pathways [24–27]. Importantly, a recent investigation pointed out that certain semisynthetic cycloastragenol derivatives impair inflammation-carcinogenesis by regulating the NF-KB signaling pathway [15].

Consistently, compound **4**, which has already been purified from the leaf extract of *A. membranaceus*, was described as a potentially anti-inflammatory molecule, because it was found to exert an inhibitory activity on the nitric oxide production in macrophages [21]. Recently, our group identified compound **4** as a metabolite responsible for the cytotoxicity of the *A. boeticus* extract. Here, this species underwent a further phytochemical investigation to understand whether analogues of compound **4** exert cytotoxicity as well. As it was already anticipated above, we demonstrated that compounds **1** and **4** were the active cycloartane glycosides isolated from *A. boeticus*.

In an attempt to further validate our findings, we compared the cytotoxicity of **4** (active compound) and **3** (inactive compound) with astragaloside IV (AS-IV), a commercially-available cycloartane glycoside extensively recognized as one of the main active components of several *Astragalus* spp. Results from these experiments confirmed the notable cytotoxicity of compound **4**, while no effect was found for AS-IV, at least in our experimental conditions (Figure S10).

From a structural point of view, these insights proved that the C3-xylopyranosyl, along with the C6-acetoxy group and the C25-free hydroxyl function, were essential structural requirements for the cytotoxic activity of these triterpenoids. As already discussed, when compound **1** was in water solutions, such as a cellular environment, it converted into compound **4** by losing the C4′ malonyl. Thereby, it was demonstrated that compound **4** was the real bioactive structure. Compounds **2**, **3**, **5** and AS-IV present the C3-xylopyranosyl, while none of them has either the C6-acetoxy group or the C25-free hydroxyl function. In accordance with previous investigations, acylation of the C-3 and C-6 secondary alcohols of diverse cycloartane derivatives resulted in a higher cytotoxic activity. This evidence led researchers to hypotheses that acylated cycloartane glycosides could lose the acyl substituents to modify proteins that play a key role in cellular signaling, whose deregulation is involved in carcinogenesis. Specifically, the acyl groups can be covalently attached to the amino acid side chains regulating the protein functions and impairing cancer progression [15].

In our study, a detailed analysis of the cytotoxic effect unveiled a differential response of Caco-2, HT-29 and HCT-116 to the treatment with compound **4**. These insights could be interpreted by describing the human colon cancer cells employed in our experimental setting. Caco-2 cell line was the wild type for the KRAS, NRAS, BRAF, PIK3CA genes; thus representing an ideal cellular model to study metastatic CRCs sensitive to anti-EGFR agents. By contrast, HT-29 and HCT-116 harbored a BRAF and some KRAS/PIK3CA mutations, respectively—therefore identifying metastatic CRCs with intrinsic resistance to the anti-EGFR treatments [28,29].

Herein, the in vitro cytotoxic screening revealed as compound **4** was clearly more effective in treating HT-29 (3 μM) than HCT-116 (40 μM) and Caco-2 (50 μM) cell lines (Figure 4).

In clinics, the BRAF mutation status is a strong indicator of a very poor prognosis for mCRC patients; indeed, they showed a worse outcome for the therapies compared with those whose tumors were wild type [30–32]. Of interest, the inhibition of BRAF oncoprotein by the small-molecule drug PLX4032 (Vemurafenib) is highly effective in the treatment of melanoma [33], whilst metastatic CRC patients associated with the same mutation showed a very limited response to this drug [34]. In fact, Vemurafenib treatment induces EGFR feedback activation, causing continued proliferation in the presence of BRAF (V600E) inhibition. Unlike CRCs, melanomas express low levels of EGFR, and thus, they are not subject to this kind of feedback activation [35].

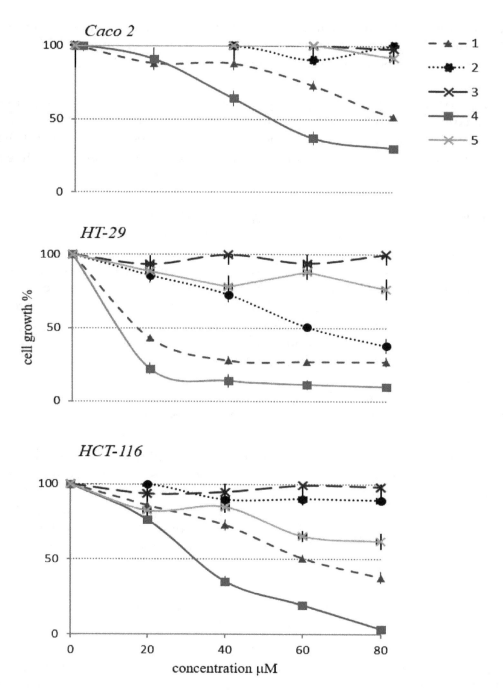

Figure 4. Cytotoxic activity of compounds **1–5** towards Caco-2, HT-29 and HCT-116 human colon cancer cell lines.

3. Materials and Methods

3.1. General Experimental Procedures

Analytical TLC was performed on Merck Kieselgel (Darmstadt, Germany) 60 F254 or RP-8 F254 plates with a 0.2 mm film thickness. Spots were visualized by UV light, or by spraying with $H_2SO_4/AcOH/H_2O$ (1:20:4), and then heating at 120 °C for 5 min. Preparative TLC was performed on Merck Kieselgel 60 F254 plates with a 0.5 or 1.0 mm film thickness.

Column chromatography (CC) was performed on Fluka (Seelze, Germany) Amberlite XAD-4 and XAD-7, on Pharmacia (Stockholm, Sweden) Sephadex LH-20, on Merck Kieselgel 60 (70–240 mesh), or on Baker (Deventer, Netherlands) RP-8. Nuclear magnetic resonance (NMR) spectra were recorded at 300 (^{1}H) and 75 MHz (^{13}C) on a Varian Mercury 300 FT-NMR spectrometer in CD_3OD

or pyridine-d$_5$ solutions at 25 °C. Chemical shifts are reported in δ (ppm), and referenced to the residual solvent signal; J (coupling constant) are given in Hz. Standard pulse sequences and phase cycling from Varian library were used for ^{1}H, ^{13}C, DEPT, DQF-COSY, COSY, TOCSY, NOESY, HSQC, H2BC, HMBC and CIGAR–HMBC experiments. ^{1}H NMR spectra were acquired over a spectral window from 14 to −2 ppm, with 1.0 s relaxation delay, 1.70 s acquisition time (AQ), and 90° pulse width = 13.8 μs. The initial matrix was zero-filled to 64 K. ^{13}C NMR spectra were recorded in ^{1}H broadband decoupling mode, over a spectral window from 235 to −15 ppm, 1.5 s relaxation delay, 90° pulse width = 9.50 μs, and AQ = 0.9 s. The number of scans for both ^{1}H and ^{13}C NMR experiments were chosen, depending on the concentration of the samples. With regards to the homonuclear and heteronuclear 2D-NMR experiments, the data points, number of scans and increments were adjusted according to the sample concentrations. Correlation spectroscopy (COSY) and double quantum filtered COSY (DQF-COSY) spectra were recorded with gradient-enhanced sequence at spectral widths of 3000 Hz in both f2 and f1 domains; the relaxation delays were of 1.0 s. The total correlation spectroscopy (TOCSY) experiments were performed in the phase-sensitive mode with a mixing time of 90 ms. The spectral width was 3000 Hz. Nuclear Overhauser effect spectroscopy (NOESY) experiments were performed in the phase-sensitive mode. The mixing time was 500 ms, and the spectral width was 3000 Hz. For all the homonuclear experiments, the initial matrix of 512 × 512 data points was zero-filled to give a final matrix of 1 k × 1 k points. Proton-detected heteronuclear correlations were also measured. Heteronuclear single-quantum coherence (HSQC) experiments (optimized for 1J(H,C) = 140 Hz) were performed in the phase sensitive mode with field gradient. The spectral width was 12,000 Hz in f1 (^{13}C) and 3000 Hz in f2 (1H) and 1.0 s of relaxation delay; the matrix of 1 k × 1 k data points was zero-filled to give a final matrix of 2 k × 2 k points. Heteronuclear 2 bond correlation (H2BC) spectra were obtained with T = 30.0 ms, and a relaxation delay of 1.0 s; the third order low-pass filter was set for 130 < 1J(C,H) < 165 Hz. A heteronuclear multiple bond coherence (HMBC) experiment (optimized for 1J(H,C) = 8 Hz) was performed in the absolute value mode with field gradient; typically, ^{1}H–^{13}C gHMBC were acquired with spectral width of 18,000 Hz in f1 (^{13}C) and 3000 Hz in f2 (1H) and 1.0 s of relaxation delay; the matrix of 1 k × 1 k data points was zero-filled to give a final matrix of 4 k × 4 k points. Constant time inverse-detected gradient accordion rescaled heteronuclear multiple bond correlation spectroscopy (CIGAR–HMBC) spectra (8 > nJ(H,C) > 5) were acquired with the same spectral width used for HMBC. Heteronuclear single quantum coherence-total correlation spectroscopy (HSQC-TOCSY) experiments were optimized for nJ(H,C) = 8 Hz, with a mixing time of 90 ms. For accurate mass measurements, the purified compounds were analyzed by an electrospray hybrid quadrupole orthogonal acceleration time-of-flight mass spectrometer (Q-TOF), fitted with a Z-spray electrospray ion source (Waters S.p.A.). All analyses were carried out in positive ion mode. The capillary source voltage and the cone voltage were set at 3500 V and 35 V, respectively. The source temperature was kept at 80 °C, and nitrogen was used as a drying gas (flow rate about 50 l/h). The time-of-flight analyzer of the mass spectrometer was externally calibrated, with GFP from m/z 50–1600. Accurate mass data were collected by directly infusing samples (1.5 pmol/μL in CH_3CN/H_2O, 1:1) into the system at a flow rate of 15 μL/min. The acquisition and processing of data were performed with the MassLynx 4.1 software (Waters S.p.A., Manchester, UK). GC-MS analyses were carried out using an HP 6890 GC instrument (Zebron ZB-5MS column, He flow 1.0 mL/min), coupled with a 5973 N mass spectrometer, equipped with an electron ionization source (EIMS), and operating with an electron energy of 70 eV. Full-scan mass spectra were collected between 0 and 600 amu at 2 scan/s. The MS was operated in the electron impact (EI) ionization mode, with an electron energy of 70 eV. The ion source and quadrupole temperatures were maintained at 230 and 150 °C, respectively. For the analyses of the acetylated alditols, the column head pressure was set at 7.41 p.s.i.

AS-IV was purchased from Shanghai Tauto Biotech Co., LTD. (Shanghai, China).

3.2. GC–MS Analysis of the Sugar Moieties

The GC-MS analysis of the sugar moieties has been previously described by Scognamiglio et al. [31]. Briefly, each metabolite (0.5 mg) was subjected to an acid hydrolysis with 2 N TFA (150 µL) at 120 °C for 1 h, obtaining the sugar moiety. This was dried under N2 flow, and reduced by adding MeOH (150 µL) and $NaBH_4$ (1.0 mg). The solution was incubated at room temperature for 1 h and then dried under N_2 flow after treatment with glacial AcOH and MeOH. The obtained alditol was acetylated by using anhydrous pyridine (200 µL) and Ac_2O (200 µL). This mixture was incubated for 20 min at 120 °C. Then, 500 µL of H_2O was added, and the product was extracted with CH_2Cl_2 (500 µL) following centrifugation at 3500 rpm for 5 min. The organic phase was dried under N_2 flow, dissolved in CH_2Cl_2 (500 µL) and analyzed by GC-MS. Temperature conditions were as follows: Injector port at 250 °C; the initial oven temperature was 160 °C for 50 s, then linearly increased to 200 °C at 10 °C/min. A further linear increase at 2.5 C/min was performed to 300 °C, and held for 40 min. Sample solutions were injected using the split mode.

3.3. Determination of Absolute Configuration of Monosaccharides of Compound 1 and 5

Compound 1 and 5 (2 mg each) were hydrolyzed with 2 N TFA (250 µL) at 120 °C for 1 h. The reaction mixture was then dried under N_2 flow and dissolved in dry pyridine (100 µL). 100 µL of pyridine solution of L-cysteine methyl ester hydrochloride (0.06 mol/L) were added to pyridine solutions of the hydrolyzed compounds 1 and 5 and pure D-xylose, and L-xylose (0.04 mol/L). These mixtures were warmed at 60 °C for 1 h, afterwards, acetic anhydride (150 µL) was added at 120 °C for 20 min. The products were dried under N_2, dissolved in 500 µL of H_2O, and extracted with CH_2Cl_2 (500 µL) following centrifugation at 3500 rpm for 5 min. The organic phase was dried under N_2 flow, dissolved in CH_2Cl_2 (500 µL), and analyzed by GC-MS. Temperature conditions were as follows: Injector port at 250 °C; initial oven temperature 45 °C, then increased linearly to 300 °C at 20 °C/min, and then held for 25 min. Sample solutions were injected using the split mode. The retention times were: D-xylose 13.89 min, L-xylose 14.17 min.

3.4. Plant Material

Leaf samples of A. boeticus were collected at vegetative state, in April 2014 in "Castel Volturno Nature Reserve" (40°57.587′N, 14°00.105′E; southern Italy). Samples were harvested, frozen in liquid nitrogen and lyophilized. A Voucher specimen CE000016 has been deposited at the Herbarium of the Dipartimento di Scienze e Tecnologie Ambientali Biologiche e Farmaceutiche of Università degli Studi della Campania "Luigi Vanvitelli".

3.5. Extraction and Isolation of Compound 1–5

Dried leaves (24.0 g) of A. boeticus were powdered, and underwent three cycles of an ultrasound-assisted extraction with an $MeOH/H_2O$ (1:1) solution (720 mL) [36], finally obtaining a crude extract (7.1 g). This was dissolved in H_2O and separated by liquid–liquid extraction, by using EtOAc as our extracting solvent. As a result, an organic and a water fraction were obtained. The former (1g) was chromatographed by SiO_2 CC, and eluted using a solution with an increasing degree of polarity ($CHCl_3$, $Me_2CO/CHCl_3$, $MeOH/CHCl_3$). Thus, 21 fractions have been collected. Of these, number 13 was chromatographed by C18 CC, and eluted with $H_2O/MeOH$ (3:2) to give compound 1 (18.6 mg) and 2 (7.1 mg). Meanwhile, number 12 was purified by Flash-CC eluting with $MeOH/CHCl_3$ (3:100) to obtain compound 4 (28 mg). On the other hand, the water fraction was chromatographed by XAD-4 (20–50 mesh; Fluka) and XAD-7 (20–50 mesh; Fluka) CC, obtaining an alcoholic eluate (900 mg) that was in turn purified by Sephadex LH-20. Subsequently, 17 fractions were given. Of these, fraction 13 was purified through RP-18 CC by using H_2O/MeOH (4:1) as the eluting system, consequently obtaining 30 fractions. One of these was chromatographed by TLC (0,5 mm), and eluted with the organic phase of $CHCl_3$/MeOH/H_2O (13:7:2) to obtain compound 3 (11.8 mg). Finally, fraction 11 was chromatographed by TLC (0.5 mm) and eluted with the organic phase of $CHCl_3$/MeOH/H_2O (13:7:2) to give compound 5 (4.6 mg).

Compound 1: 6-O-acetyl-3-O-(4-O-malonyl)-β-D-xylopyranosylcycloastragenol. $[\alpha]_D^{25}$ = +22.8 (c = 14.97 × 10^{-3}, MeOH). ^{1}H NMR (CD_3OD) and ^{13}C NMR (CD_3OD) see Table 1; ESI/Q-TOF: m/z 773.49 $[M + Na]^+$ (calcd.773.41 Da for $C_{40}H_{62}O_{13}Na$);

Compound 2: 3-O-(4-O-malonyl)-β-D- xylopyranosylcycloastragenol. $[\alpha]_D^{25}$ = +9.70 (c = 2.06 × 10^{-3}, MeOH). ^{1}H NMR (CD_3OD) and ^{13}C NMR (CD_3OD) see Table 1; ESI/Q-TOF: m/z 731.41 $[M+Na]+$ (calcd. 731.40 Da for $C_{38}H_{60}O_{12}Na$);

Compound 3: 6-O-acetyl-25-O-β-D-glucopyranosyl-3-O-β-D-xylopyranosylcycloastragenol. $[\alpha]_D^{25}$ = +13.7 (c= 6.06 × 10^{-3}, MeOH). ^{1}H NMR (CD_3OD) and ^{13}C NMR (CD_3OD) see Table 1; ESI/Q-TOF: m/z 849.46 $[M + Na]^+$ (calcd.849.43 Da for $C_{43}H_{70}O_{15}Na$);

Compound 4: 6-acetyl-3-O-(4-O-malonyl)-β-D-xylopyranosylcycloastragenol. $[\alpha]_D^{25}$ = +7.65 (c = 5.1 × 10^{-3}, MeOH/H_2O, 2:1) [22];

Compound 5: 3-O-β-D-xylopyranosylcycloastragenol. $[\alpha]_D^{25}$ = −340.1 (c = 3.74 × 10^{-3}) MeOH/H_2O, 1:1) [23].

Table 1. 1D and 2D nuclear magnetic resonance (NMR) data of compound **1–3** in CD$_3$OD.

Position	1 δ$_C$	1 Type	1 δ$_H$ (J in Hz)	1 HMBC[a]	2 δ$_C$	2 Type	2 δ$_H$ (J in Hz)	2 HMBC[a]	3 δ$_C$	3 Type	3 δ$_H$ (J in Hz)	3 HMBC[a]
1	32.8	CH$_2$	1.85 s / 1.67 s	2, 10 / 2, 10	32.3	CH$_2$	1.84 s / 1.65 s	2, 10 / 2, 10	32.8	CH$_2$	1.29 s	
2	30.3	CH$_2$	1.98 ov / 1.64 ov	3, 4 / 3, 4	30.0	CH$_2$	1.88 ov / 1.69 ov	3, 4 / 3, 4	30.2	CH$_2$	1.99 ov	3, 4
3	89.1	CH	3.21 d (J = 1.8)	28, 29, 1$_{xyl}$	89.1	CH	3.29 ov	28, 29, 1$_{xyl}$	89.1	CH	3.21 ov	1$_{xyl}$
4	42.8	C	-		42.0	C			42.8	C		
5	51.2	CH	1.71 s	1, 4, 7, 10, 28, 29	53.9	CH	1.38 s	1, 4, 7, 10, 28, 29	51.3	CH	1.72 s	1, 4, 7, 10, 28, 29
6	72.0	CH	4.75 ov	4, 5, 7, 8, 1$_{Ac}$	68.5	CH	3.48 ov	4, 5, 7, 8	72.1	CH	4.75 ov	4, 5, 1$_{ac}$
7	34.0	CH$_2$	1.56 ov	5, 6	33.4	CH$_2$	1.46 ov	5, 6	34.1	CH$_2$	1.57	5, 6, 8, 9, 14
8	46.7	CH	1.95 s	6, 9, 10, 13, 14, 19, 30	48.0	CH	1.46 s	6, 9, 10, 13, 14, 19, 30	46.1	CH	1.94 s	6, 10, 13, 14, 15, 19
9	21.8	C			21.4	C			21.6	C		
10	29.6	C			29.2	C			29.2	C		
11	26.8	CH$_2$	1.97 m	8, 12, 19	26.4	CH$_2$	1.97 s	8, 12, 19	26.4	CH$_2$	1.97 s	12
12	34.1	CH$_2$	1.64 ov / 1.56 ov	14, 18 / 14, 18	33.4	CH$_2$	1.54 ov / 1.37 ov	14, 18 / 14, 18	34.1	CH$_2$	1.64 ov / 1.56 ov	
13	47.0	C			44.7	C			46.9	C		
14	46.4	C			47.0	C			46.6	C		
15	46.2	CH$_2$	1.87 d (J = 8.0) / 1.39 d (J = 8.0)	8, 13, 17, 30 / 8, 13, 17, 30	46.4	CH$_2$	1.98 d (J = 4.4) / 1.32 d (J = 6.8)	8, 13, 17, 30 / 8, 13, 17, 30	46.0	CH$_2$	1.86 d (J = 6.0) / 1.42 d (J = 6.4)	8, 13, 14, 17, 30 / 13, 14, 30
16	74.5	CH	4.65 m	13, 14, 15	73.9	CH	4.64 m	13, 14, 15	74.3	CH	4.65 m	13, 14, 15
17	58.9	CH	2.37 d (J = 7.8)	13, 14, 16, 20, 21, 22	58.2	CH	2.37 d (J = 7.7)	13, 14, 16, 20, 21, 22	58.7	CH	2.38 d (J = 8.0)	13, 14, 16, 20, 21, 22
18	21.4	CH$_3$	1.27 s	12, 15, 17	21.4	CH$_3$	1.23 s	12, 15, 17	21.7	CH$_3$	1.27 s	12, 15, 17
19	30.1	CH$_2$	0.61 s / 0.40 s	1, 5, 8, 9, 10 / 1, 5, 8, 9, 10, 11	31.4	CH$_2$	0.53 s / 0.37 s	1, 5, 8, 9, 10 / 1, 5, 8, 9, 10, 11	30.2	CH$_2$	0.61 s / 0.40 s	1, 5, 8, 9, 10, 11 / 1, 5, 8, 9, 10, 11
20	88.3	C	-		88.2	C	-		88.3	C	-	
21	28.4	CH$_3$	1.22 s	17, 20, 22	28.1	CH$_3$	1.25 s	17, 20, 22	28.0	CH$_3$	1.24 s	
22	35.5	CH$_2$	2.62 ov / 1.87 ov	17, 20, 21 / 17, 20, 21	34.9	CH$_2$	1.69 ov	17, 20, 21 / 17, 20, 21	35.6	CH$_2$	2.54 ov / 1.84	17 / 17
23	26.8	CH$_2$	2.02 ov / 1.73	20, 24, 25 / 17, 24, 25	26.4	CH$_2$	2.02 ov	20, 24, 25 / 17, 24, 25	26.8	CH$_2$	2.16 ov / 1.72	24, 25 / 24, 25
24	82.6	CH	3.76 m	25	81.4	CH	3.80 m	25	83.0	CH	3.82 m	1$_{glc}$

Table 1. *Cont.*

Position	1 δ_C	1 Type	1 δ_H (J in Hz)	1 HMBC [a]	2 δ_C	2 Type	2 δ_H (J in Hz)	2 HMBC [a]	3 δ_C	3 Type	3 δ_H (J in Hz)	3 HMBC [a]
25	71.2	C	-		71.2	C	-		79.9	C	-	
26	26.6	CH$_3$	1.13 s	17, 24, 25	26.5	CH$_3$	1.15 s	17, 24, 25	23.2	CH$_3$	1.22 s	20, 23, 24, 25
27	27.6	CH$_3$	1.26 s	24, 25, 26	27.1	CH$_3$	1.24 s	24, 25, 26	25.3	CH$_3$	1.38 s	23, 24, 26
28	27.2	CH$_3$	1.05 s	3, 4, 5, 29	16.1	CH$_3$	0.98 s	3, 4, 5, 29	16.5	CH$_3$	0.98 s	3, 4, 5, 28
29	16.6	CH$_3$	0.98 s	3, 4, 5, 28	27.1	CH$_3$	1.25 s	3, 4, 5, 28	27.3	CH$_3$	1.04 s	3, 4, 5, 29
30	20.3	CH$_3$	1.01 s	9, 14, 15	20.9	CH$_3$	0.96 s	9, 14, 15	20.2	CH$_3$	0.99 s	14, 15
1$_{xyl}$	105.9	CH	4.32 d (J = 7.4)	3, 5$_{xyl}$	105.9	CH	4.43 d (J = 7.4)	3, 5$_{xyl}$	107.4	CH	4.26 d (J = 7.0)	3
2$_{xyl}$	75.4	CH	3.26 ov	4$_{xyl}$	75.4	CH	3.26 ov	4$_{xyl}$	75.5	CH	3.19 ov	
3$_{xyl}$	75.2	CH	3.57 ov	4$_{xyl}$, 5$_{xyl}$	75.2	CH	3.57 ov	4$_{xyl}$, 5$_{xyl}$	78.0	CH	3.29 ov	
4$_{xyl}$	73.6	CH	4.72 m	2$_{xyl}$, 3$_{xyl}$, 5$_{xyl}$, 2$_{mal}$	73.6	CH	4.72 m	2$_{xyl}$, 3$_{xyl}$, 5$_{xyl}$, 2$_{mal}$	71.2	CH	3.46 m	
5$_{xyl}$	63.3	CH$_2$	3.28 ov / 3.96 ov	1$_{xyl}$, 3$_{xyl}$, 4$_{xyl}$ / 1$_{xyl}$, 3$_{xyl}$, 4$_{xyl}$	63.3	CH$_2$	3.28 ov / 3.96 ov	1$_{xyl}$, 3$_{xyl}$, 4$_{xyl}$ / 1$_{xyl}$, 3$_{xyl}$, 4$_{xyl}$	66.7	CH$_2$	3.18 ov / 3.82 ov	
1$_{glc}$	-	-	-		-	-	-		99.6	CH	4.51 d (J = 6.6)	25
2$_{glc}$	-	-	-		-	-	-		75.0	CH	3.18 ov	5$_{glc}$
3$_{glc}$	-	-	-		-	-	-		78.2	CH	3.32 ov	1$_{glc}$, 5$_{glc}$
4$_{glc}$	-	-	-		-	-	-		71.2	CH	3.31 ov	6$_{glc}$
5$_{glc}$	-	-	-		-	-	-		77.5	CH	3.24 ov	1$_{glc}$, 3$_{glc}$
6$_{glc}$	-	-	-		-	-	-		62.7	CH$_2$	3.65 ov / 3.79 ov	4$_{glc}$ / 4$_{glc}$
1$_{ac}$	172.2	C	-		-	-	-		172.2	C	-	
2$_{ac}$	22.2	CH$_3$	1.99 s	1$_{ac}$	-	-	-		21.8	CH$_3$	1.99 s	1$_{ac}$
1$_{mal}$	170.6	C	-	-	170.6	C	-	-	-		-	-
2$_{mal}$	51.8	CH$_2$	3.69 s	1$_{mal}$, 3$_{mal}$	51.8	CH$_2$	3.69 s	1$_{mal}$, 3$_{mal}$	-		-	-
3$_{mal}$	171.7	C	-	-	171.7	C	-	-	-		-	-

[a] HMBC correlations, optimized for 6 Hz, are from proton(s) stated to the indicated carbon; [b] obscured; *d* = doublet, *m* = multiplet, *ov* = overlapped, *s* = singlet, *t* = triplet.

3.6. Cell Lines

The human HCT-116, HT-29, Caco-2 colorectal cancer cell lines were obtained from the American Type Culture Collection (ATCC) (Manassas, VA). HCT-116, HT-29 cancer cells were cultured in RPMI 1640 medium (Lonza, Cologne, Germany) supplemented with 10% fetal bovine serum, 2 mM L-glutamine, 50 U/mL penicillin and 100 µg/mL streptomycin (Lonza, Cologne, Germany). The Caco-2 cell line was cultured in DMEM medium (Lonza, Cologne, Germany), supplemented with 10% fetal bovine serum, 2 mM L-glutamine, 1% non-essential amino acid, 50 U/mL penicillin and 100 µg/mL streptomycin (Lonza, Cologne, Germany).

3.7. Proliferation Assay

The cell proliferation assay was performed with a 3-(4,5-dimethylthiazol-2-yl)-2,5-diphenyl-tetrazolium bromide (MTT) assay. Briefly, cells in logarithmic growth phase were plated in 96-well plates and incubated for 24 h before exposure to increasing doses of DMSO-diluted compounds (20, 40, 60, and 80 µM). For compounds 1 and 4 that exerted a strong cytotoxic effect in the HT-29 cell line, a lower range of doses (2, 4, 6, and 10 µM) was also investigated. 48 h after treatment, 50 µL of 1 mg/mL (MTT) were mixed with 200 µL of medium and added to the well. 1 h after incubation at 37 °C, the medium was removed, and the purple formazan crystals produced in the viable cells were solubilized in 100 µL of dimethyl sulfoxide, and quantitated by measurement of absorbance at 570 nm with a plate reader. Results were reported as mean ± s.d. of % of cell growth, with respect to the control from six replicate analyses. The control was represented by a 0.08% DMSO treatment, which corresponded to the higher amount of DMSO used for the tests.

4. Conclusions

A plethora of previous investigation regarding the phytochemistry and the bioactive components of diverse species belonging to the *Astragalus* genus are available in literature. However, to our knowledge, there are no data regarding the phytochemical constituents of *A. boeticus*. In this study, we focused on the cycloartane derivatives present in *A. boeticus*, because of its putative cytotoxic activity.

Specifically, the targeted phytochemical study of *A. boeticus* led to the isolation of five cycloartane-type glycosides (1–5); of these, 1, 2 and 3 were isolated and characterized for the first time. The cytotoxic activity of compounds 1–5 was evaluated in vitro, disclosing a strong proliferation-reducing effect of compound 4 in the HT-29 human colon cancer cell line, which was employed as a preclinical model to study refractory mCRCs that are resistant to anti-EGFR therapies, as well as other chemotherapeutic drugs currently used in the clinical setting. Our results therefore provide a small molecule scaffold that might be potentially important for the development of new agents effective against refractory mCRCs.

Indeed, these insights pave the way to further investigations aimed to figure out whether compound 4 acts on CRC cell models resistant to EGFR inhibitors with high selectivity, and if so, to elucidate the mechanism by which the anti-proliferative activity occurs.

On the other hand, as several limitations are intrinsically associated with our in vitro experimental system, future experiments shall also be addressed to evaluate the pharmacokinetic properties, and the bioavailability of the active molecule in animal models.

Author Contributions: V.G. and M.S. designed the experiments, discussed and interpreted the results. A.E. selected and identified the plant species. V.G. and M.S. carried out the experiments. A.C. and R.R. carried out the M.S. analyses. V.G. and M.S. wrote the manuscript. A.E., B.D.A. and F.C. analyzed the experimental data. A.E.,

B.D.A. interpreted the results. T.T., N.P., A.F. designed the experiments, discussed and interpreted the results and reviewed the manuscript. All authors revised the manuscript.

References

1. Verotta, L.; El-Sebakhy, N. *Cycloartane and oleanane saponins from Astragalus sp. Studies in Natural Products Chemistry*; Elsevier: Amsterdam, The Netherlands, 2001; pp. 179–234.
2. Prohens, J.; Andújar, I.; Vilanova, S.; Plazas, M.; Gramazio, P.; Prohens, R.; Herraiz, F.J.; De Ron, A.M. Swedish coffee (Astragalus boeticus L.), a neglected coffee substitute with a past and a potential future. *Genet. Resour. Crop Evol.* **2013**, *61*, 287–297. [CrossRef]
3. Williams, M.C.; Davis, A.M. Nitro Compounds in Introduced Astragalus Species. *J. Range Manage.* **1982**, *35*. [CrossRef]
4. Cook, D.; Ralphs, M.H.; Welch, K.D.; Stegelmeier, B.L. Locoweed Poisoning in Livestock. *Rangelands* **2009**, *31*, 16–21. [CrossRef]
5. Ionkova, I.; Shkondrov, A.; Krasteva, I.; Ionkov, T. Recent progress in phytochemistry, pharmacology and biotechnology of Astragalus saponins. *Phytochem. Rev.* **2014**, *13*, 343–374. [CrossRef]
6. Rios, J.L.; Waterman, P.G. A review of the pharmacology and toxicology of Astragalus. *Phytother. Res.* **1997**, *11*, 411–418. [CrossRef]
7. Gülcemal, D.; Aslanipour, B.; Bedir, E. Secondary Metabolites from Turkish Astragalus Species. In *Plant and Human Health, Volume 2: Phytochemistry and Molecular Aspects*; Ozturk, M., Hakeem, K.R., Eds.; Springer International Publishing: Berlin, Germany, 2019; pp. 43–97.
8. Wang, Y.; Auyeung, K.K.; Zhang, X.; Ko, J.K. Astragalus saponins modulates colon cancer development by regulating calpain-mediated glucose-regulated protein expression. *BMC Complement. Altern. Med.* **2014**, *14*, 401. [CrossRef]
9. Yang, L.P.; Shen, J.G.; Xu, W.C.; Li, J.; Jiang, J.Q. Secondary metabolites of the genus Astragalus: Structure and biological-activity update. *Chem. Biodivers.* **2013**, *10*, 1004–1054. [CrossRef]
10. Shkondrov, A.; Krasteva, I.; Bucar, F.; Kunert, O.; Kondeva-Burdina, M.; Ionkova, I. A new tetracyclic saponin from Astragalus glycyphyllos L. and its neuroprotective and hMAO-B inhibiting activity. *Nat. Prod. Res.* **2018**, *23*, 1–7. [CrossRef]
11. Pistelli, L.; Bertoli, A.; Lepori, E.; Morelli, I.; Panizzi, L. Antimicrobial and antifungal activity of crude extracts and isolated saponins from Astragalus verrucosus. *Fitoterapia* **2002**, *73*, 336–339. [CrossRef]
12. Yin, X.; Zhang, Y.; Yu, J.; Zhang, P.; Shen, J.; Qiu, J.; Wu, H.; Zhu, X. The antioxidative effects of astragalus saponin I protect against development of early diabetic nephropathy. *J. Pharmacol. Sci.* **2006**, *101*, 166–173. [CrossRef]
13. Aslanipour, B.; Gulcemal, D.; Nalbantsoy, A.; Yusufoglu, H.; Bedir, E. Secondary metabolites from Astragalus karjaginii BORISS and the evaluation of their effects on cytokine release and hemolysis. *Fitoterapia* **2017**, *122*, 26–33. [CrossRef]
14. Auyeung, K.K.; Law, P.C.; Ko, J.K. Combined therapeutic effects of vinblastine and Astragalus saponins in human colon cancer cells and tumor xenograft via inhibition of tumor growth and proangiogenic factors. *Nutr. Cancer* **2014**, *66*, 662–674. [CrossRef] [PubMed]
15. Debelec-Butuner, B.; Ozturk, M.B.; Tag, O.; Akgun, I.H.; Yetik-Anacak, G.; Bedir, E.; Korkmaz, K.S. Cycloartane-type sapogenol derivatives inhibit NFkappaB activation as chemopreventive strategy for inflammation-induced prostate carcinogenesis. *Steroids* **2018**, *135*, 9–20. [CrossRef] [PubMed]
16. Auyeung, K.K.; Han, Q.B.; Ko, J.K. Astragalus membranaceus: A Review of its Protection Against Inflammation and Gastrointestinal Cancers. *Am. J. Chin. Med.* **2016**, *44*, 1–22. [CrossRef]
17. Graziani, V.; Scognamiglio, M.; Belli, V.; Esposito, A.; D'Abrosca, B.; Chambery, A.; Russo, R.; Panella, M.; Russo, A.; Ciardiello, F.; et al. Metabolomic approach for a rapid identification of natural products with cytotoxic activity against human colorectal cancer cells. *Sci. Rep.* **2018**, *8*, 5309. [CrossRef] [PubMed]

18. Malvezzi, M.; Carioli, G.; Bertuccio, P.; Rosso, T.; Boffetta, P.; Levi, F.; La Vecchia, C.; Negri, E. European cancer mortality predictions for the year 2016 with focus on leukaemias. *Ann. Oncol.* **2016**, *27*, 725–731. [CrossRef] [PubMed]

19. Baselga, J. The EGFR as a target for anticancer therapy - focus on cetuximab. *Eur. J. Cancer* **2001**, *37*, S16–S22. [CrossRef]

20. Ciardiello, F.; Tortora, G. EGFR antagonists in cancer treatment. *N. Engl. J. Med.* **2008**, *358*, 1160–1174. [CrossRef]

21. Scognamiglio, M.; D'Abrosca, B.; Fiumano, V.; Chambery, A.; Severino, V.; Tsafantakis, N.; Pacifico, S.; Esposito, A.; Fiorentino, A. Oleanane saponins from Bellis sylvestris Cyr. and evaluation of their phytotoxicity on Aegilops geniculata Roth. *Phytochemistry* **2012**, *84*, 125–134. [CrossRef]

22. Wang, Z.B.; Zhai, Y.D.; Ma, Z.P.; Yang, C.J.; Pan, R.; Yu, J.L.; Wang, Q.H.; Yang, B.Y.; Kuang, H.X. Triterpenoids and Flavonoids from the Leaves of Astragalus membranaceus and Their Inhibitory Effects on Nitric Oxide Production. *Chem. Biodivers.* **2015**, *12*, 1575–1584. [CrossRef]

23. Kitagawa, I.; Wang, H.; Saito, M.; Takagi, A.; Yoshikawa, M. Saponin and sapogenol. XXXV. Chemical constituents of astragali radix, the root of Astragalus membranaceus Bunge. (2). Astragalosides I, II and IV, acetylastragaloside I and isoastragalosides I and II. *Chem. Pharm. Bull.* **1983**, *31*, 698–708. [CrossRef]

24. Tin, M.M.; Cho, C.H.; Chan, K.; James, A.E.; Ko, J.K. Astragalus saponins induce growth inhibition and apoptosis in human colon cancer cells and tumor xenograft. *Carcinogenesis* **2007**, *28*, 1347–1355. [CrossRef] [PubMed]

25. Auyeung, K.K.; Cho, C.H.; Ko, J.K. A novel anticancer effect of Astragalus saponins: Transcriptional activation of NSAID-activated gene. *Int. J. Cancer* **2009**, *125*, 1082–1091. [CrossRef] [PubMed]

26. Ionkova, I.; Momekov, G.; Proksch, P. Effects of cycloartane saponins from hairy roots of Astragalus membranaceus Bge., on human tumor cell targets. *Fitoterapia* **2010**, *81*, 447–451. [CrossRef]

27. Auyeung, K.K.; Woo, P.K.; Law, P.C.; Ko, J.K. Astragalus saponins modulate cell invasiveness and angiogenesis in human gastric adenocarcinoma cells. *J. Ethnopharmacol.* **2012**, *141*, 635–641. [CrossRef] [PubMed]

28. Saif, M.W. Colorectal cancer in review: The role of the EGFR pathway. *Expert Opin Investig. Drugs* **2010**, *19*, 357–369. [CrossRef] [PubMed]

29. Veluchamy, J.P.; Spanholtz, J.; Tordoir, M.; Thijssen, V.L.; Heideman, D.A.; Verheul, H.M.; de Gruijl, T.D.; van der Vliet, H.J. Combination of NK Cells and Cetuximab to Enhance Anti-Tumor Responses in RAS Mutant Metastatic Colorectal Cancer. *PLoS ONE* **2016**, *11*, e0157830. [CrossRef] [PubMed]

30. Richman, S.D.; Seymour, M.T.; Chambers, P.; Elliott, F.; Daly, C.L.; Meade, A.M.; Taylor, G.; Barrett, J.H.; Quirke, P. KRAS and BRAF Mutations in Advanced Colorectal Cancer Are Associated With Poor Prognosis but Do Not Preclude Benefit From Oxaliplatin or Irinotecan: Results From the MRC FOCUS Trial. *J. Clin. Oncol.* **2009**, *27*, 5931–5937. [CrossRef]

31. Roth, A.D.; Tejpar, S.; Delorenzi, M.; Yan, P.; Fiocca, R.; Klingbiel, D.; Dietrich, D.; Biesmans, B.; Bodoky, G.; Barone, C.; et al. Prognostic role of KRAS and BRAF in stage II and III resected colon cancer: Results of the translational study on the PETACC-3, EORTC 40993, SAKK 60-00 trial. *J. Clin. Oncol.* **2010**, *28*, 466–474. [CrossRef]

32. Van Cutsem, E.; Kohne, C.H.; Lang, I.; Folprecht, G.; Nowacki, M.P.; Cascinu, S.; Shchepotin, I.; Maurel, J.; Cunningham, D.; Tejpar, S.; et al. Cetuximab plus irinotecan, fluorouracil, and leucovorin as first-line treatment for metastatic colorectal cancer: Updated analysis of overall survival according to tumor KRAS and BRAF mutation status. *J. Clin. Oncol.* **2011**, *29*, 2011–2019. [CrossRef]

33. Chapman, P.B.; Hauschild, A.; Robert, C.; Haanen, J.B.; Ascierto, P.; Larkin, J.; Dummer, R.; Garbe, C.; Testori, A.; Maio, M.; et al. Improved survival with vemurafenib in melanoma with BRAF V600E mutation. *N. Engl. J. Med.* **2011**, *364*, 2507–2516. [CrossRef] [PubMed]

34. Kopetz, S.; Desai, J.; Chan, E.; Hecht, J.R.; O'Dwyer, P.J.; Lee, R.J.; Nolop, K.B.; Saltz, L. PLX4032 in metastatic colorectal cancer patients with mutant BRAF tumors. *J. Clin. Oncol.* **2010**, *28*, 3534. [CrossRef]

35. Prahallad, A.; Sun, C.; Huang, S.D.; Di Nicolantonio, F.; Salazar, R.; Zecchin, D.; Beijersbergen, R.L.; Bardelli, A.; Bernards, R. Unresponsiveness of colon cancer to BRAF(V600E) inhibition through feedback activation of EGFR. *Nature* **2012**, *483*, 100–146. [CrossRef]

36. Scognamiglio, M.; Fiumano, V.; D'Abrosca, B.; Esposito, A.; Choi, Y.H.; Verpoorte, R.; Fiorentino, A. Chemical interactions between plants in Mediterranean vegetation: The influence of selected plant extracts on Aegilops geniculata metabolome. *Phytochemistry* **2014**, *106*, 69–85. [CrossRef] [PubMed]

5

Identification of Phytoconstituents in *Leea indica* (Burm. F.) Merr. Leaves by High Performance Liquid Chromatography Micro Time-of-Flight Mass Spectrometry

Deepika Singh *, Yin-Yin Siew, Teck-Ian Chong, Hui-Chuing Yew, Samuel Shan-Wei Ho, Claire Sophie En-Shen Lim, Wei-Xun Tan, Soek-Ying Neo and Hwee-Ling Koh *

Department of Pharmacy, Faculty of Science, National University of Singapore, 18 Science Drive 4, Singapore 117543, Singapore; yindividual@hotmail.com (Y.-Y.S.); TI_Chong90@gmail.com (T.-I.C.); youyiting1979@yahoo.com.sg (H.-C.Y.); samuel.ho.s.w@icloud.com (S.S.-W.H.); clairesophie1992@yahoo.com.sg (C.S.E.-S.L.); tweixun07@hotmail.com (W.-X.T.); phansy@nus.edu.sg (S.-Y.N.)
* Correspondence: phads@nus.edu.sg (D.S.); phakohhl@nus.edu.sg (H.-L.K.); Tel.: +65-65163120 (H.-L.K.)

Academic Editor: Pinarosa Avato

Abstract: *Leea indica* (Vitaceae) is a Southeast Asian medicinal plant. In this study, an ethyl acetate fraction of *L. indica* leaves was studied for its phytoconstituents using high-performance liquid chromatography-electrospray ionization-mass spectrometry (HPLC-ESI-microTOF-Q-MS/MS) analysis. A total of 31 compounds of different classes, including benzoic acid derivatives, phenolics, flavonoids, catechins, dihydrochalcones, coumarins, megastigmanes, and oxylipins were identified using LC-MS/MS. Among them, six compounds including gallic acid, methyl gallate, (−)-epigallocatechin-3-*O*-gallate, myricetin-3-*O*-rhamnoside, quercetin-3-*O*-rhamnoside, and 4′,6′-dihydroxy-4-methoxydihydrochalcone 2′-*O*-β-D-glucopyranoside were isolated and identified by NMR analysis. The LC-MS/MS analysis led to the tentative identification of three novel dihydrochalcones namely 4′,6′-dihydroxy-4-methoxydihydrochalcone 2′-*O*-rutinoside, 4′,6′-dihydroxy-4-methoxydihydrochalcone 2′-*O*-glucosylpentoside and 4′,6′-dihydroxy-4-methoxydihydrochalcone 2′-*O*-(3″-*O*-galloyl)-β-D-glucopyranoside. The structural identification of novel dihydrochalcones was based on the basic skeleton of the isolated dihydrochalcone, 4′,6′-dihydroxy-4-methoxydihydrochalcone 2′-*O*-β-D-glucopyranoside and characteristic LC-MS/MS fragmentation patterns. This is the first comprehensive analysis for the identification of compounds from *L. indica* using LC-MS. A total 24 compounds including three new dihydrochalcones were identified for the first time from the genus *Leea*.

Keywords: *Leea indica*; HPLC-ESI-microTOF-Q-MS/MS; phenolics; dihydrochalcones

1. Introduction

Leea indica (Burm. f.) Merr. (Vitaceae), commonly known as Bandicoot berry, is an evergreen perennial shrub or a small tree of 2 to 16 m in height. It is distributed throughout Bangladesh, China, India, Malaysia, Singapore, North Australia, Thailand, and Vietnam [1–3]. Traditionally, *L. indica* is used as a remedy during pregnancy, for birth control, body pain, skin problems, and relief from dizziness [4,5]. *L. indica* is reported to possess various pharmacological activities, e.g., analgesic, anti-angiogenesis, anti-oxidant, anti-inflammatory, anti-microbial, anti-proliferative, hepatoprotective, sedative, and anxiolytic activities [3,5–12]. The plant contains different classes of compounds including phenolics, terpenoids, phthalic acid derivatives, and steroids [13–15]. Currently, there are very few reports available on the phytochemistry of *L. indica*.

The objective of the present study was to isolate and identify chemical constituents from an ethyl acetate fraction of *L. indica* leaves. The comprehensive chemical identification was carried out by high performance liquid chromatography coupled to electrospray ionization and quadrupole time-of-flight mass spectrometry (HPLC-ESI-microTOF-Q-MS) analysis along with the isolation of compounds **1, 5, 10, 14, 18,** and **27** from ethyl acetate fraction. The structures of the isolated compounds were identified using NMR and MS analyses. A total of 31 compounds belonging to different classes including benzoic acid derivatives, flavonoids, coumarins, megastigmanes, catechins, dihydrochalcones, and oxylipins were identified. Here we report the identification of three novel dihydrochalcones along with 28 known compounds from the ethyl acetate fraction of *L. indica* leaves. In total, 24 compounds, including three novel dihydrochalcones, are reported for the first time in the genus *Leea*.

2. Results and Discussion

2.1. Isolation and Identification of Compounds

The methanolic extract of *L. indica* leaves was fractionated with hexane, dichloromethane and ethyl acetate. The dried yields were 0.005%, 0.027% and 1.32% respectively. Purification of the major organic ethyl acetate fraction by repeated column chromatography led to the isolation of compounds **1, 5, 10, 14, 18,** and **27**. The compounds were identified as gallic acid (**1**) [16], methyl gallate (**5**) [17], epigallocatechin-3-*O*-gallate (**10**) [18], myricetin-3-*O*-rhamnoside (**14**) [19], quercetin-3-*O*-rhamnoside (**18**), [19] and 4′,6′-dihydroxy-4-methoxydihydrochalcone 2′-*O*-β-D-glucopyranoside (**27**) [20] by comparing their analytical data (^{1}H, ^{13}C and 2D-NMR, and LC-MS) with those reported in the literature [16–20].

2.2. Identification of Dihydrochalcones by LC-ESI-MS/MS Analysis

The ethyl acetate fraction of *L. indica* leaves was analyzed by the LC-ESI-MS/MS method. Figure 1 shows the base peak chromatogram (BPC) of the ethyl acetate fraction of *L. indica* leaves at 254 nm. Figure 2 shows the structures of the 31 compounds identified. In total, 31 compounds were identified of which ten compounds (**1, 4, 5, 8, 9, 10, 14, 15, 18** and **21**) were verified by comparison with reference standards. Seven compounds were tentatively identified as dihydrochalcone derivatives: 3-hydroxyphloridzin **17**, phloridzin **21**, 4′,6′-dihydroxy-4-methoxydihydrochalcone 2′-*O*-rutinoside **25** (m/z 595), 4′,6′-dihydroxy-4-methoxydihydrochalcone 2′-*O*-glucosyl pentoside **26** (m/z 581), 4′,6′-dihydroxy-4-methoxydihydrochalcone 2′-*O*-β-D-glucopyranoside **27**, 4′,6′-dihydroxy-4-methoxydihydrochalcone 2′-*O*-(6″-*O*-galloyl)-β-D-glucopyranoside **29** (m/z 601) and 2′,4′,6′-trihydroxy-4-methoxydihydrochalcone (3-methylphloretin) **31**. Compounds **25, 26** and **29** are reported for the first time. While dihydrochalcone phloridzin has been previously reported in *L. indica* [13], the other six dihydrochalcone derivatives have not been previously reported in the same plant species. The observed MS peaks including retention time, observed mass, calculated mass, molecular formula, ppm error, and MS/MS data are presented in Table 1.

Table 1. Identification of compounds from ethyl acetate fraction of *L. indica* by HPLC-ESI-microTOF-Q-MS/MS at 254 nm in negative ionization mode.

Peak no.	RT (min)	Observed [M − H]$^{-}$	Calculated [M − H]$^{-}$	Error (ppm)	Molecular Formula	Fragment Ions (m/z)	Identified Compound
1	10.9	169.0146	169.0142	−2.2	$C_7H_6O_5$	125.0444	Gallic acid
2	15.9	305.0668	305.0667	−0.4	$C_{15}H_{14}O_7$	261.0623, 219.0682, 179.0279, 167.0371, 165.0179, 151.1024	Gallocatechin [†]
3	20.6	327.0726	327.0722	−1.4	$C_{14}H_{16}O_9$	312.0487, 234.0173, 207.0298, 206.0222, 192.0079	Bergenin

Table 1. *Cont.*

Peak no.	RT (min)	Observed [M − H]⁻	Calculated [M − H]⁻	Error (ppm)	Molecular Formula	Fragment Ions (*m/z*)	Identified Compound
4	21.4	305.0668	305.0667	−0.4	$C_{15}H_{14}O_7$	287.059, 261.076, 219.0694, 221.0473, 179.0362, 167.0387, 165.0199	Epigallocatechin [†]
5	24.5	183.0304	183.0299	−2.7	$C_8H_8O_5$	169.0107	Methyl gallate [†]
6	26.3	913.1455	913.1469	1.6	$C_{44}H_{34}O_{22}$	761.1369, 743.1264, 609.1287, 591.1153, 573.1038, 447.0733, 423.0709, 285.0410, 169.0143	Theasinensin A (isomer 1) [†]
7	27.0	913.1471	913.1469	−0.2	$C_{44}H_{34}O_{22}$	761.131, 743.1255, 609.1205, 591.1148, 573.1104, 447.0721, 423.0752, 285.0422, 169.0178	Theasinensin A (isomer 2) [†]
8	28.5	285.0399	285.0405	2.1	$C_{15}H_{10}O_6$	243.0291, 217.0528, 199.0420, 175.047	Kaempferol
9	28.8	289.0721	289.0718	−1.0	$C_{15}H_{14}O_6$	221.0795, 203.0724, 175.0323	Epicatechin
10	29.8	457.0784	457.0776	−1.6	$C_{22}H_{18}O_{11}$	305.0660, 261.0803, 219.0637, 169.0142	Epigallocatechin-3-*O*-gallate [†]
11	31.0	911.1315	911.1312	−0.2	$C_{44}H_{32}O_{22}$	759.1258, 741.1135, 589.1027, 571.0861, 441.0556, 423.0727, 305.0618, 301.0453, 285.0431, 169.0135	Theasinensin A quinone [†]
12	32.2	897.1515	897.1520	0.5	$C_{44}H_{34}O_{21}$	745.1526, 727.1485, 575.1195, 557.1, 449.0938, 423.0693, 287.0576, 269.0482, 169.0127	Theasinensin F [†]
13	33.7	177.0191	177.0193	1.2	$C_9H_6O_4$	148.9428, 132.9003, 105.9031	Esculetin [†]
14	36.4	463.0886	463.0882	−0.8	$C_{21}H_{20}O_{12}$	317.029, 316.0226, 287.0199, 271.0247, 179.0012, 135.8248	Myricetin 3-*O*-rhamnoside (myricitrin)
15	36.9	300.9989	300.9990	0.2	$C_{14}H_6O_8$	283.9927, 245.0151, 229.0091, 201.0309, 200.0171, 173.0194	Ellagic acid [†]
16	38.3	441.0831	441.0827	−0.9	$C_{22}H_{18}O_{10}$	289.0701, 271.06, 245.9752, 169.0132	Catechin gallate (isomer) [†]
17	41.2	451.1254	451.1246	−1.7	$C_{21}H_{24}O_{11}$	289.0724, 271.1548, 167.0353	3-Hydroxyphloridzin [†]
18	41.7	447.0931	447.0933	0.4	$C_{21}H_{20}O_{11}$	301.0325, 300.0271, 255.0296, 179.0009	Quercetin 3-*O*-rhamnoside (Quercitrin)
19	43.2	417.0833	417.0827	−0.6	$C_{20}H_{18}O_{10}$	284.0316, 257.0446, 255.0304, 227.0339	Kaempferol 3-*O*-arabinoside [†]
20	45.0	615.1001	615.0992	−1.5	$C_{28}H_{24}O_{16}$	463.0903, 317.0319, 297.0616, 178.9989, 169.0188	Myricetin-*O*-(*O*-galloyl)-3-rhamnopyranoside (isomer 1) [†]
21	46.0	435.1299	435.1297	−0.5	$C_{21}H_{24}O_{10}$	273.0758, 167.0349	Phloridzin
22	46.5	615.0988	615.0992	0.6	$C_{28}H_{24}O_{16}$	463.0817, 317.0332, 297.0677, 178.9976, 169.011	Myricetin-*O*-(*O*-galloyl)-3-rhamnopyranoside (isomer 2) [†]
23	46.8	315.0146	315.0146	0.1	$C_{15}H_8O_8$	299.9902, 270.9912, 243.9987, 151.0037	Methyl-*O*-ellagic acid [†]
24	50.4	599.1048	599.1042	−1.0	$C_{28}H_{24}O_{15}$	447.0893, 301.0369, 169.0125, 151.8637	Quercitrin 2″-*O*-gallate [†]
25	51.4	595.2031	595.2032	0.2	$C_{28}H_{36}O_{14}$	433.1347, 329.1078, 308.2508, 287.0929, 167.0376	4′,6′-Dihydroxy-4-methoxy dihydrochalcone 2′-*O*-rutinoside [†]

Table 1. *Cont.*

Peak no.	RT (min)	Observed [M − H]⁻	Calculated [M − H]⁻	Error (ppm)	Molecular Formula	Fragment Ions (*m/z*)	Identified Compound
26	52.1	581.1889	581.1876	−0.5	$C_{27}H_{34}O_{14}$	419.1210, 329.102, 311.0951, 293.0907, 287.0926, 273.0953, 243.1026, 167.0355	4′,6′-Dihydroxy-4-methoxy dihydrochalcone 2′-*O*-glucosylpentoside [†]
27	53.6	449.1452	449.1453	0.4	$C_{22}H_{26}O_{10}$	329.1080, 287.0921, 273.0744, 272.0683, 243.1032, 181.017, 167.0298, 166.0275, 151.0067	4′,6′-Dihydroxy-4-methoxy dihydrochalcone 2′-*O*-β-D-glucopyranoside [†]
28	54.5	327.2171	327.2177	1.8	$C_{18}H_{32}O_5$	309.2164, 298.9867, 291.1998, 239.1283, 229.1447, 211.1327, 183.0131, 171.103	9,12,13-Trihydroxy octadecadienoic acid [†]
29	55.0	601.1595	601.1563	−5.3	$C_{29}H_{30}O_{14}$	439.0901, 329.1098, 313.0559, 287.0914, 271.0502, 243.1106, 211.0199, 169.0167	4′,6′-Dihydroxy-4-methoxy dihydrochalcone 2′-*O*-(3″-*O*-galloyl)-β-D-glucopyranoside [†]
30	57.7	221.1186	221.1183	−1.4	$C_{13}H_{18}O_3$	149.0978	Dehydrovomifoliol [†]
31	58.6	287.0926	287.0925	−0.2	$C_{16}H_{16}O_5$	243.1034, 167.037, 151.0043	2′,4′,6′-Trihydroxy-4-methoxy dihydrochalcone (3-Methylphloretin) [†]

[†] Compounds identified for the first time in the genus *Leea*.

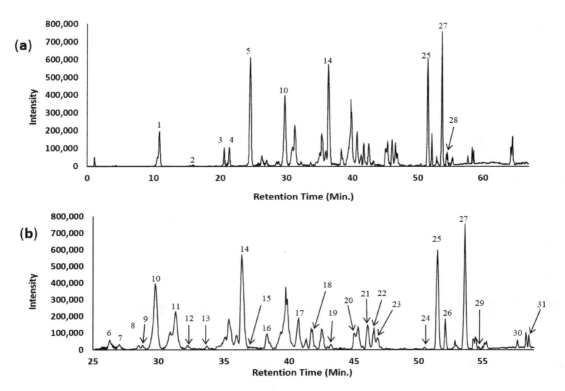

Figure 1. (a) Base peak chromatogram (BPC) of *L. indica* ethyl acetate fraction by HPLC-ESI-MS in negative ionization mode; (b) Expanded BPC. Peak labeling represents the compounds identified.

The structural identification of three new dihydrochalcones **25**, **26** and **29** was based on the relevance of the LC-MS/MS fragmentation patterns with the isolated compound 4′,6′-dihydroxy-4-methoxy dihydrochalcone 2′-*O*-β-D-glucopyranoside **27**. The MS/MS spectra of compounds **25**, **26**, **27** and **29**, showed a common base ion peak at *m/z* 287 for 2′,4′,6′-trihydroxy-4-methoxydihydrochalcone, which is a characteristic ion formed by the loss of glycoside(s) and/or galloyl glycoside moieties.

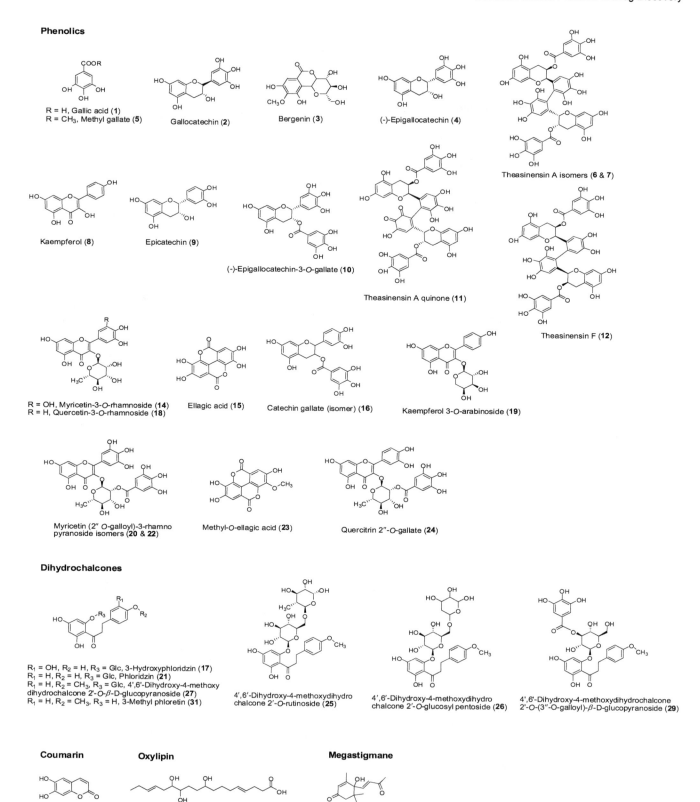

Figure 2. Structures of compounds identified in *L. indica* according to their chemical classes.

In LC-MS spectra, peaks **25**, **26** and **29** eluted at retention times (RT) 51.4, 52.1 and 55.0 min, and showed precursor ions $[M - H]^-$ at m/z 595.2031, 581.1889 and 601.1595, respectively. Peaks **25** (m/z 595) and **26** (m/z 581) showed a mass difference of 146 Da (rhamnose) and 132 Da (arabinose/xylose) respectively compared to the isolated dihydrochalcone **27** (m/z 449).

Also, peak **26** (m/z 581) was found to be 14 Da lighter than peak **25** (m/z 595), indicating the presence of a pentose sugar. In agreement with mass analysis data, peaks **25** and **26** were tentatively characterized as 4′,6′-dihydroxy-4-methoxydihydrochalcone 2′-O-rutinoside (m/z 595) and 4′,6′-dihydroxy-4-methoxydihydrochalcone 2′-O-glucosylpentoside (m/z 581) respectively.

Peak **25** displayed a molecular ion [M − H]$^-$ at m/z 595.2031 ($C_{28}H_{36}O_{14}$) and fragment ions at m/z 433, 329 and 287 (Scheme 1 and Figure S1). In the MS/MS spectrum, a characteristic fragment ion at m/z 287 as base peak suggested that this compound corresponded to a 2′,4′,6′-trihydroxy-4-methoxydihydrochalcone linked to a rutinose moiety, where the neutral loss of 308 Da is characteristic of the loss of a rutinose moiety [21]. The fragments at m/z 433 [M − $C_{10}H_{10}O_2$ − H]$^-$ and 329 [M − $C_{10}H_{18}O_8$ − H]$^-$ were obtained by the cleavage of the C-C bond of chalcone and sugar moiety respectively (Scheme 1). The fragment ion at m/z 329 [M − H − $C_9H_{13}O_7$ − H_2O − CH_3]$^-$ was obtained by the cleavage of a glucose moiety, with the loss of a water molecule and further by losing a methyl group. Based on these deductions, peak **25** was tentatively identified as 4′,6′-dihydroxy-4-methoxydihydrochalcone 2′-O-rutinoside, a new dihydrochalcone.

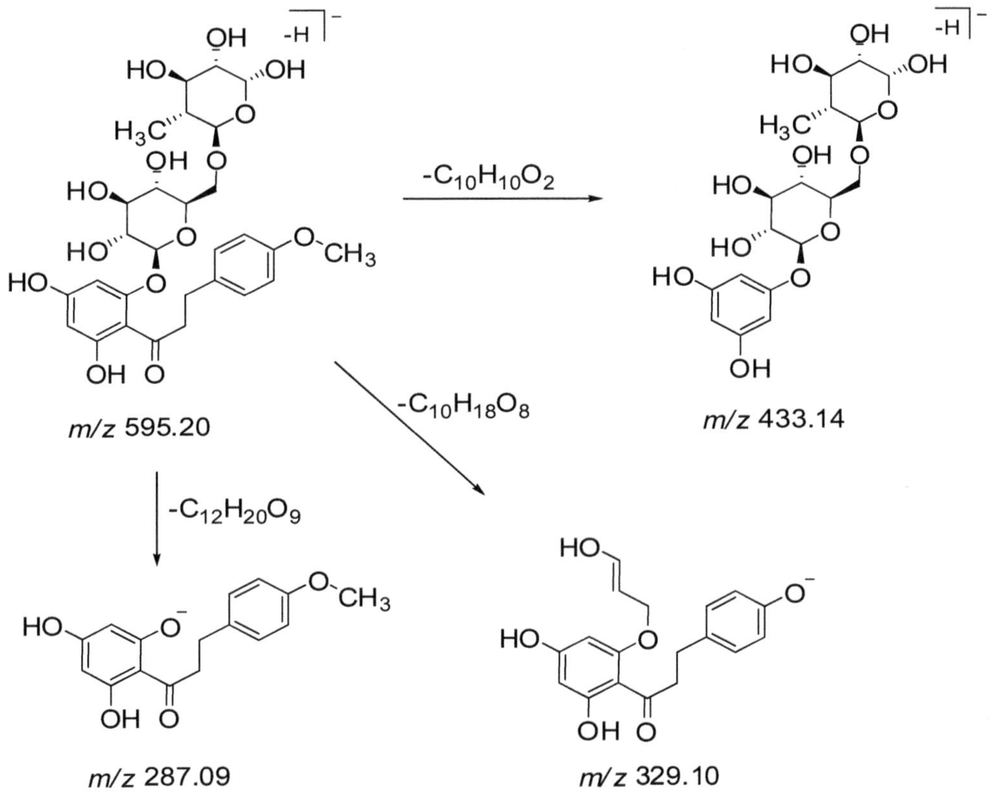

Scheme 1. Proposed MS/MS fragmentation of compound **25**.

Peak **26** exhibited a precursor ion [M − H]$^-$ at m/z 581.1889 ($C_{27}H_{34}O_{14}$) and fragment ions at m/z 419, 311, 293, and 243 (Scheme 2 and Figure S2). The MS/MS spectrum showed product ion at m/z 287 ($C_{16}H_{16}O_5$) [M − H − 162 Da − 132 Da]$^-$ as base peak by the loss of a glucosylpentoside moiety, suggesting to possess a basic skeleton of isolated dihydrochalcone **27**. The cleavage of a C-C bond gave a fragment ion at m/z 419 due to the loss of a $C_{10}H_{10}O_2$ moiety. The neutral loss of 312 Da showed the presence of a glucosyl pentoside moiety, losing a molecule of water to generate a product ion at m/z 293 (Scheme 3). Therefore, compound **26** was plausibly identified as 4′,6′-dihydroxy-4-methoxydihydrochalcone 2′-O-glucosylpentoside and found as first occurrence in nature.

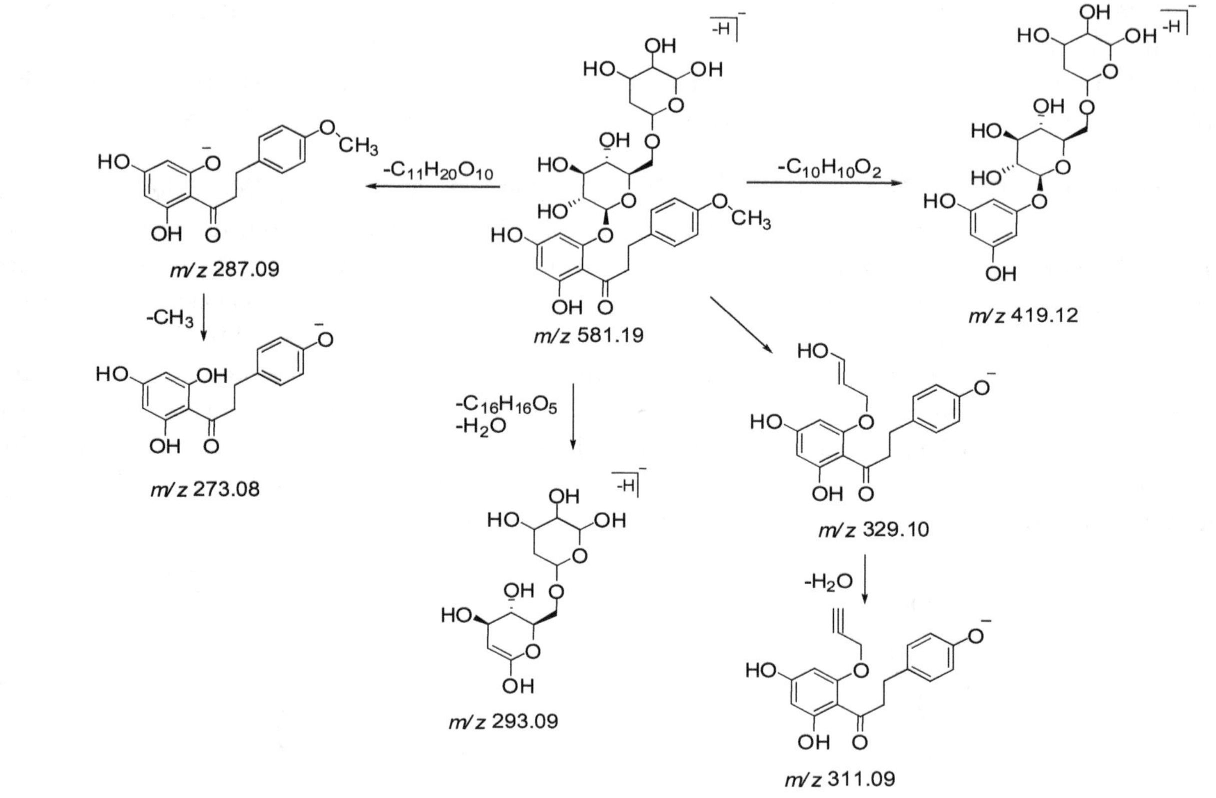

Scheme 2. Proposed MS/MS fragmentation of compound **26**.

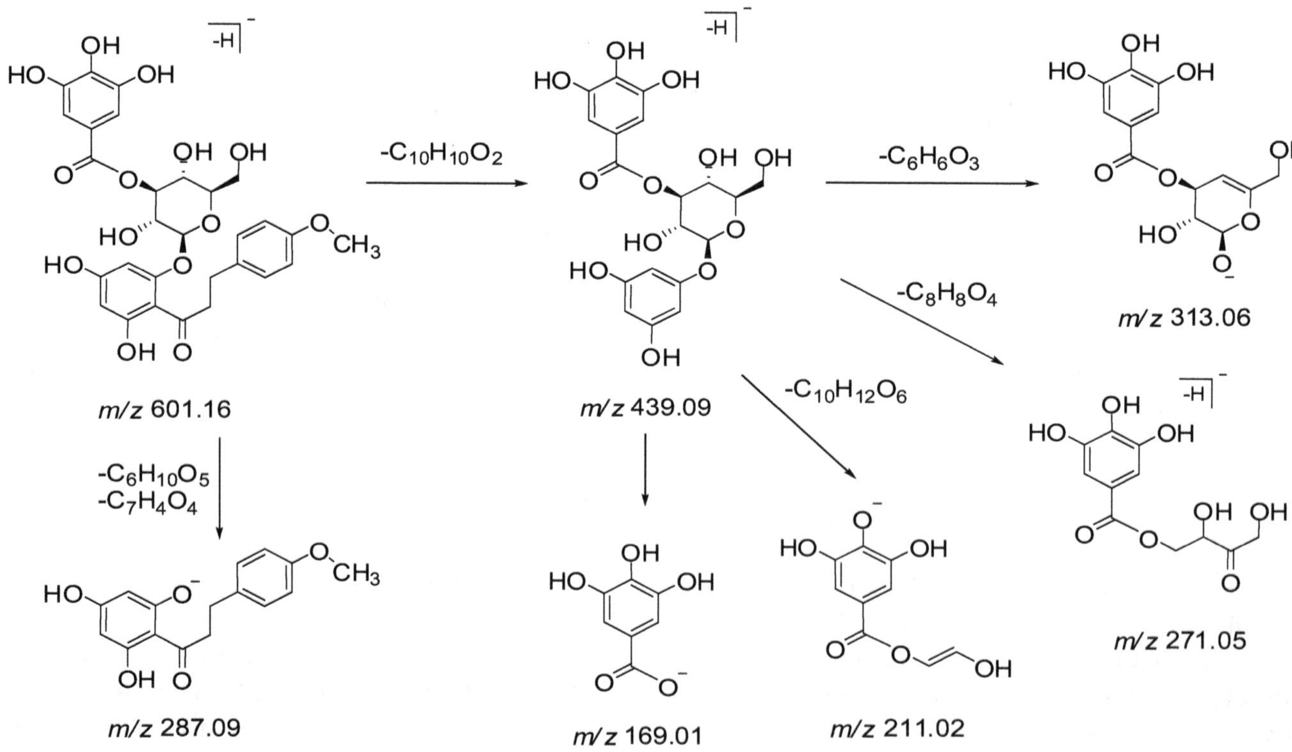

Scheme 3. Proposed MS/MS fragmentation of compound **29**.

Peak **29** showed a precursor ion $[M - H]^-$ at m/z 601.1595 ($C_{29}H_{30}O_{14}$) and fragment ions at m/z 439, 313, 287, 271, 211, and 169 in the MS/MS spectrum. A base ion peak at m/z 287 $[M - C_6H_{10}O_5 - C_7H_4O_4 - H]^-$ was observed due to the loss of glucose (162 Da) and galloyl (153 Da) moieties. Fragment ions at m/z 169 and m/z 313 indicate the presence of a galloyl and a galloylglucose moiety respectively. Monogalloylglucose can exist as five possible isomers namely, 1-O-galloylglucose, 2-O-galloylglucose, 3-O-galloylglucose, 4-O-galloylglucose, and 6-O-galloylglucose [22]. The characteristic fragment ions at m/z 271 and 211 suggest that the substitution of the galloyl group could be at the C-3 position of the glucose moiety (Scheme 3 and Figure S3). Product ion detected at m/z 439 suggested the cleavage of the C-C bond (loss of $C_{10}H_{10}O_2$ moiety) in the MS/MS spectrum. Thus, the compound corresponding to peak **29** was tentatively identified as a new dihydrochalcone 4′,6′-dihydroxy-4-methoxydihydrochalcone 2′-O-(3″-O-galloyl)-β-D-glucopyranoside. It is also a gallic acid derivative of the isolated dihydrochalcone **27**.

The isolated dihydrochalcone **27** exhibited a precursor ion [M − H]$^-$ at m/z 449.1452 ($C_{22}H_{26}O_{10}$). The MS/MS spectrum showed product ions at m/z 287 [M − $C_6H_{10}O_5$ −H]$^-$ and 273 [M − $C_6H_{10}O_5$ − CH_3 − H]$^-$ due to the loss of glucose (162 Da) and methyl groups (15 Da) (Figure S4). Compound **27** was isolated and identified as 4′,6′-dihydroxy-4-methoxydihydrochalcone 2′-O-β-D-glucopyranoside.

The LC-MS fragmentation patterns of the three novel dihydrochalcones (**25**, **26** and **29**) were compared to the isolated dihydrochalcone (**27**), and we noted that the observed HR-MS data were in good agreement with the calculated masses. Further isolation of the peaks **25**, **26** and **29** and spectroscopic analyses would be required to unambiguously confirm the proposed structures of these dihydrochalcones.

3. Materials and Methods

3.1. Plant Materials

Fresh ground leaves of *L. indica* were collected in Singapore. A voucher specimen (no. LI-0109) was deposited at the herbarium of the National University of Singapore (NUS) Medicinal Plant Research Group.

3.2. Chemicals and Reagents

Standards gallic acid, methyl gallate, myricitrin, quercitrin, epigallocatechin-3-O-gallate, ellagic acid, epicatechin, and kaempferol were purchased from Sigma-Aldrich (St. Louis, MO, USA). Phloridzin and epigallocatechin were purchased from TCI Co. Ltd. (Tokyo, Japan). LC-MS grade solvents (acetonitrile, methanol and formic acid) were purchased from MERCK (Darmstadt, Germany) and water used in LC analysis was obtained using Milli-Q advanced system (Millipore, Milford, MA, USA).

3.3. Extraction and Isolation

The fresh ground leaves of *L. indica* (2.8 kg) were macerated with 70% v/v MeOH at room temperature. The extract was filtered and concentrated under vacuum, yielding a crude methanolic extract. The dried methanolic extract was dissolved in water and partitioned with different solvents, concentrated under vacuum to give hexane (0.005%), dichloromethane (0.027%) and ethyl acetate (1.32%) fractions.

The ethyl acetate fraction (37.0 g) was chromatographed over silica gel using 25% EtOAc–hexane as eluent, yielding a white solid, which was recrystallized in $CHCl_3$-MeOH as white needles of methyl gallate (60 mg). Fractions obtained from repeated silica gel column chromatography of EtOAc fraction using 6–10% MeOH-$CHCl_3$ as eluent were further purified by Sephadex (LH-20) and reversed phase cartridge yielding two compounds gallic acid (140 mg) and 4′,6′-dihydroxy-4-methoxydihydrochalcone 2′-O-β-D-glucopyranoside (12 mg). The estimated concentration of gallic acid in the fresh leaves was 0.005–0.011% w/w. Pooled fractions obtained from silica gel column chromatography of the EtOAc fraction using 10–20% MeOH-$CHCl_3$ were further subjected to Sephadex (LH-20) column chromatography. At an eluent concentration of 50% MeOH-water, a mixture of two compounds was obtained. It was further purified by silica gel column chromatography eluting with 8% MeOH-$CHCl_3$

and 10–12% MeOH-CHCl₃ to yield quercetin-3-*O*-rhamnoside (5 mg) and myricetin-3-*O*-rhamnoside (650 mg) respectively. Epigallocatechin-3-*O*-gallate (64 mg) was obtained from the silica gel column chromatography using 2–5% methanol in dichloromethane. The structures of isolated compounds **1, 5, 10, 14, 18,** and **27** were confirmed by NMR and LC-MS analyses.

3.4. General Information

NMR spectra were recorded on a Bruker Avance-400 Spectrometer (Fallanden, Switzerland), ^{1}H at 400 MHz and ^{13}C at 100 MHz in deuterated solvents using tetramethylsilane (TMS) as an internal reference. Deuterated solvents, methanol-d_4 and dimethyl sulfoxide-d_6 for NMR were purchased from Sigma-Aldrich (USA).

Silica-gel (60–120, 100–200, 70–230 mesh; Merck, Germany), Sephadex LH-20 (Sigma, Uppsala, Sweden) and reversed phase C18 (77.9 µm) cartridge column from Waters (Ireland) were used for chromatographic separation. Thin layer chromatography was performed on pre-coated Si-gel 60 F₂₅₄ plates (Merck, Germany) using a visualizing reagent.

The LC-MS analysis was carried out using a Dionex Ultimate 3000 VWD system coupled with a VWD and a micro-TOF-Q mass detector (Bruker Daltonics Inc., Billerica, MA, USA). Chromatographic separation was performed on an RP-C₁₈ column (3.0 × 150 mm; particle size 2.7 µM; Agilent Poroshell 120, New Castle, DE, USA), operated at 25 °C. Analysis was carried out using a gradient elution program of 0.1% formic acid in water (A) and 0.1% formic acid in acetonitrile (B) as a mobile phase at a flow rate of 0.5 mL/min. The following gradient system was used: 0–45 min, 5–30% B; 45–60 min 30–100% B and 60–65 min 100% B. UV detection was performed by scanning the samples at 210, 254, 280, and 360 nm. Electrospray ionization mass spectra (ESI-MS) were recorded in negative ionization mode. The mass range of m/z 50–2000 was scanned. For MS/MS analysis, collision energies were set automatically.

4. Conclusions

This study presents the comprehensive identification of chemical constituents of an ethyl acetate fraction of *L. indica* leaves using HPLC-ESI-microTOF-Q-MS/MS analysis. Here we identified 31 compounds, among them six phenolic compounds were isolated by column chromatography. Three novel dihydrochalcones derivatives were tentatively identified as 4',6'-dihydroxy-4-methoxydihydrochalcone 2'-*O*-rutinoside, 4',6'-dihydroxy-4-methoxydihydro chalcone 2'-*O*-glucosylpentoside and 4',6'-dihydroxy-4-methoxydihydrochalcone 2'-*O*-(3''-*O*-galloyl)-β-D-glucopyranoside. A total of 24 compounds are reported for the first time in the genus *Leea*. Our results indicated that *L. indica* is a good source of diverse phenolic contents including phenolic acids (gallic acid and methyl gallate), polyphenolic (ellagic acid), flavan-3-ols (gallocatechin, epigallocatechin and epigallocatechin-3-*O*-gallate), flavonoids/flavonoid glycosides (kaempferol, quercitrin, myricitrin), dihydrochalcones (phloridzin and its derivatives), and dimeric catechins (theasinensin A dimers and theasinensin F). The wide range of potential bioactive compounds supports the diverse pharmacological activities of *L. indica*. Further research to identify and develop useful therapeutics and health supplements from *L. indica* is warranted.

Author Contributions: D.S.: isolation and identification of compounds, data analysis, preparation and correction of manuscript; Y.-Y.S., T.-I.C.: extraction of plant materials, isolation and identification of compounds; H.-C.Y., S.S.-W.H., C.S.E.-S.L. and W.-X.T.: extraction of plant materials; S.-Y.N.: correction of manuscript; H.-L.K.: conception of study and correction of manuscript.

Acknowledgments: The authors are grateful to Steven Yuan Cheng Hui, Dept. of Chemistry, NUS for technical support and Kim-Chuan Ng of the Nanyang Technological University Community Herb Garden, Singapore for his kind support.

References

1. Ridsdale, C.E. Leeaceae. In *Flora Malesiana, Series I—Spermatophyta Flowering Plants*; Noordhoff International Publishing: Leiden, The Netherlands, 1976; Volume 7, pp. 755–782.

2. The Angiosperm Phylogeny Group. An update of the Angiosperm Phylogeny Group classification for the orders and families plants: APG III. *Bot. J. Linn. Soc.* **2009**, *161*, 105–121. [CrossRef]

3. Siew, Y.Y.; Yew, H.C.; Neo, S.Y.; Seow, S.V.; Lew, S.M.; Lim, S.W.; Lim, C.S.E.S.; Ng, Y.C.; Seetoh, W.G.; Ali, A.; et al. Evaluation of anti-proliferative activity of medicinal plants used in Asian Traditional Medicine to treat cancer. *J. Ethnopharmacol.* **2019**, *235*, 75–87. [CrossRef] [PubMed]

4. Bourdy, G.; Walter, A. Maternity and medicinal plants in Vanuatu I. The cycle of reproduction. *J. Ethnopharmacol.* **1992**, *37*, 179–196. [CrossRef]

5. Singh, D.; Siew, Y.Y.; Yew, H.C.; Neo, S.Y.; Koh, H.L. Botany, phytochemistry and pharmacological activities of *Leea* species. In *Medicinal Plants: Chemistry, Pharmacology, and Therapeutic Applications*; Swamy, M.K., Patra, J.K., Rudramurthy, G.R., Eds.; CRC Press Taylor & Francis Group: Boca Raton, FL, USA, 2019; in press.

6. Wiart, C.; Mogana, S.; Khalifah, S.; Mahan, M.; Ismail, S.; Buckle, M.; Narayana, A.K.; Sulaiman, M. Antimicrobial screening of plants used for traditional medicine in the state of Perak, Peninsular Malaysia. *Fitoterapia* **2004**, *75*, 68–73. [CrossRef] [PubMed]

7. Raihan, M.O.; Habib, M.R.; Brishti, A.; Rahman, M.M.; Saleheen, M.M.; Manna, M. Sedative and anxiolytic effects of the methanolic extract of *Leea indica* (Burm. f.) Merr. Leaf. *Drug Discov. Ther.* **2011**, *5*, 185–189. [CrossRef] [PubMed]

8. Wong, Y.H.; Kadir, H.A. *Leea indica* ethyl acetate fraction induces growth-inhibitory effect in various cancer cell lines and apoptosis in Ca Ski human cervical epidermoid carcinoma cells. *Evid. Based Complement Alternat. Med.* **2011**. Available online: http://dx.doi.org/10.1155/2011/293060 (accessed on 18 January 2019).

9. Reddy, N.S.; Navanesan, S.; Sinniah, S.K.; Wahab, N.A.; Sim, K.S. Phenolic content, antioxidant effect and cytotoxic activity of *Leea indica* leaves. *BMC Complement Altern. Med.* **2012**, *12*, 128. Available online: http://dx.doi.org./10.1186/1472-6882-12-128 (accessed on 18 January 2019). [CrossRef] [PubMed]

10. Rahman, M.A.; Imran, T.B.; Islam, S. Antioxidative, antimicrobial and cytotoxic effects of the phenolics of *Leea indica* leaf extract. *Saudi J. Biol. Sci.* **2013**, *20*, 213–225. [CrossRef] [PubMed]

11. Avin, B.R.V.; Thirusangu, P.; Ramesh, C.K.; Vigneswarana, V.; Kumar, M.V.P.; Mahmood, R.; Prabhakar, B.T. Screening for the modulation of neovessel formation in non-tumorigenic and tumorigenic conditions using three different plants native to Western ghats of India. *Biomed. Aging Pathol.* **2014**, *4*, 343–348. [CrossRef]

12. Mishra, G.; Khosa, R.L.; Singh, P.; Jha, K.K. Hepatoprotective activity of ethanolic extract of *Leea indica* (Burm. f.) Merr. (Leeaceae) stem bark against paracetamol induced liver toxicity in rats. *Niger. J. Exp. Clin. Biosci.* **2014**, *2*, 59–63. [CrossRef]

13. Saha, K.; Shaari, K.; Lajis, N.H. Phytochemical study on *Leea indica* (Burm. F.) Merr. (Leeaceae). *J. Bangladesh Chem. Soc.* **2007**, *20*, 139–147.

14. Srinivasan, G.V.; Ranjith, C.; Vijayan, K.K. Identification of chemical compounds from the leaves of *Leea indica*. *Acta Pharm.* **2008**, *58*, 207–214. [CrossRef] [PubMed]

15. Wong, Y.H.; Kadir, H.A.; Ling, S.K. Bioassay-guided isolation of cytotoxic cycloartane triterpenoid glycosides from the traditionally used medicinal plant *Leea indica*. *Evid. Based Complement Alternat. Med.* **2012**. Available online: http://dx.doi.org/10.1155/2012/164689 (accessed on 18 January 2019).

16. Liu, J.X.; Di, D.L.; Shi, Y.P. Diversity of chemical constituents from *Saxifraga montana* H. *J. Chinese Chem. Soc.* **2008**, *55*, 863–870. [CrossRef]

17. Ekaprasada, M.T.; Nurdin, H.; Ibrahim, S.; Dachriyanus, H. Antioxidant activity of methyl gallate isolated from the leaves of *Toona sureni*. *Indones. J. Chem.* **2009**, *9*, 457–460. [CrossRef]

18. Zhong, Y.; Shahidi, F. Lipophilized epigallocatechin gallate (EGCG) derivatives as novel antioxidants. *J. Agric. Food Chem.* **2011**, *59*, 6526–6533. [CrossRef]

19.   Aderogba, M.A.; Ndhlala, A.R.; Rengasamy, K.R.R. Antimicrobial and selected in vitro enzyme inhibitory effects of leaf extracts, flavonols and indole alkaloids isolated from *Croton menyharthii*. *Molecules* **2013**, *18*, 12633–12644. [CrossRef]

20.   Silva, D.H.S.; Yoshida, M.; Kato, M.J. Flavonoids from *Iryanthera sagotiana*. *Phytochemistry* **1997**, *46*, 579–582. [CrossRef]

21.   Zhang, M.; Duan, C.; Zang, Y.; Huang, Z.; Liu, G. The flavonoid composition of flavedo and juice from the pummel cultivar (*Citrus grandis* (L.) Osbeck) and the grapefruit cultivar (*Citrus paradise*). *Food Chem.* **2011**, *129*, 1530–1536. [CrossRef]

22.   Fathoni, A.; Saepudin, A.; Cahyanal, H.; Rahayu, D.U.C.; Haib, J. Identification of nonvolatile compounds in clove (*Syzygium aromaticum*) from Manado. *AIP Conf. Proc.* **2017**, *1862*. [CrossRef]

6

Squalene Found in Alpine Grassland Soils under a Harsh Environment in the Tibetan Plateau, China

Xuyang Lu [1,2], Shuqin Ma [3,*], Youchao Chen [4], Degyi Yangzom [5] and Hongmao Jiang [1,6]

[1] Institute of Mountain Hazards and Environment, Chinese Academy of Sciences, Chengdu 610041, China; xylu@imde.ac.cn (X.L.); jianghongmao@163.com (H.J.)
[2] Key Laboratory of Mountain Surface Processes and Ecological Regulation, Chinese Academy of Sciences, Chengdu 610041, China
[3] College of Tourism, Henan Normal University, Xinxiang 453007, China
[4] Wuhan Botanical Garden, Chinese Academy of Sciences, Wuhan 430074, China; chenyouchao@wbgcas.cn
[5] Ecological Monitoring & Research Center, Tibetan Environment Monitoring Station, Lhasa 850000, China; dejiyangzong09@126.com
[6] University of Chinese Academy of Sciences, Beijing 100049, China
* Correspondence: mashuqin@htu.edu.cn;

Abstract: Squalene is found in a large number of plants, animals, and microorganisms, as well as other sources, playing an important role as an intermediate in sterol biosynthesis. It is used widely in the food, cosmetics, and medicine industries because of its antioxidant, antistatic, and anti-carcinogenic properties. A higher natural squalene component of lipids is usually reported as being isolated to organisms living in harsh environments. In the Tibetan Plateau, which is characterized by high altitude, strong solar radiation, drought, low temperatures, and thin air, the squalene component was identified in five alpine grasslands soils using the pyrolysis gas chromatography–mass spectrometry (Py-GC/MS) technique. The relative abundance of squalene ranged from 0.93% to 10.66% in soils from the five alpine grasslands, with the highest value found in alpine desert and the lowest in alpine meadow. Furthermore, the relative abundance of squalene in alpine grassland soils was significantly negatively associated with soil chemical/microbial characteristics. These results indicate that the extreme environmental conditions of the Tibetan Plateau may stimulate the microbial biosynthesis of squalene, and the harsher the environment, the higher the relative abundance of soil squalene.

Keywords: squalene; alpine grassland; Py-GC/MS; soil microorganism; Tibetan Plateau

1. Introduction

Squalene is named after the shark family Squalidae, and is a triterpene with the formula $C_{30}H_{50}$. It is an intermediate in the biosynthesis of sterols and hopanoids in the plant, animal, human, and microorganism worlds [1,2]. From the moment life appeared on Earth, squalene appeared in microorganisms. The cell membranes of higher organisms from the Precambrian contained great proportions of squalene, which was an essential substance for their survival in the hostile oxygen-free environment [2]. Squalene and its related compounds such as oxidosqualene and bis-oxidosqualene are precursors of thousands of bioactive triterpenoids and are also a carbon source which can be utilized by some microorganisms [3].

Squalene itself has several beneficial properties and values. For instance, it is a hydrophilic natural antioxidant which serves in health-promoting functions including skin hydration and tumor-suppression. It has cardio-protective, antibacterial/antifungal, immunity-boosting, and cholesterol-lowering effects. It can also be used as a drug delivery agent, and has been used as a feasible source of biofuels [4,5]. Thus, squalene has recently attracted a great deal of attention due to its industrial value as a lubricant, health-promoting agent, and/or as a form of biofuel.

The richest known source of squalene in the living world is the liver of certain species of fish, especially sharks living in the deep sea [1,6]. As the main organ for lipid storage, as an energy source, and for adjusting buoyancy, the liver of sharks comprises 50–80% unsaponifiable matter, with the great majority thereof being squalene. For example, *Centrophorus artomarginatus* deep-sea sharks can survive in waters with a depth of 600–1000 m, where with the environmental characteristics include lack of sunlight, consistently high pressure, and very poor oxygen supply. This survival is due to squalene from their liver, which accounts for 25–30% of their total body weight [2,7].

Squalene was also identified in many plant oils over broad ranges. The first vegetable oil in which it was found was olive oil, with a concentration of 5.64–5.99 g kg^{-1}. In other vegetable oils, it is also quite prominent in soybean, grape seed, hazelnuts, peanuts, corn, pumpkin, rice bran, amaranth, and camellia oils [2,8]. Human serum also contains 10–13% squalene as one of its major constituents [3,9]. In addition, microbial squalene production has become a promising alternative in recent years due to the advantages of fast and massive growth, although microorganisms do not accumulate as much squalene as plants or shark livers [10–12].

The Tibetan Plateau, as the roof of the world, is considered to be the third "pole" of the world. The plateau is peculiarly cold due to its latitude, and is colder than anywhere else outside the polar regions. It has an average elevation of 4 km above sea level, and possesses one of the largest ice masses on Earth [13–15]. The plants, animals, and microorganisms living in the Tibetan Plateau endure extreme circumstances, characterized by high altitude, strong solar radiation, drought, low temperatures, thin air, and so on [16–18]. Low temperature and low oxygen pose key physiological challenges for those living in these harsh conditions on the plateau, a situation which is to some extent similar to that of sharks living within a deep-sea environment.

Squalene has been identified from some Tibetan plant components, including the lipophilic extracts from flowers (0.29–0.77%) and leaves (0.56–1.16%) of *Lamiophlomis rotate*, and the volatile oil from roots (1.73%) of *Rhodiola crenulata* [19,20]. The Tibetan yak can thrive well at altitudes of 2000–5000 m above sea level, and provides meat, milk, and other necessities for the local people. The highest squalene content in lipids was reported to exist in the longissimus muscle (20.99 mg/100 g), the biceps femoris muscle (59.82 mg/100 g), the liver (6.94 mg/100 g), the subcutaneous adipose tissue (7.06 mg/100 g), and the abdominal adipose tissue (7.06 mg/100 g) of the Tibetan yak [21]. Therefore, the chemical component of squalene has been found in some plants and animals on the Tibetan Plateau. Could this component also be identified from some microorganisms which likewise live in high-altitude, low-temperature, low-oxygen alpine conditions? As a variety of microorganisms were found to distributed in alpine soils of the Tibetan Plateau [22–24], in the present study alpine soils from five types of alpine grassland were analyzed by using pyrolysis gas chromatography–mass spectrometry (Py-GC/MS) to identify the squalene component. The aim of this study was to compare squalene content among different alpine grassland soils and further to explore the relationships between the squalene content and the soil environmental factors in the harsh conditions on the Tibetan Plateau.

2. Materials and Methods

2.1. Study Area

Tibet covers a total area of more than 1.2 million km^2 and represents is approximately one-eighth of the total area of China, with an average altitude higher than 4000 m. It regulates climate change and water resources in China and eastern Asia due to its geomorphological uniqueness in the world [25,26]. Because of its extensive territory and highly dissected topography, this region has a diverse range of climate and vegetation zones. Solar radiation is strong, with annual radiation varying between 140 and 190 kcal cm^{-2}. Due to the geographical conditions and atmospheric circulation, the average annual temperature is rather low, with the temperature varying from 18 to −4 °C, decreasing gradually from the southeast to the northwest. The average annual precipitation is less than 1000 mm in most areas of Tibet; annual precipitation rates can reach up to 2817 mm in the east and drop down to approximately 70 mm in the west [27].

Alpine grasslands are the most dominant ecosystems in Tibet, covering more than 70% of the whole plateau's area. It ranks first among all Chinese provinces and autonomous regions in the diversity of its grassland ecosystems, comprising 17 types of grassland based on the classification system used for the whole country [28,29]. Among all grassland types, alpine meadow (AM) is composed of perennial mesic and mesoxeric herbs under cold and wet climate conditions, occupying approximately 31.3% of the total grassland area of Tibet. Alpine steppe (AS) is composed of drought-tolerant perennial herbs or small shrubs under cold and arid/semiarid climate conditions, representing approximately 38.9% of the total Tibetan grassland area. Alpine desert (AD) is a grassland type developed and controlled by cold and extreme drought conditions, covering 6.71% of the total grassland area. Alpine meadow steppe (AMS) is a transitional type of alpine grassland from the meadow to the steppe, and alpine desert steppe (ADS) is a transitional type of alpine grassland from the steppe to the desert, covering 7.32% and 10.7% of the total grassland area in Tibet, respectively [27].

2.2. Soil Sampling

In this research, the study area was located at 30.75°–33.43° N, 79.75°–92.07° E, and the sampling sites were located in 10 counties from east to west in the Tibet Autonomous Region of China. Five sampling sites were selected at each of the three main natural grassland types, including AM, AS, and ADS. Three sampling sites were selected from the relatively small natural grassland area, including AMS and AD, in August 2016. At each sample site, three 1 m × 1 m quadrats were laid out at intervals of approximately 50 m. In total, 63 quadrats of alpine grassland in Tibet were sampled with 45 quadrats (15 sites × 3 quadrats) for AM, AS, and ADS and 18 quadrats (6 sites × 3 quadrats) for AMS and AD, respectively. At each quadrat, all aboveground plants and litter were removed from the soil surface before the sampling. Five soil samples were obtained for each quadrat at depths of 0–15 cm, and five soil samples were mixed as a soil sample for the soil chemical and microbial properties analysis. All soils were transported to the lab with cooler, and stored in sealed containers at 4 °C before the measurement. For the determination of soil bulk density, soil cores (5.4 cm in diameter) were also taken from each layer using a stainless-steel cylinder. In addition, the location and elevation of each site were measured using Global Positioning System (GPS) (Garmin MAP62CSX made in Garmin Ltd., Olathe, KS, USA).

2.3. Soil Analyses

In the lab, soil samples for soil chemical and microbial properties analyses were sieved to pass through a 2-mm-mesh sieve, and roots and stones were removed by hand. Then the samples were divided into three sub-samples. One sub-sample was air-dried and the squalene component was identified by pyrolysis gas chromatography–mass spectrometry (Py-GC/MS); the second was stored at 4 °C prior to determine soil microbial phospholipid fatty acids (PLFAs); and the third was sieved through 250-μm mesh for analysis of soil pH, soil organic carbon (SOC), dissolved organic carbon (DOC), total nitrogen (TN), and total inorganic nitrogen (TIN) contents.

Py-GC/MS tests were performed in a pyrolyzer (CDS5200). For this, 25 mg of soil was placed in quartz tubes (2 cm in length, 2 mm inside diameter) and quantified using a Mettler microbalance (Mettler–Toledo, Greifensee, Switzerland). The pyrolysis chamber was full of He. The soil samples were heated from ambient to 700 °C at a rate of 20 °C/ms and kept for 15 s. The pyrolyzer was coupled with PerkinElmer Clarus680GC-SQ8MS Systems (PerkinElmer, Santa Clara, CA, USA), and the carrier gas was He. For operation, the temperature program of the capillary column (HP-5, 0.25 mm) of GC was as follows: 3 min at 40 °C, then temperature was increased to 280 °C at a rate of 10 °C/min and kept at 280 °C for 5 min. The injector temperature was 280 °C. The MS indicator was operated in the electron impact mode at electron energy of 70 eV, and the ion source temperature was kept at 250 °C. The pyrolysis products were identified using identifications of the NIST 2014 library and the report by other researchers. Pyrolysis products were quantified by using the surface of two characteristics ion fragments of each product. The relative percentage of squalene compound was calculated according to peak height above baseline. For each sample, the relative peak height of squalene compound was calculated by normalizing results to the largest peak measured in the chromatogram. The percentage of squalene compound reported herein, therefore, is the relative percentage of that compound with respect to the largest peak compounds identified, not the absolute abundance of compounds of squalene in soils.

The soil microbial community was characterized by PLFA analysis. Lipids were extracted from soils by using one-phase chloroform, methanol, and water extractant, then fractionated into neutral lipids, glycolipids, and phospholipids on a silicic acid column. The quantification of PLFAs was performed by GC chromatography (GC Agilent 6890-Agilent Technology, Santa Clara, CA, USA) using a flame ionization detector (FID), split injector, and an HP7673 auto sampler. He as a carrier gas was operated with a flow rate at 0.8 mL min^{-1} and a pressure of 35 psi. The injector and detector temperatures were 250 °C and 300 °C, respectively [30]. PLFAs were designated $X:Y\omega Z$. X: the total number of carbon atoms; Y: the number of unsaturated olefinic bond; ω: the end of methyl; Z: the location of the keys or cyclopropane chain; a (anteriso) and i (iso): branching chain; 10Me: a methyl group tenth at the end of the pitch molecule carbon atoms; and cy: a cyclopropyl group on the carbon chain [31].

The absolute abundance of PLFAs is expressed as nmol/g dry soil, and the sum of absolute abundances of PLFAs was the microbial biomass [31]. The PLFAs, which were present in <3 samples at very low concentrations, were discarded from analysis. The bacterial PLFAs were estimated as the sum of general bacteria and non-specific bacteria. PLFA biomarkers included i13:0, 14:0, i14:0, i15:0, a15:0, i15:1 G, 16:0, i16:0, 16:1 2OH, 16:1G, 16:1ω5c, 16:1ω9c, i17:0, a17:0, cy17:0, 17:1ω8c, 18:1ω5c, 18:0, and cy19:0ω8c [32–36]. Actinomycete bacteria are represented by 10Me17:0 and 10Me18:0 [37]. Fungal groups included 18:1ω9c [37].

Soil pH was measured electrochemically (Model PHS-3E Meter, Leici Instruments Co. Ltd., Shanghai, China) in H_2O at a soil: solution ratio of 1:2.5 [38]. Soil organic carbon content was detected by the potassium dichromate sulfuric acid oxidation technique [39]. Total nitrogen was detected by the Kjeldahl method [40]. Total inorganic nitrogen and dissolved organic carbon content were detected by extracting 5 g fresh-weight soil with 25 mL 0.5 mol K_2SO_4; then the soil extraction was passed through filter paper, with filtrates then analyzed by an Autosampler (SEAL XY-2 Sampler, Bran & Luebbe, Sydney, Australia) [41].

2.4. Data Analysis and Statistics

One-way ANOVA followed by Duncan's multiple comparisons was employed to test the differences in soil chemistries, including squalene relative abundance, SOC, DOC, TIN, and TN among soils collected from the AM, AS, AMS, ADS, and AD grassland types. The squalene relative abundance and soil chemical/microbial characteristics were subjected to principal component analysis (PCA), based on linear combinations of the original variables on independent orthogonal axes, while the squalene relative abundance and soil chemical/microbial traits were subjected to redundancy analysis (RDA), performed using Canoco 5 (Microcomputer Power, Ithaca, NY, USA, 2012). All statistical analyses were conducted using SPSS 20.0 (IBM, Chicago, IL, USA, 2011) with a significance level of $p < 0.05$. All figures were made by Sigmaplot® Version 10 software (Systat Software Inc., Chicago, IL, USA, 2007).

3. Results

3.1. Squalene Relative Abundance

The squalene component was identified from the soils in all five alpine grasslands, including AM, AS, AMS, ADS, and AD in the Tibetan Plateau using Py-GC/MS (Figure 1). There were significant differences in the squalene relative abundance of the soils among five alpine grassland types (Figure 2).

The relative abundance of squalene of the soils in AD was the highest, with a value of 10.66 ± 2.07%, and that of the soils in ADS was the second highest, with a value of 5.42 ± 1.38%. The squalene relative abundances of the soils in AM, AS, and AMS were significantly lower than those of the soils in AD, with values of 0.93 ± 0.22%, 3.12 ± 1.23%, 1.61 ± 0.52%, respectively.

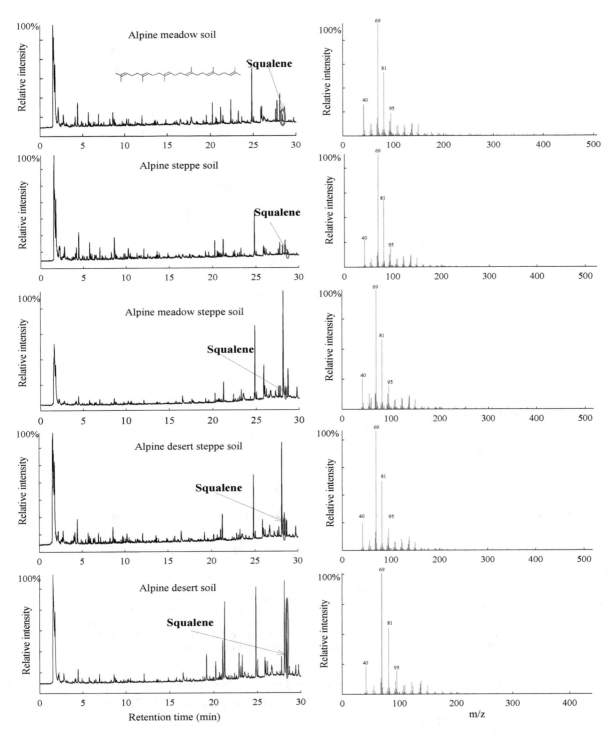

Figure 1. The squalene chromatograms (**left**) and mass spectrums (**right**) obtained from alpine grassland soils by pyrolysis gas chromatography–mass spectrometry (Py-GC/MS) in the Tibetan Plateau. m/z: mass-to-charge ratio.

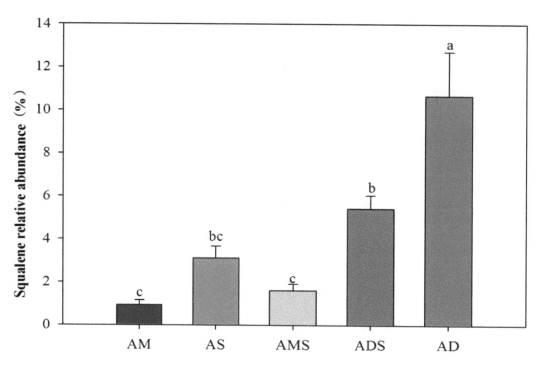

Figure 2. Squalene relative abundance in alpine grassland soils in the Tibetan Plateau. AM: alpine meadow, AS: alpine steppe, AMS: alpine meadow steppe, ADS: alpine desert steppe, AD: alpine desert.

3.2. Soil Chemical/Microbial Characteristics

Soil pH of the soils in five alpine grasslands was in the range of 7.57–9.52, with the highest value in the AMS soil and the lowest in the AS soil. Significant differences in the soil chemical characteristics were observed among the five types of alpine grassland in northern Tibet (Table 1). The SOC, DOC, TN, and TIN contents were the highest in the AM soil (34.97 ± 2.89 g kg^{-1}, 98.39 ± 27.30 mg kg^{-1}, 1.18 ± 0.24 g kg^{-1}, 39.65 ± 6.68 mg kg^{-1}, respectively); these values were 8.02, 4.63, 7.87, and 14.58 times those of the AD soil, respectively, which had the lowest indexes.

Table 1. The soil chemical characteristics of alpine grasslands in the Tibetan Plateau.

Soil Chemical Indexes	pH	SOC (g kg^{-1})	DOC (mg kg^{-1})	TN (g kg^{-1})	TIN (mg kg^{-1})
AM	8.00 ± 0.15 [c]	34.97 ± 2.89 [a]	98.39 ± 27.30 [a]	1.19 ± 0.54 [a]	39.65 ± 6.68 [a]
AS	7.57 ± 0.03 [d]	17.26 ± 2.48 [b]	66.21 ± 9.03 [ab]	0.75 ± 0.32 [ab]	14.52 ± 2.39 [b]
AMS	9.52 ± 0.21 [a]	9.75 ± 5.58 [bc]	41.91 ± 12.84 [b]	0.42 ± 0.20 [bc]	13.58 ± 1.16 [b]
ADS	8.46 ± 0.29 [b]	8.74 ± 1.99 [c]	36.38 ± 6.28 [b]	0.34 ± 0.12 [bc]	5.72 ± 2.71 [b]
AD	8.16 ± 0.11 [bc]	4.36 ± 0.58 [c]	21.24 ± 2.73 [b]	0.15 ± 0.10 [c]	2.72 ± 1.48 [b]

AM: alpine meadow, AS: alpine steppe, AMS: alpine meadow steppe, ADS: alpine desert steppe, AD: alpine desert, SOC: soil organic carbon, DOC: dissolved organic carbon, TN: total nitrogen, TIN: total inorganic nitrogen. Values are mean values of soil chemical characteristics $\pm$ standard error (S.E.) in alpine grasslands. Values within the same row followed by the same letter are not significantly different at $p < 0.05$.

The absolute abundance of PLFAs in five grassland type soils showed that the richness order of soil samples was as follows: total PLFA, bacteria, fungi, and actinomycetes (Table 2). The total PLFA values were the highest in the AM soils (23.58 ± 2.76 nmol g soil^{-1}), at 2.00, 2.37, 5.30 and 6.45 times those of the AS, AMS, ADS and AD soils. The bacterial PLFAs showed a generally similar pattern to that of total PLFAs. The predominant bacteria were most prevalent in the AM soils (22.84 ± 2.95 nmol g soil^{-1}) of these five grassland types, and were least prevalent in AD soil (2.57 ± 0.69 nmol g soil^{-1}). The amounts of the fungi and actinomycetes were also the highest in the AM soil, at 3.70 ± 0.54 nmol g soil^{-1}, and 1.96 ± 0.27 nmol g soil^{-1}, respectively, but the lowest values were found in the ADS soils at 0.96 ± 0.15 nmol g soil^{-1} and 0.37 ± 0.15 nmol g soil^{-1}, respectively.

Table 2. The soil microbial composition characteristics of alpine grasslands in the Tibetan Plateau.

PLFAs (nmol g^{-1})	Bacteria	Fungi	Actinomycetes	Total
AM	22.84 ± 2.95 [a]	3.70 ± 0.54 [a]	1.96 ± 0.27 [a]	23.58 ± 2.76 [a]
AS	11.32 ± 1.43 [b]	2.03 ± 0.31 [b]	1.22 ± 0.15 [b]	11.81 ± 1.41 [b]
AMS	9.23 ± 1.22 [bc]	1.86 ± 0.30 [b]	0.84 ± 0.18 [bc]	9.96 ± 1.27 [bc]
ADS	3.72 ± 0.93 [cd]	0.96 ± 0.15 [b]	0.36 ± 0.15 [c]	4.45 ± 0.98 [cd]
AD	2.57 ± 0.69 [d]	1.05 ± 0.25 [b]	0.55 ± 0.11 [c]	3.66 ± 0.93 [d]

PLFAs: phospholipid fatty acids, AM: alpine meadow, AS: alpine steppe, AMS: alpine meadow steppe, ADS: alpine desert steppe, AD: alpine desert. Values are mean values of soil microbial PLFA characteristics ± standard error (S.E.) in alpine grasslands. Values within the same row followed by the same letter are not significantly different at $p < 0.05$.

3.3. Relationships between Squalene Relative Abundance and Soil Chemical/Microbial Characteristics

Two principal components were used as tools to distinguish the different grassland ecosystems (AM, AS, AMS, ADS, and AD), considering all properties together (SOC, DOC, TN, TIN, pH, PLFAs, and relative abundance of squalene). The cumulative variation in the distribution of the selected variable was 74.86% and 86.04% for the sum of the principal components PC1 and PC2 in the evaluation performed with soil chemical traits and PLFAs (Figure 3). The analysis of the interaction showed an integrated effect of the grassland ecosystem, soil chemical characteristics, and PLFAs on the relative abundance of soil squalene. For soil chemical characteristics, the relative abundance of squalene had a negative correlation with SOC ($r = -0.616$, $p < 0.01$), DOC ($r = -0.510$, $p < 0.05$), TN ($r = -0.612$, $p < 0.01$), and TIN ($r = -0.579$, $p < 0.01$). Nevertheless, the squalene relative abundance was not in correlation with soil pH. For soil microbial characteristics, the relative abundance of squalene was also significantly negatively correlated with soil PLFA quantity, including soil total PLFA ($r = -0.642$, $p < 0.01$), bacteria PLFAs ($r = -0.650$, $p < 0.01$), fungi PLFAs ($r = -0.576$, $p < 0.01$), and Actinomycete PLFAs ($r = -0.583$, $p < 0.01$).

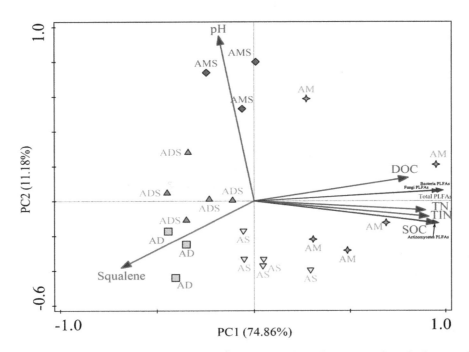

Figure 3. The relationships between squalene relative abundances and soil chemical/microbial characteristics in alpine grassland in the Tibetan Plateau. AM: alpine meadow, AS: alpine steppe, AMS: alpine meadow steppe, ADS: alpine desert steppe, AD: alpine desert, PLFAs: phospholipid fatty acids, SOC: soil organic carbon, DOC: dissolved organic carbon, TN: total nitrogen, TIN: total inorganic nitrogen.

4. Discussion

Squalene is a natural triterpene known to be an important intermediary of cholesterol/phytosterol biosynthesis in animals, plants, humans, and microorganisms. It is used widely in the food, cosmetic, and medicine industries due to its multiple functions [2,4]. Scientists have discovered that when squalene is found in great proportions in some animals and microorganisms, it is likely to be essential to their survival in extreme environments, especially hostile environments free of oxygen. Some animals include sharks, which live in the deep sea with dark, cold, high-pressure, and oxygen-poor conditions [6]. Other examples include moles, which inhabit a damp environment [42], and yaks, which thrive at altitudes of 2000–5000 m above sea level [21]. Squalene is absorbed and distributed to different organs from many biological sources, and is present in varying quantities [5]. In recent years, the bioavailability of squalene has been well established in cell cultures, animal models, and in humans, and further progress has been made concerning on the intracellular transport of this lipophilic molecule. Squalene accumulates in the animal liver and decreases levels of hepatic cholesterol and triglycerides, with these actions being exerted via a complex network of changes in gene expression at both transcriptional and post-transcriptional levels [5].

The Tibetan Plateau, the highest and most extensive highland in the world, is characterized by a harsh environment and fragile ecosystems at high altitude, with strong solar radiation, drought, low temperatures, and poor levels of oxygen [43]. In the present study, the squalene component was identified from five alpine grassland soils in the Tibetan Plateau by using the Py-GC/MS technique. Py-GC/MS served as a valuable analytical technique because pyrolysis products could be separated by gas chromatography and detected by mass spectrometry. The data by Py-GC/MS do not provide insight into the absolute abundance of compounds across samples, an approach that would require multiple internal standards. However, it is an efficient tool for revealing chemical characteristics in the organic matter of soils through semi-quantitative analyses with a comparison of abundance ratios of selected pyrolysis products [44–46]. A squalene component was found from all the soils in the five alpine grasslands, with relative abundance ranging from 0.93% to 10.66% in the Tibetan Platea, as shown using the Py-GC/MS technique (Figures 1 and 2). Nevertheless, at present the squalene component has only been found in very few soils in other regions, such as tropical rainforest soils in Indonesia [47], temperate broadleaved forest soils in Belgium [48], Mediterranean forest soil located in Spain [49], and agricultural soil in Canada [50]. For most of the soils, the squalene component was not obtained using the same technique [50–54].

In the Tibetan Plateau, squalene was identified in all the alpine grassland soils and some distribution characteristics are shown in Figure 3. The points were scattered among different alpine grassland types, while the points were concentrated in same grassland type. That is to say, the squalene relative abundances were different among different alpine grassland types, while they were similar in the same alpine grassland type (Figure 3). Comparing the five alpine grassland types, the squalene relative abundance was the highest in alpine desert soils, with a value of $10.66 \pm 2.07\%$, and it was the lowest in alpine meadow soils, with the value $0.93 \pm 0.22\%$ (Figure 2). Thus, the relative abundance of squalene relative in alpine desert soils was 11.5 times that of alpine meadow soils. This could be attributed to the different environmental conditions in two alpine grassland types. Alpine deserts are distributed in harsher environments; they are the highest and driest grassland type in China and the world [55]. The average annual temperature ranges from $-10\,°C$ to $-8\,°C$, the average annual precipitation from 20.6 mm to 53.8 mm, and the vegetation total cover from 5% to 14% in the alpine desert area. In the alpine meadow area, the average annual temperature is around $0\,°C$, the average annual precipitation ranges from 450 mm to 600 mm, and the total vegetation cover is from 50% to 90% [55–57].

In general, the squalene relative abundance was significantly negatively correlated with soil chemical/microbial characteristics in the Tibetan Plateau (Figure 3). This indicated that the relative abundance of squalene is higher in soils with low microbial quantities and confirmed that squalene is a product of biological adaptation to extreme environments. Soil microbial PLFA quantities in alpine grasslands were positively associated with mean annual temperature, mean annual precipitation, soil organic carbon, and aboveground biomass, and negatively associated with elevation, indicating that the harsh environmental conditions may not benefit the survival of soil microorganisms in the Tibetan Plateau [22,58,59]. Thus, microorganisms may adapt to harsh environmental conditions by increasing the levels of squalene in their bodies. It has been reported that each molecule of squalene could be formed by fusing two molecules of farnesyl diphosphate in microorganisms, and that some special mechanism exists to allow certain microorganisms to independently adapt to extreme environments [3,60]. For instance, prokaryotic hopanoid biosynthesis does not require molecular oxygen as a substrate, and the squalene is directly cyclized by the enzyme squalene-hopene cyclase in hypoxic environments [60]. Squalene has a role in facilitating tighter packing of archaeal lipid mixtures and also influences spatial organization in archaeal membranes of *Halobacterium salinarum*, an extremely halophilic archaeon [61]. Soil organic matter provides energy and the nitrogen elements constituting the nutrients required for the life activity process for microorganisms [62,63]. Therefore, the relationships between squalene abundance and soil chemical characteristics were consistent with its relationships to soil microbes in the Tibetan Plateau (Figure 3).

5. Conclusions

Squalene, which is attracting great biological interest due to its beneficial properties and is generally considered to be a product of biological adaptation to extreme environments, was found in all the soils in five alpine grasslands in the Tibetan Plateau using the Py-GC/MS technique. The relative abundance of squalene is higher in soil with low microbial quantities, which in the harsh environmental conditions may not benefit the survival of soil microorganisms in the Tibetan Plateau. This suggests that squalene is possibly a bioactive component for microorganisms in alpine grassland soils to adapt to harsh environmental conditions, especially in oxygen-poor environments. Furthermore, the relative abundance of squalene in alpine grassland soils had a significantly negative correlation with soil chemical/microbial characteristics. Therefore, the harsher the environment, the higher the relative abundance of squalene needed to adapt to this environment in the Tibetan Plateau.

In general, the present study represents preliminary research for squalene in alpine grassland soils; we still do not know which species or populations of microorganisms could biosynthesize squalene, what the mechanism of squalene biosynthesis is in the body of microorganisms, and why and how the extreme environmental conditions stimulate the production of squalene in the soils. In addition, Py-GC/MS is an analytic technique that uses semi-quantitative analyses with a comparison of abundance ratios of selected pyrolysis products. The absolute content of squalene in soils needs to be determined by using an authenticated external standard of squalene. Thus, further in-depth studies concerning squalene distribution, its biosynthesis mechanism, and its relationship with environmental factors are still needed in the Tibetan Plateau.

Author Contributions: Conceptualization, X.L. and S.M.; Methodology, X.L. and Y.C.; Software, Y.C. and H.J.; Validation, X.L., S.M., Y.C., D.Y. and H.J.; Formal Analysis, D.Y.; Investigation, S.M.; Resources, X.L.; Data Curation, X.L. and Y.C.; Writing—Original Draft Preparation, X.L.; Writing—Review and Editing, X.L. and S.M.; Funding Acquisition, X.L. and D.Y.

References

1. Amarowicz, P. Squalene: A natural antioxidant? *Eur. J. Lipid Sci. Technol.* **2009**, *111*, 411–412. [CrossRef]
2. Popa, O.; Bsbeanu, N.E.; Popa, I.; Nitã, S.; Dinu-Pârvu, C.E. Methods for obtaining and determination of squalene from natural sources. *BioMed Res. Int.* **2015**, *2015*, 367202. [CrossRef] [PubMed]
3. Spanova, M.; Daum, G. Squalene—Biochemistry, molecular biology, process biotechnology, and applications. *Eur. J. Lipid Sci. Technol.* **2011**, *113*, 1299–1320. [CrossRef]

4. Katabami, A.; Li, L.; Iwasaki, M.; Furubayashi, M.; Saito, K.; Umeno, D. Production of squalene by squalene synthases and their truncated mutants in *Escherichia coli. J. Biosci. Bioeng.* **2015**, *119*, 165–171. [CrossRef] [PubMed]

5. Lou-Bonafonte, J.M.; Martínez-Beamonte, R.; Sanclemente, T.; Surra, J.C.; Herrera-Marcos, L.V.; Sanchez-Marco, J.; Arnal, C.; Osada, J. Current insights into the biological action of squalene. *Mol. Nutr. Food Res.* **2018**, *62*, e1800136. [CrossRef] [PubMed]

6. Hall, D.W.; Marshall, S.N.; Gordon, K.C.; Killee, D.P. Rapid quantitative determination of squalene in shark liver oils by Raman and IR spectroscopy. *Lipids* **2016**, *51*, 139–147. [CrossRef] [PubMed]

7. Vadalà, M.; Laurino, C.; Palmieri, L.; Palmieri, B. Shark derivatives (Alkylglycerols, Squalene, Cartilage) as putative nutraceuticals in oncology. *Eur. J. Oncol.* **2017**, *22*, 5–20.

8. Yuan, C.; Xie, Y.; Jin, R.; Ren, L.; Zhou, L.; Zhu, M.; Ju, Y. Simultaneous analysis of tocopherols, phytosterols, and squalene in vegetable oils by high-performance liquid chromatography. *Food Anal. Methods* **2017**, *10*, 3716–3722. [CrossRef]

9. Fooshee, D.R.; Aiona, P.K.; Laskin, A.; Laskin, J.; Nizkorodov, S.A.; Baldi, P.F. Atmospheric oxidation of squalene: Molecular study using COBRA modeling and high-resolution mass spectrometry. *Environ. Sci. Technol.* **2015**, *49*, 13304–13313. [CrossRef] [PubMed]

10. Ghimire, G.P.; Thuan, N.H.; Koirala, N.; Sohng, J.K. Advances in biochemistry and microbial production of squalene and its derivatives. *J. Microbiol. Biotechnol.* **2016**, *26*, 441–451. [CrossRef] [PubMed]

11. Xu, W.; Ma, X.; Wang, Y. Production of squalene by microbes: An update. *World J. Microbiol. Biotechnol.* **2016**, *32*, 195. [CrossRef] [PubMed]

12. Fagundes, M.B.; Vendruscolo, R.G.; Maroneze, M.M.; Barin, J.S.; de Menezes, C.R.; Zepka, L.Q.; Jacob-Lopes, E.; Wagner, R. Towards a sustainable route for the production of squalene using cyanobacteria. *Waste Biomass Valorization* **2018**, *3*, 1–8. [CrossRef]

13. Qiu, J. China: The third pole. *Nature* **2008**, *454*, 393–396. [CrossRef] [PubMed]

14. Yao, T.; Thompson, L.G.; Mosbrugger, V.; Zhang, F.; Ma, Y.; Luo, T.; Xu, B.; Yang, X.; Joswiak, D.R.; Wang, W.; et al. Third Pole Environment (TPE). *Environ. Dev.* **2012**, *3*, 52–64. [CrossRef]

15. Yang, Y.; Gao, Y.; Wang, S.; Xu, D.; Yu, H.; Wu, L.; Lin, Q.; Hu, Y.; Li, X.; He, Z.; et al. The microbial gene diversity along an elevation gradient of the Tibetan grassland. *ISME J.* **2014**, *8*, 430–440. [CrossRef] [PubMed]

16. Guo, G.; Kong, W.; Liu, J.; Zhao, J.; Du, H.; Zhang, X.; Xia, P. Diversity and distribution of autotrophic microbial community along environmental gradients in grassland soils on the Tibetan Plateau. *Appl. Microbiol. Biotechnol.* **2015**, *99*, 8765–8776. [CrossRef] [PubMed]

17. Pugnaire, F.I.; Zhang, L.; Li, R.; Luo, T. No evidence of facilitation collapse in the Tibetan plateau. *J. Veg. Sci.* **2015**, *26*, 233–242. [CrossRef]

18. Pan, S.; Zhang, T.; Rong, Z.; Hu, L.; Gu, Z.; Wu, Q.; Dong, S.; Liu, Q.; Lin, Z.; Deutschova, L.; et al. Population transcriptomes reveal synergistic responses of DNA polymorphism and RNA expression to extreme environments on the Qinghai-Tibetan Plateau in a predatory bird. *Mol. Ecol.* **2017**, *26*, 2993–3010. [CrossRef] [PubMed]

19. Liu, J.; Nan, P.; Wang, L.; Wang, Q.; Tsering, T.; Zhong, Y. Chemical variation in lipophilic composition of *Lamiophlomis rotata* from the Qinghai-Tibetan Plateau. *Chem. Nat. Compd.* **2006**, *42*, 525–528. [CrossRef]

20. Yuan, L.; Zhong, G.; Quan, H.; Tian, F.; Zhong, Z.; Lan, X. GC-MS study on chemical components of volatile oil from roots of *Rhodiola crenulata* growing in Tibet. *Chin. J. Exp. Tradit. Med. Formulae* **2012**, *18*, 67–70. (In Chinese with English Abstract).

21. Liu, C.; Jin, G.; Luo, Z.; Li, S.; Sun, S.; Li, Y.; Ma, M. Chinese yak and yellow cattle exhibit considerable differences in tissue content of squalene, tocopherol, and fatty acids. *Eur. J. Lipid Sci. Technol.* **2015**, *117*, 899–902. [CrossRef]

22. Chen, Y.L.; Ding, J.Z.; Peng, Y.F.; Li, F.; Yang, G.B.; Liu, L.; Qin, S.Q.; Fang, K.; Yang, Y.H. Patterns and drivers of soil microbial communities in Tibetan alpine and global terrestrial ecosystems. *J. Biogeogr.* **2016**, *43*, 2027–2039. [CrossRef]

23. Qi, Q.; Zhao, M.; Wang, S.; Ma, X.; Wang, Y.; Gao, Y.; Lin, Q.; Li, X.; Gu, B.; Li, G.; et al. The biogeographic pattern of microbial functional genes along an altitudinal gradient of the Tibetan pasture. *Front. Microbiol.* **2017**, *8*, 976. [CrossRef] [PubMed]

24. Yang, T.; Adams, J.M.; Shi, Y.; He, J.S.; Jing, X.; Chen, L.; Tedersoo, L.; Chu, H. Soil fungal diversity in natural grasslands of the Tibetan Plateau: Associations with plant diversity and productivity. *New Phytol.* **2017**, *215*, 756–765. [CrossRef] [PubMed]

25. Immerzeel, W.W.; Beek, L.P.H.; Bierkens, M.F.P. Climate change will affect the Asian water towers. *Science* **2010**, *328*, 1382–1385. [CrossRef] [PubMed]

26. Bibi, S.; Wang, L.; Li, X.; Zhou, J.; Chen, D.; Yao, T. Climatic and associated cryospheric, biospheric, and hydrological changes on the Tibetan Plateau: A review. *Int. J. Climatol.* **2018**, *38*, e1–e17. [CrossRef]

27. Lu, X.; Yan, Y.; Sun, J.; Zhang, X.; Chen, Y.; Wang, X.; Cheng, G. Carbon, nitrogen, and phosphorus storage in alpine grassland ecosystems of Tibet: Effects of grazing exclusion. *Ecol. Evol.* **2015**, *5*, 4492–4504. [CrossRef] [PubMed]

28. Gai, J.P.; Christie, P.; Cai, X.B.; Fan, J.Q.; Zhang, J.L.; Feng, G.; Li, X.L. Occurrence and distribution of arbuscular mycorrhizal fungal species in three types of grassland community of the Tibetan Plateau. *Ecol. Res.* **2009**, *24*, 1345–1350. [CrossRef]

29. Lu, X.; Yan, Y.; Sun, J.; Zhang, X.; Chen, Y.; Wang, X.; Cheng, G. Short-term grazing exclusion has no impact on soil properties and nutrients of degraded alpine grassland in Tibet, China. *Solid Earth* **2015**, *6*, 1195–1205. [CrossRef]

30. Prayogo, C.; Jones, J.E.; Baeyens, J.; Bending, G.D. Impact of biochar on mineralisation of C and N from soil and willow litter and its relationship with microbial community biomass and structure. *Biol. Fertil. Soils* **2014**, *50*, 695–702. [CrossRef]

31. Hannam, K.D.; Quideau, S.A.; Kishchuk, B.E. Forest floor microbial communities in relation to stand composition and timber harvesting in northern Alberta. *Soil Biol. Biochem.* **2006**, *38*, 2565–2575. [CrossRef]

32. Pankhurst, C.E.; Yu, S.; Hawke, B.G.; Harch, B.D. Capacity of fatty acid profiles and substrate utilization patterns to describe differences in soil microbial communities associated with increased salinity or alkalinity at three locations in South Australia. *Biol. Fertil. Soils* **2001**, *33*, 204–217. [CrossRef]

33. Arthur, M.A.; Bray, S.R.; Kuchle, C.R.; McEwan, R.W. The influence of the invasive shrub, *Lonicera maackii*, on leaf decomposition and microbial community dynamics. *Plant Ecol.* **2012**, *213*, 1571–1582. [CrossRef]

34. McMahon, S.; Schimel, J.P. Shifting patterns of microbial N-metabolism across seasons in upland Alaskan tundra soils. *Soil Biol. Biochem.* **2017**, *105*, 96–107. [CrossRef]

35. Sun, S.Q.; Liu, T.; Wu, Y.H.; Wang, G.X.; Zhu, B.; DeLuca, T.H.; Wang, Y.Q.; Luo, J. Ground bryophytes regulate net soil carbon efflux: Evidence from two subalpine ecosystems on the east edge of the Tibet Plateau. *Plant Soil* **2017**, *417*, 363–375. [CrossRef]

36. Jílková, V.; Cajthaml, T.; Frouz, J. Relative importance of honeydew and resin for the microbial activity in wood ant nest and forest floor substrate—A laboratory study. *Soil Biol. Biochem.* **2018**, *117*, 1–4. [CrossRef]

37. Yang, B.; Pang, X.Y.; Hu, B.; Bao, W.K.; Tian, G.L. Does thinning-induced gap size result in altered soil microbial community in pine plantaton in eastern Tibetan Plateau? *Ecol. Evol.* **2017**, *7*, 2986–2993. [CrossRef] [PubMed]

38. Jiao, F.; Shi, X.R.; Han, F.P.; Yuan, Z.Y. Increasing aridity, temperature and soil pH induce soil C-N-P imbalance in grasslands. *Sci. Rep.* **2016**, *6*, 1–9. [CrossRef] [PubMed]

39. Chen, Q.Q.; Sun, Y.M.; Shen, C.D.; Peng, S.L.; Yi, W.X.; Li, Z.A.; Jiang, M.T. Organic matter turnover rates and CO_2 flux from organic matter decomposition of mountain soil profiles in the subtropical area, south China. *Catena* **2002**, *49*, 217–229. [CrossRef]

40. Liang, B.; Yang, X.Y.; He, X.H.; Zhou, J.B. Effects of 17-year fertilization on soil microbial biomass C and N and soluble organic C and N in loessial soil during maize growth. *Biol. Fertil. Soils* **2011**, *47*, 121–128. [CrossRef]

41. Kalbitz, K.; Geyer, S. Different effects of peat degradation on dissolved organic carbon and nitrogen. *Org. Geochem.* **2002**, *33*, 319–326. [CrossRef]

42. Downing, D.T.; Stewart, M.E. Skin surface lipids of the mole *Scalopus aquaticus*. *Comp. Biochem. Physiol. Part B Comp. Biochem.* **1987**, *86*, 667–670. [CrossRef]

43. Sun, J.; Zhou, T.; Liu, M.; Chen, Y.; Shang, H.; Zhu, L.; Shedayi, A.A.; Yu, H.; Cheng, G.; Liu, G.; et al. Linkages of the dynamics of glaciers and lakes with the climate elements over the Tibetan Plateau. *Earth-Sci. Rev.* **2018**, *185*, 308–324. [CrossRef]

44. Dai, X.Y.; Ping, C.L.; Michaelson, G. J. Characterizing soil organic matter in Arctic tundra soil by different analytical approaches. *Org. Geochem.* **2002**, *33*, 407–419. [CrossRef]

45. Grandy, A.; Sinsabaugh, R.; Neff, J.; Stursova, M.; Zak, D. Nitrogen deposition effects on soil organic matter chemistry are linked to variation in enzymes, ecosystems and size fractions. *Biogeochemistry* **2008**, *91*, 37–49. [CrossRef]

46. Ma, S.Q.; Chen, Y.C.; Lu, X.Y.; Wang, X.D. Soil Organic Matter Chemistry: Based on Pyrolysis-Gas Chromatography- Mass Spectrometry (Py-GC/MS). *Mini-Rev. Org. Matter* **2018**, *15*, 389–403. [CrossRef]

47. Yassir, I.; Buurman, P. Soil organic matter chemistry changes upon secondary succession in Imperata Grasslands, Indonesia: A pyrolysis–GC/MS study. *Geoderma* **2012**, *173–174*, 94–103. [CrossRef]

48. Vancampenhout, K.; De Vos, B.; Wouters, K.; Swennen, R.; Buurman, P.; Deckers, J. Organic matter of subsoil horizons under broadleaved forest: Highly processed or labile and plant-derived? *Soil Biol. Biochem.* **2012**, *50*, 40–46. [CrossRef]

49. Campo, J.; Nierop, K.G.J.; Cammeraat, E.; Andreu, V.; Rubio, J.L. Application of pyrolysis-gas chromatography/mass spectrometry to study changes in the organic matter of macro- and microaggregates of a Mediterranean soil upon heating. *J. Chromatogr. A* **2011**, *1218*, 4817–4827. [CrossRef] [PubMed]

50. Jeannottea, R.; Hamela, C.; Jabaji, S.; Whalena, J.K. Pyrolysis-mass spectrometry and gas chromatography-flame ionization detection as complementary tools for soil lipid characterization. *J. Anal. Appl. Pyrolysis* **2011**, *90*, 232–237. [CrossRef]

51. Dai, X.Y.; White, D.; Ping, C.L. Comparing bioavailability in five Arctic soils by pyrolysis-gas chromatography/mass spectrometry. *J. Anal. Appl. Pyrolysis* **2002**, *62*, 249–258. [CrossRef]

52. Buurman, P.; Peterse, F.; Martin, G.A. Soil organic matter chemistry in allophanic soils: A pyrolysis-GC/MS study of a Costa Rican Andosol catena. *Eur. J. Soil Sci.* **2007**, *58*, 1330–1347. [CrossRef]

53. Grandy, A.S.; Strickland, M.S.; Lauber, C.L.; Bradford, M.A.; Fierer, N. The influence of microbial communities, management, and soil texture on soil organic matter chemistry. *Geoderma* **2009**, *150*, 278–286. [CrossRef]

54. Carr, A.S.; Boom, A.; Chase, B.M.; Meadows, M.E.; Roberts, Z.E.; Britton, M.N.; Cumming, A.M.J. Biome-scale characterisation and differentiation of semi-arid and arid zone soil organic matter compositions using pyrolysis–GC/MS analysis. *Geoderma* **2013**, *200–201*, 189–201. [CrossRef]

55. Land Management Bureau of Tibet. *Grassland Resources in Tibet Autonomous Region*; Sciences Press: Beijing, China, 1994. (In Chinese)

56. Yu, G.; Tang, L.; Yang, X.; Ke, X.; Harrison, S.P. Modern pollen samples from alpine vegetation on the Tibetan Plateau. *Glob. Ecol. Biogeogr.* **2001**, *10*, 503–520. [CrossRef]

57. Yan, Y.; Lu, X. Is grazing exclusion effective in restoring vegetation in degraded alpine grasslands in Tibet, China? *PeerJ* **2015**, *3*, e1020. [CrossRef] [PubMed]

58. Xu, M.; Li, X.; Cai, X.; Gai, J.; Li, X.; Christie, P.; Zhang, J. Soil microbial community structure and activity along a montane elevational gradient on the Tibetan Plateau. *Eur. J. Soil Biol.* **2014**, *64*, 6–14. [CrossRef]

59. Liu, X.; Cong, J.; Lu, H.; Xue, Y.; Wang, X.; Li, D.; Zhang, Y. Community structure and elevational distribution pattern of soil Actinobacteria in alpine grasslands. *Acta Ecol. Sin.* **2017**, *37*, 213–218. [CrossRef]

60. Takishita, K.; Chikaraishi, Y.; Leger, M.M.; Kim, E.; Yabuki, A.; Ohkouchi, N.; Roger, A.J. Lateral transfer of tetrahymanol-synthesizing genes has allowed multiple diverse eukaryote lineages to independently adapt to environments without oxygen. *Biol. Direct* **2012**, *7*, 5. [CrossRef] [PubMed]

61. Gilmore, S.F.; Yao, A.I.; Tietel, Z.; Kind, T.; Facciotti, M.T.; Parikh, A.N. Role of squalene in the organization of monolayers derived from lipid extracts of *Halobacterium salinarum*. *Langmuir* **2013**, *29*, 7922–7930. [CrossRef] [PubMed]

62. Yang, Y.; Zhang, N.; Xue, M.; Lu, S.T.; Tao, S. Effects of soil organic matter on the development of the microbial polycyclic aromatic hydrocarbons (PAHs) degradation potentials. *Environ. Pollut.* **2011**, *159*, 591–595. [CrossRef] [PubMed]

63. Kuzyakov, Y.; Xu, X. Competition between roots and microorganisms for nitrogen: Mechanisms and ecological relevance. *New Phytol.* **2013**, *198*, 656–669. [CrossRef] [PubMed]

7

Studies on the Design and Synthesis of Marine Peptide Analogues and their Ability to Promote Proliferation in HUVECs and Zebrafish

Yinglin Zheng, Yichen Tong, Xinfeng Wang, Jiebin Zhou and Jiyan Pang *

School of Chemistry, Sun Yat-Sen University, Guangzhou 510275, China; zhengylin6@mail2.sysu.edu.cn (Y.Z.); tongych3@mail2.sysu.edu.cn (Y.T.); tomorrow1996@163.com (X.W.); sysuzhoujieb@163.com (J.Z.)
* Correspondence: cespjy@mail.sysu.edu.cn;

Academic Editor: Pinarosa Avato

Abstract: In our previous studies, tripeptide **1** was found to induce angiogenesis in zebrafish embryos and in HUVECs. Based on the lead compound **1**, seven new marine tripeptide analogues **2–8** have been designed and synthesized in this paper to evaluate the effects on promoting cellular proliferation in human endothelial cells (HUVECs) and zebrafish. Among them, compounds **5–7** possessed more remarkable increasing proliferation effects than other compounds, and the EC_{50} values of these and the leading compound **1** were 1.0 ± 0.002 μM, 1.0 ± 0.0005 μM, 0.88 ± 0.0972 μM, and 1.31 ± 0.0926 μM, respectively. Furthermore, **5–7** could enhance migrations (58.5%, 80.66% and 60.71% increment after culturing 48 h, respectively) and invasions (49.08%, 47.24% and 56.24% increase, respectively) in HUVECs compared with the vehicle control. The results revealed that the tripeptide including L-Tyrosine or D-Proline fragments instead of L-Alanine of leading compound **1** would contribute to HUVECs' proliferation. Taking the place of the original (L-Lys-L-Ala) segment of leading compound **1**, a new fragment (L-Arg-D-Val) expressed higher performance in bioactivity in HUVECs. In addition, compound **7** could promote angiogenesis in zebrafish assay and it was more interesting that it also could repair damaged blood vessels in PTK787-induced zebrafish at a low concentration. The above data indicate that these peptides have potential implications for further evaluation in cytothesis studies.

Keywords: marine peptides; proliferation; migration; angiogenesis; zebrafish

1. Introduction

Marine peptides are mainly obtained from diverse marine organisms. Marine organisms play an important role as sources of nitrogen and amino acids, which have numerous potential physiological functions [1]. Because of their special marine environment, marine peptides have unique structures, such as rare coded amino acids, special connection bonds and highly modified amino acid residues. The structural diversity of marine peptides results in various bioactivities, such as neurotoxicity [2], anticancer [3], antivirus [4], antimicrobial [5], and antioxidant [6] effects.

Cellular proliferation is not only one of the most indispensable characteristics of the cell cycle, but the foundation of organism growth, inheritance and evolution. Proliferation plays an important role in physiology and pathology. It is a tightly regulated process and a normal occurrence in numerous biological processes, such as embryogenesis, tissue remodeling, bone development, the ovarian cycle and wound healing [7]. Over the past few years, researchers have started to focus more on cellular proliferation, which has a prominent role to play in the treatment of common diseases. For example, acute dermal wounds heal quickly in healthy individuals but turn into deep sores in diabetics, leading to severe infections in underlying tissues. Therefore, it is vital for promoting faster cellular proliferation and wound healing [8]. In bone repair and regeneration, osteogenic growth peptide (OGP) is a biologically active peptide that affects immune functions, proliferation and differentiation [9]. Furthermore, the significance of promoting proliferation has focused on therapeutic angiogenesis in recent years. Therapeutic angiogenesis, which can re-establish blood perfusion and rescue ischemic tissue, is used to treat ischemic diseases such as peripheral vascular occlusive disease (PVOD), a common manifestation of atherosclerosis with a high rate of morbidity [10]. Zebrafish embryo are recognized as a suitable model to explore the formation of blood vessel because their vascular system can be easily described in the developing embryo. Numerous pathways involved in angiogenesis in mammals are highly conserved in this model.

In our earlier work, novel marine cyclopeptide analogue xyloallenoide A (Figure 1) was isolated from the mangrove fungus *Xylaria* sp. 2508 in the South China Sea [11]. According to the structure of xyloallenoide A, a *t*-Butyloxy carbonyl (Boc)-protected cyclotripeptide (X-13) was synthesized [12], and it could dose-dependently induce angiogenesis in zebrafish embryos and human umbilical vein endothelial cells (HUVECs), which consisted of Boc-L-Lys, D-N-MeVal and D-N-MeAla. The compound X-13 expressed potent angiogenic properties and is very promising for development as a novel class of pro-angiogenic agents for angiotherapy [13]. Considering the complex structure and hard synthesis of cyclopeptides, a series of linepeptides were designed and synthesized [13]. Among them, tripeptide **1** with the group of D-Val, Boc-L-Lys and L-Ala had the strongest induced angiogenesis effect, both in vivo and in vitro. The effect of tripeptide **1** on angiogenesis wasmore significant than that of the compound X-13 [14]. Previous structure–activity relationship (SAR) analysis revealed that linear tripeptides and tetrapeptides, including Val, Lys and Ala amino acid segments, displayed favorable activities.

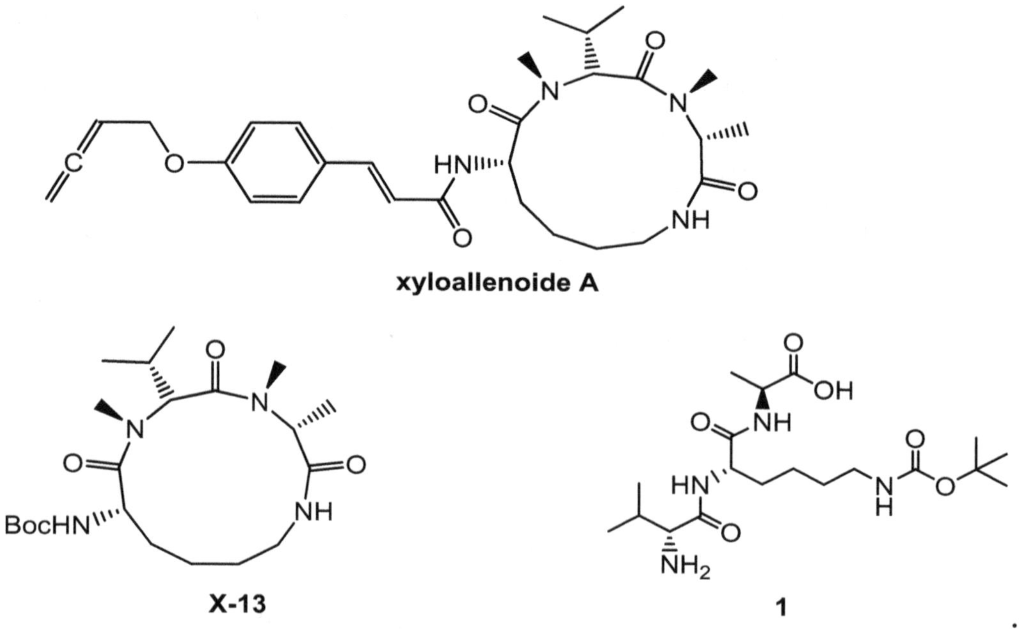

xyloallenoide A

X-13   **1**

1.

Figure 1. The structures of xyloallenoide A, X-13 and

In this paper, to explore more leading bioactive compounds resembling compound **1**, we designed a series of new tripeptides. Based on lead compound **1**, more tripeptides **2**–**8** (Figure 2), including a variety of different amino acids and substituents, were synthesized. Further promoting cellular proliferations were performed on HUVECs to identify more new candidate drugs and discuss the SAR. Moreover, the further proliferative and angiogenesis effects of selected compound were evaluated on normal and damaged zebrafish models.

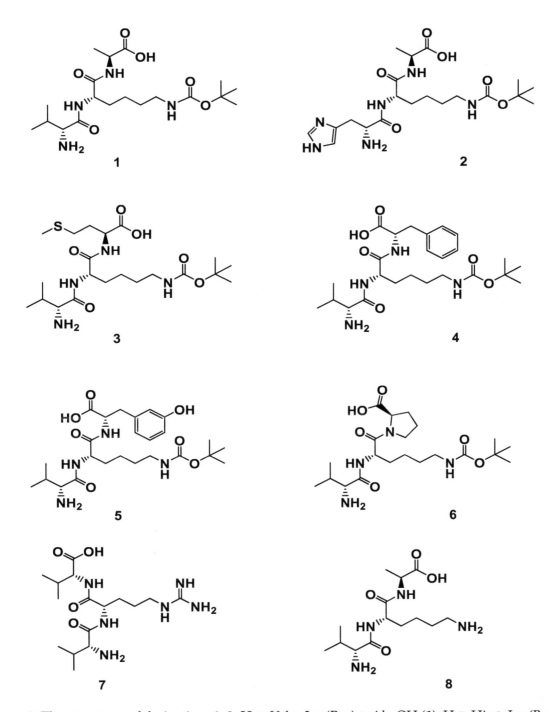

Figure 2. The structures of derivatives **1–8**. H-D-Val-L-Lys(Boc)-L-Ala-OH (**1**); H-D-His-L-Lys(Boc)-L-Ala-OH (**2**); H-D-Val-L-Lys(Boc)-L-Met-OH (**3**); H-D-Val-L-Lys(Boc)-L-Phe-OH (**4**); H-D-Val-L-Lys(Boc)-L-Tyr-OH (**5**); H-D-Val-L-Lys(Boc)-D-Pro-OH (**6**); H-D-Val-L-Arg-D-Val-OH (**7**); H-D-Val-L-Lys-L-Ala-OH (**8**).

2. Results and Discussion

2.1. Chemistry

To assess the cellular bioactivities of different modifications of compound **1**, a series of analogues **2–8** were designed, with modification focused on the different amino acids and the lipophilic/hydrophilic and acidity/alkaline properties of compounds. With the aim of studying the steric effect, compounds **4** and **8** were designed. Compound **2** was synthesized to explore the bioactivity of unsaturated alkaline amino acid, with D-Histidine instead of D-Valine. Compounds **3** and

6 were focused on the effect of the structure of the methylthio group and tetrahydropyrrole on cellular bioactivities. Furthermore, acidity and hydrophily are probably related to activity, so compound **5** was designed. Due to the Arg-Gly-Asp (RGD) sequence relating to angiogenesis [15], compound **7** containing an RGD moiety was synthesized.

The line peptide compounds **1–8** were prepared by our previous method [12] (Scheme 1). Generally, Cbz-D-Val-OH, Cbz-D-His-OH, H-L-Lys(Boc)-OMe and H-L-Arg(Pbf)-OMe were used as starting materials and coupled with another amino acid by coupling reagents (HOBt, HBTU and DIEA) to obtain the corresponding dipeptide and tripeptide. The dipeptide and tripeptide were demethylated using LiOH in THF/H_2O. All Cbz-groups were removed by H_2 with Pd/C-catalyzed. All the target molecules were purified through flash column chromatography, and the structures were fully characterized by ^1H NMR, ^{13}C NMR and HR-EI-MS. The purity of all target compounds was $\geq 95\%$ as determined by HPLC analysis.

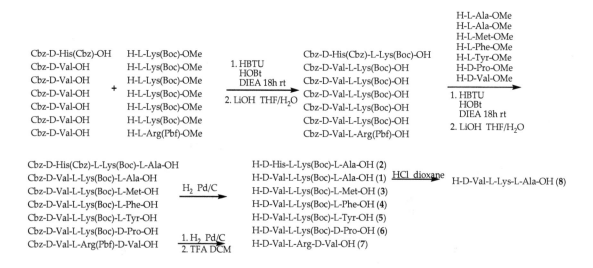

Scheme 1. Synthetic route of compounds **1–8**. All peptides were synthesis by HBTU, HOBt and DIEA as coupling reagents at room temperature 18 h. The dipeptide and tripeptide were demethylated using LiOH in THF/H_2O. All Cbz-groups were removed by H_2 with Pd/C-catalyzed.

2.2. Effects of Compounds **1–8** on HUVEC Proliferation

The endothelial cell's proliferation is an important phase in the process of normal life. Human umbilical vein endothelial cells (HUVECs) are frequently used to measure the angiogenic property in vitro. HUVECs are usually used as a laboratory model system for the study of the function and pathology of endothelial cells such as angiogenesis [16] and hypertension [17]. Like human umbilical artery endothelial cells, they exhibit a cobblestone phenotype when lining vessel walls. To evaluate the cellular bioactivity in vitro, compounds **1–8** were studied on the HUVECs with different concentrations: 0.0625 μM, 0.125 μM, 0.25 μM, 0.5 μM, 1 μM, 2 μM, 5 μM, 10 μM, and 50 μM. A quantity of 20 ng/mL VEGF was used as a positive control. The results are shown in Figure 3 and Table 1.

Lead compound **1** clearly showed a notable proliferative effect on HUVECs with EC$_{50}$ value of 1.3 ± 0.0926 μM in a concentration-dependent manner. Compounds **5–7** possessed better proliferation effects with respect to HUVECs than other compounds, and the EC$_{50}$ values were 1.0 ± 0.002 μM, 1.0 ± 0.0005 μM and 0.88 ± 0.0972 μM, respectively.

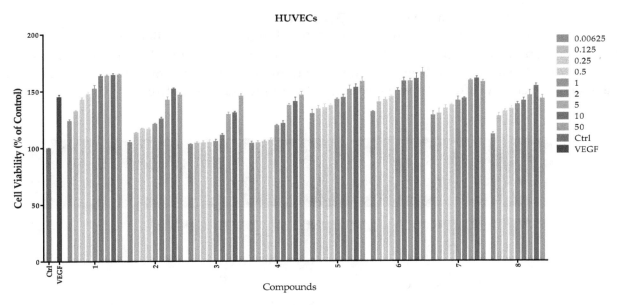

Figure 3. Effects of compounds **1–8** on proliferation of HUVECs. HUVECs were cultured with different concentrations (0–50 μM) of compounds. Cellular proliferation was assessed using the thiazolyl blue tetrazolium bromide (MTT) assay after 48 h. Data are expressed as the mean ± SEM ($n = 4$) of three individual experiments. The x-axis represents different compounds and the y-axis represents the cell viability (the control as 100%); different column colors represent different concentrations from 0.0625 μM to 50 μM.

Table 1. Values EC_{50} (μM) of compounds with respect to HUVEC proliferation.

Compounds	EC_{50} (μM)
1	1.31 ± 0.0926
2	57.55 ± 6.10
3	>200.00
4	76.02 ± 0.205
5	1.00 ± 0.002
6	1.00 ± 0.0005
7	0.88 ± 0.0972
8	1.33 ± 0.201

In view of the assays of promoting proliferation, the SAR analysis revealed that:

(a) the D-histidine fragment of compound **2** replaced the D-valine of compound 1, or L-methionine fragment of compound **3** replaced the L-alanine fragment of compound 1; both reduced cellular bioactivity, which might indicate that cellular proliferation was depressed due to steric hindrance of the substrates;

(b) secondly, the L-Tyrosine with phenol group (compound **5**) or D-proline with tetrahydropyrrole fragment (compound **6**) substituting for L-alanine also increased proliferation in HUVECs probably through hydrogen-bonding interaction;

(c) to our surprise, compound **7** exerted strong effects on HUVECs, which revealed that the L-Arg-D-Val fragment resembles the Lys(Boc)-L-Ala-OH in cytoactive terms;

(d) compared with compound **1** and **8**, we found that the *t*-Butyloxy carbonyl group was not a determinant factor in increasing cellular proliferation of HUVECs.

2.3. Migration Assays–Wound Healing of Compounds **5–7**

Cellular migration is a central process in the development of multicellular organisms. The wound healing method was used to evaluate the effects of compounds on HUVEC migration. Based on the results of proliferative assay on HUVECs, compounds **1** and **5–7** were chosen to evaluate the effects of reconstruction and migration at 50 μM. DMSO served as a control. The states of cellular growth at 0 h, 12 h, 24 h, 36 h and 48 h are presented in Figure 4. No significant endothelial cellular migrations were found in compound-treated groups and the vehicle control HUVEC before 12 h. However, compounds **1, 5, 6** and **7** treated groups all showed an increase in migration (58.5%, 80.66%, 60.71%, and 80.63% increment, respectively) after 48 h when compared with the vehicle control.

(A)

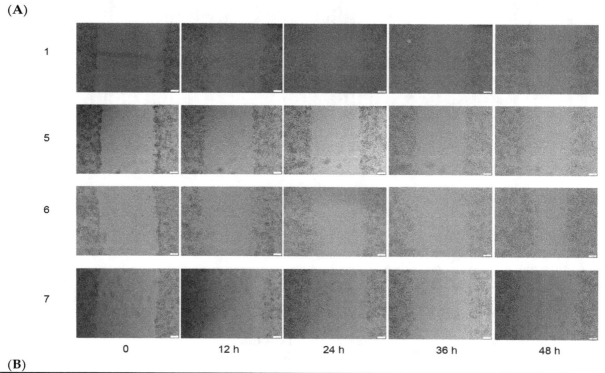

(B)

Compounds	Cellular Migration %				
	0 h	12 h	24 h	36 h	48 h
Control	0	12.12 ± 2.64	17.67 ± 1.92	23.76 ± 0.41	32.10 ± 1.23
1	0	33.55 ± 1.05	47.78 ± 1.01	70.48 ± 1.14	80.63 ± 0.54*
5	0	18.19 ± 0.90	23.56 ± 1.27	30.83 ± 0.43	58.53 ± 1.21*
6	0	27.46 ± 1.80	34.76 ± 1.22	38.86 ± 3.77	80.66 ± 0.68*
7	0	15.33 ± 1.51	25.23 ± 2.77	31.45 ± 1.03	60.71 ± 1.87*

(C)

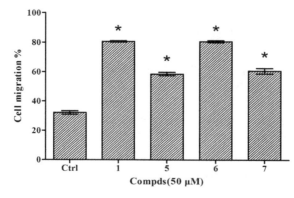

Figure 4. Effects of compounds **1** and **5–7** on HUVEC migration. (**A**) Observation of the effect of compounds on HUVEC migration; (**B**) The values of the compound-induced HUVEC migration at 0–48 h post-wounding; (**C**) Quantitative evaluation of the migration of HUVECs. Cellular migration was assessed at 48 h post-wounding. Data are expressed as the mean ± SEM (*n* = 4) of three individual experiments. Values vs control group: * *p* < 0.01 versus control.

2.4. Invasion Assays of Compounds 5–7 in HUVECs

Cellular proliferation, migration and invasion are clear characteristics of cytothesis in organisms. Therefore, transwell assays were utilized to determine the invasion of compounds 1 and 5–7 in HUVECs. There were 49.08%, 47.24%, 56.24%, and 53.17% increases in the invasion of HUVECs treated with compound 1 and 5–7 at 50 μM, respectively (Figure 5). The results indicated that compounds 5–7 were capable of inducing HUVEC migration similar to compound 1. The above results suggest that these three tripeptides possess potential in the application of cytothesis studies.

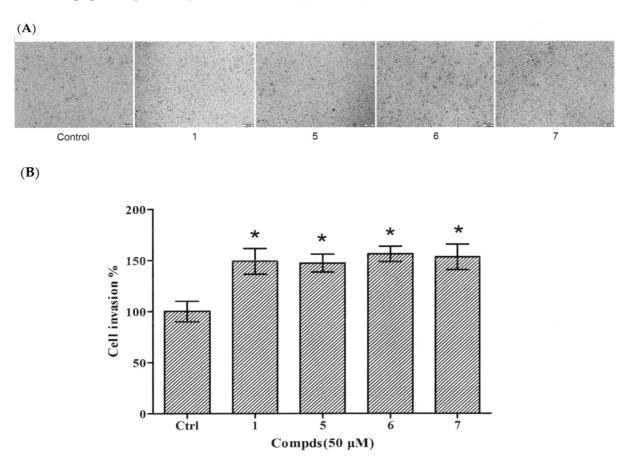

Figure 5. Effects of compounds 1 and 5–7 on HUVEC invasion. (**A**) Observation of the effect of compounds on HUVEC invasion; (**B**) Quantitative evaluation of the compound-induced HUVEC invasion. Cellular invasion was assessed at 24 h. Data are expressed as the mean ± SEM ($n = 3$) of three individual experiments. Values vs control group: * $p < 0.01$ versus control.

2.5. The Angiogenic Activity of Compound 6 in Zebrafish

It is meaningful to explore new candidate drugs for angiogenic therapy. An increasing number of studies are now available on the zebrafish model due to its short life cycle, availability and low cost. Based on the above assays, the proliferative effect of compound 7 was the most of significant on HUVEC proliferation. To further explore the effect of angiogenesis and restoration of blood vessel injury of compound 7, the zebrafish assay was performed. The angiogenesis effects of compound 7 on normal zebrafish and PTK787-induced zebrafish blood vessel injury are presented in Figures 6 and 7, respectively. The results indicated that compound 7 could promote angiogenesis in zebrafish. It was more interesting that compound 7 could relieve the injuries of damaged sub-intestinal vein (SIV) on PTK787-induced zebrafish at a low concentration at 5 μM ($p < 0.05$), indicating that it can repair damaged blood vessels.

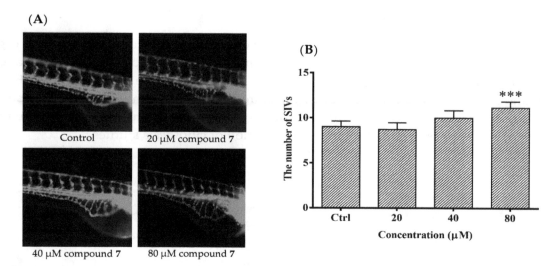

Figure 6. The effects of compound **7** on the angiogenesis formation in transgenic Tg (fli1: EGFP) zebrafish. Zebrafish embryos (24 hpf) were treated with test solution for 48 h and were evaluated using a microscope. (**A**) Representative images of blood vessel formation of zebrafish larvae at 72 hpf; (**B**) Quantitative analysis of the number of subintestinal vessel plexus (SIVs). Data are expressed as the means ± SEM (*n* = 10), and statistical significance was assessed by one-way ANOVA. Values vs control group: *** $p < 0.001$.

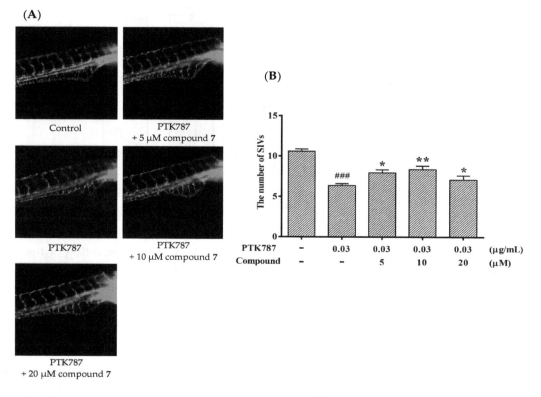

Figure 7. Compound **7** relieved the injuries of damaged SIVs in zebrafish. Zebrafish embryos (24 hpf) were treated with PTK787 for 24 h, then continually incubated with mixed solution of PTK787 and compound until 72 hpf. Zebrafish embryos were evaluated using a microscope. (**A**) Representative images of blood vessel formation of zebrafish larvae at 72 hpf; (**B**) Quantitative analysis of the regenerating caudal fin. Data are plotted as the mean ± SEM (*n* = 20), and statistical significance was assessed by one-way ANOVA. Values vs control group: ### $p < 0.001$; values vs model group: * $p < 0.05$ and ** $p < 0.01$.

3. Experimental Section

3.1. Chemistry

All reagents and solvents were of commercial quality. NMR data were recorded in methanol or DMSO, using TMS as an internal reference on a Varian Inova 500 MB NMR spectrometer (^{1}H, 500 MHz; ^{13}C, 125 MHz, Varian Medical Systems, Inc., Palo Alto, CA, USA), Bruker Avance 400 MB NMR spectrometer (^{1}H, 400 MHz; ^{13}C, 101 MHz, Bruker Corporation, Billerica, MA, USA). HREIMS were measured using Thermo MAT95XP High Resolution mass spectrometry (Thermo Fisher Scientific Inc. Waltham, MA, USA). EI were recorded on a Thermo DSQ EI-mass spectrometer. Column chromatography was carried out on silica gel (200–300 mesh, Qingdao Haiyang Chemical Co. Ltd., Qingdao, China). High-performance liquid chromatography (HPLC) was performed on a, Shimadzu LC-2010c (Shimadzu Corporation, Kyoto, Japan) equipped with UV detector. The purity of all compounds synthesized in this study was ≥95% as determined by HPLC analysis. Compounds **2–8** were first reported. The HPLC of compounds were shown in the Supplementary Flies (Tables S1–S9).

3.2. General Procedure for the Synthesis of Compounds **1–8**

All the tested compounds were synthesized according to the literature [12]. Generally, amino acids Cbz-D-Val-OH and H-L-Lys(Boc)-OMe were used to starting materials and HBTU, HOBt and DIEA as coupling reagents. The mixtures were dissolved in DCM and stirred for 18 h at room temperature, followed by demethylation to form Cbz-D-Val-L-Lys(Boc)-OH. Coupling Cbz-D-Val-L-Lys(Boc)-OH and the O-methylation of L-alanie, L-methionine, L-phenylanaline, L-typrosine, and D-proline, respectively, in the same way and then demethylating with LiOH in THF/H$_2$O to form compounds **1**, **3**, **4**, **5** and **6**. Tripeptide **8** was obtained by removal of the Boc group of compound **1** in HCl/dioxane. Similarly, tripeptide **2** was obtained by coupling Cbz-D-His(Cbz)-OH, H-L-Lys(Boc)-OMe and H-L-Ala-OMe. Compound **7** was prepared by coupling Cbz-D-Val-OH, H-L-Arg(Pbf)-OMe and H-D-Val-OMe. The intermediate was then stirred in TFA/DCM to remove the Pbf-group to yield tripeptide **7**. The NMR spectrum of compounds were shown in the Supplementary Flies (Figures S1–S15).

H-D-Val-L-Lys(Boc)-L-Ala-OH (**1**). White solid. ^{1}H NMR (500 MHz, MeOD) δ 8.54 (d, *J* = 8.2 Hz, 1H), 8.37 (d, *J* = 7.3 Hz, 1H), 6.68 (s, *J* = 8.4, 5.5 Hz, 1H), 4.21 (p, *J* = 7.4 Hz, 1H), 3.68 (d, *J* = 5.2 Hz, 1H), 2.88 (dd, *J* = 13.1, 6.7 Hz, 2H), 2.51 (dt, *J* = 3.6, 1.8 Hz, 7H), 2.18–1.98 (m, 1H), 1.73–1.45 (m, 2H), 1.30 (s, 11H), 1.29 (d, *J* = 7.3 Hz, 4H), 0.94 (dd, *J* = 11.8,6.9 Hz, 6H). ^{13}C NMR (125 MHz, MeOD) δ 174.26, 171.33, 168.10, 156.00, 77.81, 57.78, 52.63, 47.88, 30.35, 29.52, 28.74, 22.94, 18.86, 17.82, 17.52. EI-MS: *m/z* 417.5 (M$^+$); HR-EI-MS calcd. for C$_{19}$H$_{36}$O$_6$N$_4$: 417.5257 (M$^+$), found: 417.5228.

H-D-His-L-Lys(Boc)-L-Ala-OH (**2**). White solid. ^{1}H NMR (500 MHz, MeOD) δ 8.72 (s, 1H), 7.38 (s, 1H), 4.42–4.34 (m, 1H), 4.31 (dd, *J* = 8.7,5.3 Hz, 1H), 4.17 (t, *J* = 7.1 Hz, 1H), 3.25 (m, *J* = 15.0, 6.6 Hz, 1H), 3.00 (t, *J* = 7.2 Hz, 2H), 1.77 (dt, *J* = 13.8, 7.4 Hz, 1H), 1.69–1.58 (m, 1H), 1.40 (d, *J* = 7.3 Hz, 4H). ^{13}C NMR (125 MHz, MeOD) δ 174.25, 172.15, 167.32, 161.62, 157.30, 134.85, 128.41, 117.50, 110.01, 53.35, 52.24, 39.74, 31.43, 29.22, 27.38, 26.83, 22.58, 16.05. EI-MS: *m/z* 455.10 (M$^+$); HR-EI-MS calcd. for C$_{20}$H$_{35}$O$_6$N$_6$: 455.2612 (M$^+$), found: 455.2611.

H-D-Val-L-Lys(Boc)-L-Met-OH (**3**). White solid. ^{1}H NMR (500 MHz, MeOD) δ 4.59 (dd, *J* = 9.5, 4.3 Hz, 1H), 4.34 (dd, *J* = 9.0, 5.2 Hz, 1H), 3.82 (d, *J* = 3.6 Hz, 2H), 3.80 (d, *J* = 3.5 Hz, 3H), 3.77 (d, *J* = 7.8 Hz, 5H), 3.73–3.67 (m, 5H), 3.67–3.56 (m, 6H), 3.10–2.98 (m, 2H), 2.63 (ddd, *J* = 13.5, 8.5, 5.0 Hz, 1H), 2.53 (dt, *J* = 13.5, 7.9 Hz, 1H),2.23–2.13 (m, 2H), 2.09 (s, 4H), 1.96 (ddd, *J* = 14.2, 8.8, 4.3 Hz, 1H), 1.87 (dt, *J* = 12.7, 6.1 Hz, 1H), 1.77–1.63 (m, 1H), 1.45 (m, *J* = 55.4, 14.3, 7.2 Hz, 16H), 1.06 (dd, *J* = 6.8, 5.1 Hz, 7H). ^{13}C NMR (125 MHz, MeOD) δ 174.81, 174.47, 169.67, 158.59, 79.93, 73.03, 71.40, 65.15, 59.87, 54.90, 52.21, 32.76, 32.19, 31.42, 31.18, 30.54, 28.79, 24.25, 19.03, 18.03, 15.11. EI-MS: *m/z* 477.05 (M$^+$); HR-EI-MS calcd. for C$_{21}$H$_{39}$O$_6$N$_4$S: 475.2595 (M$^-$), found: 475.2597.

H-D-*Val*-L-*Lys(Boc)*-L-*Phe*-OH (**4**). White solid. ^{1}H NMR (500 MHz, MeOD) δ 7.32–7.24 (m, 1H), 7.23–7.14 (m, 1H), 4.63 (dd, J = 8.2, 5.2 Hz, 1H), 4.34 (dd, J = 9.1, 4.8 Hz, 1H), 3.63 (d, J = 6.2 Hz, 1H), 3.19 (dd, J = 14.0, 5.3 Hz, 1H), 3.02 (ddd, J = 8.4, 7.4, 4.4 Hz, 1H), 2.17 (dq, J = 13.6, 6.8 Hz, 1H), 1.8 (ddd, J = 14.3, 10.8, 5.9 Hz, 1H), 1.73–1.60 (m, 1H), 1.51–1.32 (m, 3H), 1.05 (t, J = 7.4 Hz, 1H). ^{13}C NMR (125 MHz, MeOD) δ 173.14, 172.67, 168.12, 157.18, 136.98, 128.98, 128.05, 126.39, 78.51, 88.49, 53.99, 53.38, 39.66, 36.85, 31.57, 29.99, 29.12, 27.38, 22.84, 17.65, 16.55. EI-MS: m/z 493.10 (M$^+$); HR-EI-MS calcd. for $C_{25}H_{39}O_6N_4$: 491.2875 (M$^-$), found: 491.2877.

H-D-*Val*-L-*Lys(Boc)*-L-*Tyr*-OH (**5**). White solid. ^{1}H NMR (500 MHz, MeOD) δ 7.07 (d, J = 8.5 Hz, 1H), 4.56 (dd, J = 8.0, 5.1 Hz, 1H), 4.34 (dd, J = 9.0, 4.5 Hz, 1H), 3.86–3.73 (m, 9H), 3.73–3.67 (m, 4H), 3.66–3.57 (m, 5H), 3.14–2.80 (m, 2H), 2.17 (dd, J = 13.4, 6.7 Hz, 1H), 1.80 (dd, J = 14.3, 8.2 Hz, 1H), 1.72–1.61 (m, 1H), 1.05 (dd, J = 8.3, 7.1 Hz, 3H). ^{13}C NMR (125 MHz, MeOD) δ 155.92, 150.16, 129.99, 114.80, 71.63, 70.00, 63.75, 58.50, 54.25, 53.39, 36.11, 31.59, 29.99, 29.13, 27.38, 22.84, 17.66, 16.54. EI-MS: m/z 509.05 (M$^+$); HR-EI-MS calcd. for $C_{25}H_{39}O_7N_4$: 507.2824 (M$^-$), found: 507.2825.

H-D-*Val*-L-*Lys(Boc)*-D-*Pro*-OH (**6**). White solid. ^{1}H NMR (500 MHz, MeOD) δ 5.05 (t, J = 5.5 Hz, 1H), 4.71 (dd, J = 8.9, 4.9 Hz, 2H), 4.47–4.39 (m, 2H), 4.35 (dd, J = 9.7, 4.2 Hz, 1H), 3.91 (dd, J = 10.8, 6.0 Hz, 2H), 3.64 (dt, J = 9.5, 4.7 Hz, 4H), 3.49 (ddd, J = 19.1, 11.3, 6.0 Hz, 1H), 3.10–2.95 (m, 4H), 2.32–2.24 (m, 2H), 2.22–2.14 (m, 2H), 2.11–2.00 (m, 5H), 1.94 (dd, J = 15.0, 7.6 Hz, 1H), 1.8 (dd, J = 16.2, 7.0 Hz, 2H), 1.67 (ddd, J = 14.0, 11.6, 6.8 Hz, 2H), 1.13 0 0.97 (m, 14H). ^{13}C NMR (125 MHz, MeOD) δ 173.93, 171.00, 167.96, 157.19, 78.48, 59.62, 59.22, 58.49, 58.31, 39.50, 30.57, 29.14, 28.83, 27.38, 24.20, 22.74, 22.03, 17.69, 16.54. EI-MS: m/z 443.05 (M$^+$); HR-EI-MS calcd. for $C_{21}H_{37}O_6N_4$: 441.2718 (M$^-$), found: 441.2720.

H-D-*Val*-L-*Arg*-D-*Val*-OH (**7**). White solid. ^{1}H NMR (500 MHz, MeOD) δ 4.58 (dd, J = 7.9, 6.0 Hz, 1H), 4.32 (d, J = 5.6 Hz, 1H), 3.85–3.77 (m, 2H), 3.77 (s, 1H), 3.69 (q, J = 5.7 Hz, 2H), 3.63 (dd, J = 11.1, 5.9 Hz, 1H), 3.26–3.14 (m, 3H), 2.19 (dqd, J = 13.7, 6.9, 4.0 Hz, 2H), 1.94–1.81 (m, 1H), 1.81–1.53 (m, 4H), 1.06 (dd, J = 8.6, 7.0 Hz, 7H), 0.98 (dd, J = 6.8, 4.2 Hz, 8H). ^{13}C NMR (125 MHz, MeOD) δ 171.95, 168.26, 157.24, 71.63, 70.01, 63.75, 58.43, 57.90, 40.56, 30.39, 30.03, 29.42, 25.21, 16.29, 17.60, 16.54. EI-MS: m/z 373.10 (M$^+$); HR-EI-MS calcd. for $C_{16}H_{33}O_4N_6$: 373.2557 (M$^+$), found: 373.2557.

H-D-*Val*-L-*Lys*-L-*Ala*-OH (**8**). White solid. ^{1}H NMR (400 MHz, MeOD) δ 4.41 (dd, J = 11.8, 6.0 Hz, 1H), 3.71 (d, J = 6.2 Hz, 1H), 2.92 (t, J = 7.5 Hz, 1H), 2.20 (dq, J = 13.4, 6.6 Hz, 1H), 1.90 (tq, J = 14.0, 7.4 Hz, 1H), 1.74 (ddd, J = 23.2, 15.0, 7.8 Hz, 2H), 1.54 (dd, J = 15.0, 7.5 Hz, 1H), 1.39 (dd, J = 36.4, 19.5 Hz, 2H), 1.16–0.97 (m, 3H). EI-MS: m/z 317.20 (M$^+$); HR-EI-MS calcd. for $C_{14}H_{29}O_4N_4$: 317.2183 (M$^+$), found: 317.2178.

3.3. Cellular Culture and Drug Treatment

Human umbilical vein endothelial cellular (HUVEC) cells were obtained from ScienCell Research Laboratories, Inc. (San Diego, CA, USA). (CAT. 8000). HUVECs were cultured in M199 medium with 100 µg/mL penicillin-streptomycin, 30 µg/mL endothelial cellular growth supplement and 10% FBS in 75 cm^2 tissue culture flasks at 37 °C in a humidified atmosphere of 5% CO_2. Compounds were dissolved in DMSO to make a 200 µM stock solution and were then diluted to different concentrations as needed.

3.4. Proliferative Assays

HUVECs were seeded onto 96-well gelatin coated plates at a density of 10^4 cells/well. In order to achieve a quiescent state, complete medium was replaced after 24 h incubation with low serum (0.5% FBS) medium and re-incubated for 24 h. After this, the medium was replaced with various drug treatments diluted in low serum (0.5% FBS) medium. DMSO (0.1%) and VEGF (20 ng/mL) served as negative and positive controls, respectively. In accordance with the manufacturer's protocol, plates were incubated for an additional 48 h and cellular proliferation was assessed by the MTT, which is widely used to observe the growth of cell. The spectrophotometric absorbance of each well was measured. The wavelengths used to measure absorbance of the formazan product were 570 nm and 630 nm. The results were expressed as the percentage of proliferating cells.

3.5. Migration Assays

HUVEC migration assays were performed using the wound healing method. The HUVECs (3×10^5 cells) were seeded into each well of a 24-well plate and incubated with complete medium at 37 °C and 5% CO_2. After 24 h of incubation, cells were starved for additional 24 h by low serum (0.5% FBS) medium. The HUVECs were then scraped away horizontally in each well using a P100 pipette tip. Three randomly selected views along the scraped line were photographed on each well using an Olympus ix53 microscope (Olympus, Tokyo, Japan) and the CCD camera attached to the microscope at $10\times$ magnification. The medium was then changed to fresh low serum (1% FBS) medium with compounds **1** and **5–7** (50 μM) or with DMSO. After incubation (0 h, 12 h, 24 h, 36 h and 48 h), another set of images were taken by the same method. Image analysis for signs of migration was performed by Metamorph Imaging Series (Molecular Devices, LLC., San Jose, CA, USA). The average scraped area of each well under each condition was measured and subtracted from that of the before-treatment condition. Data are expressed as percentage wound closure relative to the wound closure area in the control medium. The wound closure area of the control cells was set at 100%.

3.6. Invasion Assay

HUVEC invasion assay was carried out following previous methods [13]. Briefly, the effect of compounds **1** and **5–7** on HUVEC invasion was measured using the 10 mm tissue culture insert (transwell permeable supports, Corning Incorporated, Tewksbury, MA, USA) with polycabonate membarane (8 mm pores) and 24-well companion plate. The upper side and lower side of the membrane were pre-coated with 1:30 (v/v) of Matrigel (Corning Incorporated, Tewksbury, MA, USA). The HUVECs were resuspended in low serum (1% FBS) medium and seeded onto the culture inserts at 5×10^4 cells per insert in triplicate. They were then deposited into the 24-well companion plate with 500 μL of low serum (1% FBS) medium containing compounds (50 μM) in the presence. In addition, the wells of the companion plate, containing DMSO (0.1%), served as a vehicle control. The inserts were removed after 8 h of incubation and were then washed with PBS. Non-invasive cells on the upper surface of the membrane were removed by wiping with cotton swabs. The inserts were fixed in paraformaldehyate, stained with DAPI and mounted on a microscope and a CCD camera. Following this, HUVECs per insert were examined with the software Metamorph Imaging Series (Molecular Devices, Tokyo, Japan).

3.7. Zebrafish Assay of Compound **7**

Zebrafish embryos were used to examine the effect of different compounds on embryonic angiogenesis. Compound **7** was added to embryo water from 24 hpf. Zebrafish embryos were generated by natural pairwise mating and raised at 28.5 °C in embryo water. Embryos were maintained in embryo water at 28 °C. Three embryos were placed into each well of a 96-well plate containing 200 μL embryo water with or without the drug. The blood vessel development using an inverted Olympus DP70 epifluorescence microscope (Olympus, Tokyo, Japan). Because the fish embryo receives nourishment from an attached yolk ball for the duration of the experiment, no additional maintenance was required during the duration of the experiments. After 72 hpf, the embryos were anesthetized using 0.05% 2-phenoxyethanol in embryo water, and each embryo was examined for the presence of ectopic vessels in the subintestinal vessel plexus (SIV). The experiments of zebrafish were conducted according to the guidelines for animal care and use of China and were approved by the animal ethics committee of the Chinese Academy of Medical Science (Beijing, China).

PTK787 is frequently used as angiogenesis inhibitors [18]. In order to test the effect of compound **7** on damaged zebrafish, we evaluated a quantitative assay in transgenic zebrafish using angiogenesis inhibitor PTK787. The 24 hpf embryos were cultured and collected. The inhibitor, PTK787 (0.03 μg/mL) was added into embryo water and the embryo were cultured 24 h. Subsequently, compound **7** was added into embryo water afer removing the PTK787 and cultured for 24 h. After 72 hpf, the embryos were anesthetized using 0.05% 2-phenoxyethanol in embryo water, and each embryo was examined for the presence of ectopic vessels in the subintestinal vessel plexus (SIV).

3.8. Statistical Analysis

Statistical analysis was performed using SPSS Statistics 21 software (IBM corporation, Armonk, NY, USA). Survival curves were analyzed by the life table method and evaluation of the effects of compounds on the mean survival time was done by the Wilcoxon rank sum test. All the curves and column diagrams were drawn using GraphPad Prism 6 software (GraphPad Software, Inc., San Diego, CA, USA). Data are expressed as the mean $\pm$ SEM. Statistical comparisons between groups were performed using one-way ANOVA followed by Dunnett's *t*-test using non-treatment as the control group. $p < 0.05$ was considered statistically significant.

4. Conclusions

In summary, seven compounds have been designed and synthesized to evaluate the proliferation, migration and invasion of HUVECs by MTT assays, based on the lead compound **1**, which was demonstrated significantly stimulate angiogenesis both in vivo and in vitro. Among these analogues, compounds **5–7** possess remarkable proliferations, migrations and invasions of HUVECs compared with the lead compound 1. The results show that hydrophilic, alkaline group, L-Tyrosine and D-Proline fragment substituting for L-alanine may greatly contribute to proliferation of HUVECs. To our surprise, compound **7** exerted a significant effect on HUVECs, which revealed that the L-Arg-D-Val fragment resembles Lys(Boc)-L-Ala-OH in terms of cytoactivity. With its good proliferation, compound **7** can promote angiogenesis in zebrafish and can repair blood vessels in PTK787-induced zebrafish at a low concentration. These small molecular peptides could be easily prepared compared the macromolecule proteins. Because of the briefness of their strutures, they would eventually develop into a promising drug candidate for the treatment of damage repair and related diseases.

Supplementary Materials: Figure S1: ^{1}H NMR (MeOD, 500 MHz) of Compound **1**, Figure S2: ^{13}C NMR (MeOD, 125 MHz) of Compound **1**, Figure S3: ^{1}H NMR (MeOD, 500 MHz) of Compound **2**, Figure S4: ^{13}C NMR (MeOD, 125 MHz) of Compound **2**, Figure S5: ^{1}H NMR (MeOD, 500 MHz) of Compound **3**, Figure S6: ^{13}C NMR (MeOD, 125 MHz) of Compound **3**, Figure S7: ^{1}H NMR (MeOD, 500 MHz) of Compound **4**, Figure S8: ^{13}C NMR (MeOD, 125 MHz) of Compound **4**, Figure S9: ^{1}H NMR (MeOD, 500 MHz) of Compound **5**, Figure S10: ^{13}C NMR (MeOD, 125 MHz) of Compound **5**, Figure S11: ^{1}H NMR (MeOD, 500 MHz) of Compound **6**, Figure S12: ^{13}C NMR (MeOD, 125 MHz) of Compound **6**, Figure S13: ^{1}H NMR (MeOD, 500 MHz) of Compound **7**, Figure S14: ^{13}C NMR (MeOD, 125 MHz) of Compound **7**, Figure S15: ^{1}H NMR (MeOD, 400 MHz) of Compound **8**, Table S1: Purities and retention times of all tested compounds, Table S2: HPLC chromatography of compound **1**, Table S3: HPLC chromatography of compound **2**, Table S4: HPLC chromatography of compound **3**, Table S5: HPLC chromatography of compound **4**, Table S6: HPLC chromatography of compound **5**, Table S7: HPLC chromatography of compound **6**, Table S8: HPLC chromatography of compound **7**, Table S9: HPLC chromatography of compound **8**.

Author Contributions: Conceptualization, Y.P. and Y.Z.; methodology, Y.Z. and X.W.; software, J.Z.; validation, J.P., Y.Z. and Y.C.; formal analysis, Y.Z.; investigation, Y.Z. and Y.T.; resources, X.W.; data curation, Y.T.; writing—original draft preparation, Y.Z.; writing—review and editing, J.P.; visualization, Y.Z.; supervision, J.P.; project administration, J.P.; funding acquisition, J.P.

Acknowledgments: This work was supported by the National Natural Science Foundation of China (21172271), the Natural Science Foundation of Guangdong Province, China (Grant No. S2011020001231 and 2017A030313064) and the Major Scientific and Technological Special Project of Administration of Ocean and Fisheries of Guangdong Province (GDME-2018C013).

References

1.   Zhou, X.; Liu, J.; Yang, B.; Lin, X.; Yang, X.W.; Liu, Y. Marine natural products with anti-HIV activities in the last decade. *Curr. Med. Chem.* **2013**, *20*, 953–973. [PubMed]

2.   Edwards, D.J.; Marquez, B.L.; Nogle, L.M. Structure and biosynthesis of the jamaicamides, new mixed polyketide-peptide neurotoxins from the marine cyanobacterium *Lyngbya majuscula*. *Am. Math. Soc.* **2004**, *11*, 817–833. [CrossRef] [PubMed]

3.   Huang, H.N.; Rajanbabu, V.; Pan, C.Y. A cancer vaccine based on the marine antimicrobial peptide pardaxin (GE33) for control of bladder-associated tumors. *Biomaterials* **2013**, *34*, 10151–10159. [CrossRef] [PubMed]

4.   Jang, I.S.; Sun, J.P. Hydroxyproline-containing collagen peptide derived from the skin of the Alaska pollack inhibits HIV-1 infection. *Mol. Med. Rep.* **2016**, *14*, 5489–5494. [CrossRef] [PubMed]

5.   Chopra, L.; Singh, G.; Choudhary, V. Sonorensin: An antimicrobial peptide, belonging to the heterocycloanthracin subfamily of bacteriocins, from a new marine isolate, *Bacillus sonorensis* MT93. *Appl. Environ. Microbiol.* **2014**, *80*. [CrossRef] [PubMed]

6.   Ko, S.C.; Kim, D.; Jeon, Y.J. Protective effect of a novel antioxidative peptide purified from a marine Chlorella ellipsoidea protein against free radical-induced oxidative stress. *Food Chem. Toxicol.* **2012**, *50*, 2294–2302. [CrossRef] [PubMed]

7.   Hyder, S.M.; Stancel, G.M. Regulation of angiogenic growth factors in the female reproductive tract by estrogens and progestins. *Mol. Endocrinol.* **1999**, *13*, 806–811. [CrossRef] [PubMed]

8.   Singla, R.; Soni, S.; Patial, V. Cytocompatible anti-microbial dressings of *Syzygium cumini* cellulose nanocrystals decorated with silver nanoparticles accelerate acute and diabetic wound healing. *Sci. Rep.* **2017**, *7*. [CrossRef]

9.   Suzane, C.P.; Marcell, C.M.; Sybele, S.; Joni, A.C.; Raquel, M.S.C. Role of osteogenic growth peptide (OGP) and OGP (10-14) in bone regeneration: A review. *Mol. Sci.* **2016**, *17*. [CrossRef]

10. Guo, D.; Murdoch, C.E.; Xu, H. Vascular endothelial growth factor signaling requires glycine to promote angiogenesis. *Sci. Rep.* **2017**, *7*. [CrossRef] [PubMed]

11. Lin, Y.; Wu, X.; Feng, S.; Jiang, G.; Zhou, S.; Vrijmoedb, L.L.P.; Gareth Jonesb, E.B. A novel N-cinnamoylcyclopeptide containing an allenic ether from the fungus *Xylaria* sp. (strain #2508) from the South China Sea. *Tetrahedron. Lett.* **2001**, *42*, 449–451.

12. Wang, S.Y.; Xu, Z.L.; Wang, H.; Li, C.R.; Fu, L.W.; Pang, J.Y.; Li, J.; She, Z.G.; Lin, Y.C. Total Synthesis, absolute configuration, and biological activity of xyloallenoide A. *Helv. Chim. Acta* **2012**, *95*, 973–982. [CrossRef]

13. Lu, X.L.; Xu, Z.L.; Yao, X.L. Marine cyclotripeptide X-13 promotes angiogenesis in zebrafish and human endothelial cells via PI3K/Akt/eNOS signaling pathways. *Mar. Drugs* **2012**, *10*, 1307–1320. [CrossRef] [PubMed]

14. Li, J.; Lu, X.; Wu, Q.; Yu, G.; Xu, Z.; Qiu, L.; Pei, Z.; Lin, Y.; Pang, J. Design, SAR, angiogenic activities evaluation and pro-angiogenic mechanism of new marine cyclopeptide analogs. *Curr. Med. Chem.* **2013**, *20*, 1183–1194. [CrossRef] [PubMed]

15. Byung, C.L.; Hyun, J.S.; Ji, S.K.; Kyung-Ho, J.; Yearn, S.C.; Kyung-Han, L.; Dae, Y.C. Synthesis of Tc-99m labeled glucos amino-Asp-cyclic (Arg-Gly-Asp-D-Phe-Lys) as a potential angiogenesis imaging agent. *Bioorg. Med. Chem.* **2007**, *15*, 7755–7764.

16. Park, H.J.; Zhang, Y.; Georgescu, S.P.; Johnson, K.L.; Kong, D.; Galper, J.B. Human umbilical vein endothelial cells and human dermal microvascular endothelial cells offer new insights into the relationship between lipid metabolism and angiogenesis. *Stem Cell Rev.* **2006**, *2*, 93–102. [CrossRef] [PubMed]

17. Yi, F.; Hao, Y.; Chong, X. Overexpression of microRNA-506-3p aggravates the injury of vascular endothelial cells in patients with hypertension by downregulating Beclin1 expression. *Exp. Ther. Med.* **2018**, *15*, 2844–2850. [CrossRef] [PubMed]

18. Tal, T.L.; Mccollum, C.W.; Harris, P.S. Immediate and long-term consequences of vascular toxicity during zebrafish development. *Reprod. Toxicol.* **2014**, *48*, 51–61. [CrossRef] [PubMed]

8

Discovery of Lipid Peroxidation Inhibitors from *Bacopa* Species Prioritized through Multivariate Data Analysis and Multi-Informative Molecular Networking

Tongchai Saesong [1], Pierre-Marie Allard [2], Emerson Ferreira Queiroz [2], Laurence Marcourt [2], Nitra Nuengchamnong [3], Prapapan Temkitthawon [1], Nantaka Khorana [4], Jean-Luc Wolfender [2,*] and Kornkanok Ingkaninan [1,*]

[1] Department of Pharmaceutical Chemistry and Pharmacognosy, Faculty of Pharmaceutical Sciences and Center of Excellence for Innovation in Chemistry, Naresuan University, Phitsanulok 65000, Thailand
[2] School of Pharmaceutical Sciences, EPGL, University of Geneva, University of Lausanne, CMU Rue Michel Servet 1, 1211 Geneva 4, Switzerland
[3] Science Lab Center, Faculty of Science, Naresuan University, Phitsanulok 65000, Thailand
[4] Division of Pharmaceutical Sciences, School of Pharmaceutical Sciences, University of Phayao, Phayao 56000, Thailand
* Correspondence: jean-luc.wolfender@unige.ch (J.-L.W.); k_ingkaninan@yahoo.com (K.I.)

Academic Editor: Pinarosa Avato

Abstract: A major goal in the discovery of bioactive natural products is to rapidly identify active compound(s) and dereplicate known molecules from complex biological extracts. The conventional bioassay-guided fractionation process can be time consuming and often requires multi-step procedures. Herein, we apply a metabolomic strategy merging multivariate data analysis and multi-informative molecular maps to rapidly prioritize bioactive molecules directly from crude plant extracts. The strategy was applied to 59 extracts of three *Bacopa* species (*B. monnieri*, *B. caroliniana* and *B. floribunda*), which were profiled by UHPLC-HRMS^2 and screened for anti-lipid peroxidation activity. Using this approach, six lipid peroxidation inhibitors **1–6** of three *Bacopa* spp. were discovered, three of them being new compounds: monnieraside IV (**4**), monnieraside V (**5**) and monnieraside VI (**6**). The results demonstrate that this combined approach could efficiently guide the discovery of new bioactive natural products. Furthermore, the approach allowed to evidence that main semi-quantitative changes in composition linked to the anti-lipid peroxidation activity were also correlated to seasonal effects notably for *B. monnieri*.

Keywords: metabolomics; multivariate data analysis; molecular network; *Bacopa monnieri*; LC-MS

1. Introduction

Natural products (NPs) play an important role as a source of various pharmaceuticals and biologically active substances. However, the discovery of new bioactive NPs is challenging because of the inherent complex composition of crude natural extracts. Such extracts contain hundreds, if not thousands, of chemical constituents and the purification and identification of bioactive NPs by conventional methods is a time consuming multi-step procedure. Moreover, bioactive substances can be lost during purification and effort can be wasted in the unnecessary re-isolation of known NPs. Therefore, it is important to pinpoint bioactive candidates and recognize known metabolites (dereplication) early in the purification process in order to avoid the redundant isolation of known molecules [1,2].

Recently, metabolomics combined with multivariate data analysis (MVA) has proven to be an efficient tool to predict bioactive constituents in NP research [3–7]. Metabolomics aims at providing comprehensive qualitative and quantitative analysis of the whole set of metabolites (metabolome) present in a complex biological sample [8,9]. The most used analytical techniques in metabolomics are nuclear magnetic resonance (NMR) and mass spectrometry (MS) [10]. Generally metabolite profiling of natural extracts is achieved via high resolution ultra-high performance liquid chromatography (UHPLC), coupled to high resolution tandem mass spectrometry (HRMS^2), which provides molecular formula and fragmentation information on most NPs in extracts in an untargeted manner [11]. Unsupervised or supervised multivariate data analysis such as principal components analysis (PCA) or orthogonal partial least squares (OPLS) are then needed to mine such data and highlight biomarkers. Alternative strategies have been developed to explore LC-HRMS^2 metabolite profiling datasets with the aim of highlighting structural similarities between analytes and efficiently identify new compounds with potential therapeutic interest. Molecular network analysis (MN) [12,13] is a computer-based approach allowing the organization of fragmentation spectra from MS-based metabolomics experiments in order to dereplicate and eventually prioritize natural products of interest [14–16]. MN is generated based on the similarities of fragmentation patterns and, thus, indirectly allows the grouping of analytes with closely related structures. Networks can be built using the Global Natural Product Social Molecular Networking (GNPS) platform [17] or software such as Metgem or MS-Dial [18,19].

Bacopa is a genus of aquatic plants belonging to the Plantaginaceae family. Three species occur in Thailand: *B. monnieri*, *B. caroliniana* and *B. floribunda* [20]. Among them, only *B. monnieri* (Brahmi) has been reported as a herbal medicine in Ayurvedic medicine for learning and memory improvement [21]. The safety and efficacy of Brahmi extracts in animal models [22,23] and in clinical trials [24–28] have been proven and support its traditional uses. Intake of Brahmi has been reported to exert undesirable effects on the gastrointestinal tract, such as nausea, increased stool frequency and abdominal cramps [25,29], which might be explained by a cholinergic effect [30]. In addition, severe liver toxicity has been detected in women taking Brahmi products for vitiligo disease. Nevertheless, their liver function returned to normal after discontinuation of products' usage [31]. Other reports however indicated that Brahmi possessed hepatoprotective activity [32,33]. Notwithstanding such adverse effects and considering the positive effects of the plant in relation with cognition improvements, further investigations are still worth to identify bioactive principles.

The compounds responsible for the memory enhancing effects of Brahmi have been reported to be triterpenoid saponins i.e., bacoside A$_3$, bacopaside I, bacopaside II, bacopasaponin C and bacopaside X [34,35]. They are considered as markers of Brahmi [36–41], and their level is assessed for quality control purposes. Usually, the level of plant specialized metabolites is highly variable according to environmental factors. In Brahmi, the levels of such markers were found to vary significantly depending on the part of used (leaves, stems, shoots etc.), collection area and season [42–45].

Moreover, this plant also contains other classes of NPs such as sterols [46], flavonoids [47] and phenylethanoids [48,49] that may play roles in the pharmacological activities of the plant. It has also been reported that part of the neuroprotective effects of Brahmi appeared to result from its antioxidant activities that suppress neuronal oxidative stress. Brahmi has been found to inhibit the lipid peroxidation reaction of brain homogenate in a dose-dependent manner [50].

In this study, we aimed at searching for compounds that could be involved in the memory improvement activity of Brahmi through lipid peroxidation inhibitory activity. In addition, the anti-lipid peroxidation activity of two other *Bacopa* species has been investigated. To achieve these goals, a metabolomic strategy combining multivariate data analysis (MVA) and bioactivity informed molecular maps [14] was used as a guide to highlight bioactive constituents early in the phytochemical study process and directly target their isolation.

2. Results and Discussion

Fifty-nine extracts of three *Bacopa* species from different regions of Thailand and harvested at various seasons [summer (March to June), rainy season (July to October) and winter (November to February)] were collected for this study. All extracts were profiled by UHPLC-HRMS^2 to generate data that could be used to monitor metabolite profile variations across the whole dataset and provide high quality data dependent MS^2 spectra for annotation. In parallel, all of the extracts were screened for their anti-lipid peroxidation activity. Variations in the profiles were then linked to bioactivity modulation through MVA in order to highlight possible bioactive metabolites. In addition, the MS^2 dataset was organized using the GNPS platform to generate a MN, which was visualized using Cytoscape software. The bioactivity and taxonomy of plant extracts were mapped on the MN in order to pinpoint cluster(s) of potentially bioactive metabolite(s). The lists of prioritized candidates from MVA and MN were finally compared and the common metabolites were then selected as bioactive candidates. They were annotated based on their MS^2 spectra compared with experimental or in silico MS/MS database (GNPS libraries and DNP–ISDB). Both known and possibly novel compounds were isolated to establish their bioactivities and their structures were unambiguously determined by NMR. A summary of the prioritization workflow is presented in Figure 1.

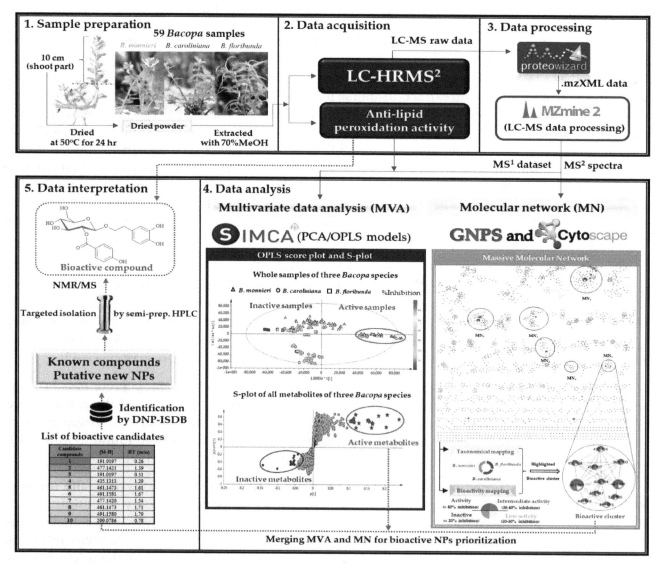

Figure 1. Schematic diagram of lipid peroxidation inhibitor discovery from LC-HRMS^2 analyses of 59 *Bacopa* extracts combining metabolomics MVA and multi-informative MN.

2.1. Lipid Peroxidation Inhibitory Activity Evaluation of the Extracts

The fifty-nine extracts of three *Bacopa* species collected from different regions of Thailand in rainy season, winter and summer were submitted to a thiobarbituric acid reactive substances (TBAR) assay. A significant variation of lipid peroxidation inhibitory activities between groups of related samples was observed (Figure 2A–C). In particular, *B. monnieri* harvested in summer (Figure 2C) exhibited stronger inhibitory effects (around 2-fold) than *B. monnieri* collected in other seasons or than other *Bacopa* species.

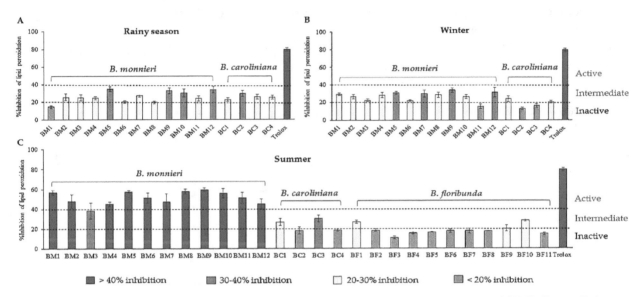

Figure 2. Anti-lipid peroxidation activities of three *Bacopa* species i.e., *B. monnieri* (BM), *B. caroliniana* (BC), and *B. floribunda* plant (BF) collected from different regions in the (**A**) rainy, (**B**) winter and (**C**) summer seasons. Samples giving >40% inhibition were considered active, 30-40% inhibition was intermediate activity, 20-30% inhibition was low activity, and those exhibiting <20% inhibition were considered inactive. Trolox (100 µg/mL) was used as a positive control.

2.2. Potential Bioactive Metabolites Prioritized through Multivariate Statistical Analysis and Molecular Networking

2.2.1. Organization and Pre–Treatment of the Metabolite Profiling Data

All extracts that were screened for bioactivity were profiled by UHPLC-HRMS^2 using a generic gradient in negative ionization (NI) mode to provide MS^1 and MS^2 data of all metabolites in the *Bacopa* samples. The NI mode was used because it provided far more molecular ion features than the positive ionization (PI) mode for the samples considered. This was in good agreement with the rich polyphenolic content of *Bacopa* species.

After profiling, the LC–HRMS^2 data was treated by MZmine [51] for mass detection, chromatogram building, deconvolution, isotopic peak grouping, alignment and gap filling. This resulted in a peaklist of 6082 features which was further filtered to a peaklist of 4191 features having associated MS^2 spectra. This peaklist of 4191 features was exported as input for the MVA (MS^1 data only) and for MN generation (MS^1 and MS^2 data). These data were correlated to the extract's bioactivity results in order to highlight bioactive compounds responsible for anti–lipid peroxidation in *Bacopa* species.

2.2.2. Multivariate Data Analysis

As a preliminary step, the whole MS^1 dataset (consisting of *m/z* values, retention times (RT), and intensities) was analyzed by principal component analysis (PCA) to investigate the differences of metabolite profiles of three *Bacopa* species and the effects on quality of regional cultivation and seasonal harvesting of BM and BC samples. The PCA scatter plot (normalized by Pareto-scaling) is presented in Figure 3A. It showed obvious discrimination among *B. monnieri* (BM), *B. caroliniana* (BC) and *B. floribunda* (BF), exhibiting 65.50% of the total variance in the dataset (46.10% of the variance for PC1 and 19.40% for PC2). This plot exhibited obvious inter–species variations, while intra–species variation of BM and BC samples could only be observed in the PCA plots generated from the individual datasets of BM and BC (Figure 3B,C). Interestingly, the PCA plot of the BM dataset showed a clear separation between BM samples collected in summer versus those harvested in the rainy season and winter (Figure 3B). For BC, the samples were clustered into three groups, according to the harvesting season (Figure 3C). These results demonstrated that the metabolite profiles of BM and BC in different seasons were different and could thus impact the bioactivity of these samples. Therefore, notably for BM, which is used as a food supplement, the harvesting season clearly needs to be taken in consideration to favor the sought-after bioactivity. On the other hand, the PCA plots indicated that the sample composition did not seem to be affected by the region of provenance.

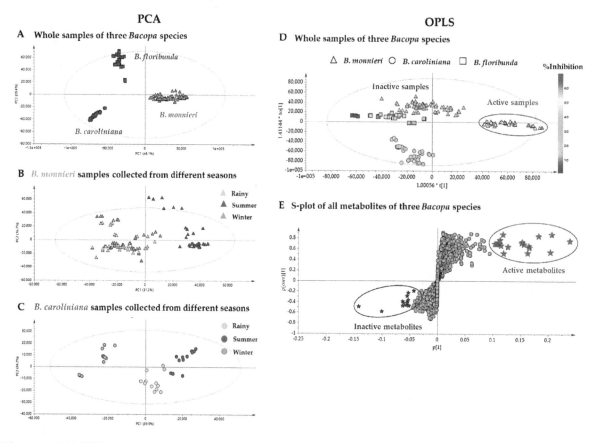

Figure 3. (**A**) PCA score plot based on chemical profiles of 59 extracts of three *Bacopa* species. (**B,C**) PCA score plots based on chemical profiles of 36 extracts of *B. monnieri* and 12 extracts of *B. caroliniana*, respectively from different sources in three seasonal collections. (**D**) OPLS score plot based on the chemical profiles and anti-lipid peroxidation activity of all *Bacopa* extracts. (**E**). S-plot presenting nineteen candidate active features with high p[1] values (red filled star) and inactive features with low p[1] value (blue filled star).

In order to correlate the variations observed in bioactivities with the metabolite profiles of all extracts, the data was analyzed by a supervised method (OPLS), which is a regression extension of PCA allowing maximization of the separation between groups of observations and pinpointing of variables contributing to the separation. The peaklist consisting of *m/z* values, RT, and intensities was used as X variables (similarly to what had been done for PCA) and the %inhibitions of lipid peroxidation were used as the Y variables. A significant separation between the active and the inactive groups was observed, as shown in the OPLS score plot (Figure 3D), where a reddish color represents a high %lipid peroxidation inhibition. As expected from the initial screening results (see Figure 2), all samples exhibiting an activity higher than 40% were grouped (BM samples collected in summer). From the S-plot of all metabolites in the *Bacopa* samples (Figure 3E), 19 features at the upper right corner (highlighted with red stars) were identified as the most discriminating features between the active and non-active samples, and were thus potentially responsible for the observed anti-lipid peroxidation effects. In contrast, the features at the lower left corner corresponded to metabolites that were likely non-actives. These nineteen features with high p[1] values were thus ranked as putative bioactive features (Table 1). Using the *m/z* and RT of each feature (labeled **F–n°** in the Table 1), we found that seventeen features corresponded to unique compounds and that two other features, **F2** and **F8** were adduct and dimer forms of **F18** and **F3**, respectively. Therefore, seventeen bioactive candidates were prioritized from the S-plot. In parallel to this MVA treatment, the same dataset was explored using the multi-informative MN strategy.

2.2.3. Multi-Informational Molecular Map

Multi-informative MN is a strategy that has previously been demonstrated to effectively prioritize bioactive compounds in natural extract collections [14]. For this, the MS^1–MS^2 peaklist was analyzed using such approach in order to visually highlight the clusters of compounds possibly responsible for the observed anti-lipid peroxidation activity. Here, the 4191 features presenting MS^2 were organized using the GNPS platform to generate a single MN. In this MN, the nodes representing each feature were grouped into 602 clusters by similarity of fragmentation patterns. A multi-informational molecular map was created by merging this MN with biological results and taxonomical information (Figure 4A). All nodes in the MN were color-labeled according to the corresponding lipid peroxidation inhibition level of the extracts (bioactive mapping). This allowed a rapid highlighting of potential bioactive molecular families. Additionally, a taxonomical mapping was applied. The species were differentiated by colored tags on the border of each node (Figure 4A). This additional layout was used to indicate the distribution of plant species for each node. If a given node was most abundantly found in bioactive species, it could be hypothesized that this node was potentially related to an NP responsible for the observed bioactivity of the extract of the corresponding species. Using such mapping, twenty putative bioactive clusters with a minimum of five nodes, corresponding to more than a hundred features were selected by visual inspection based on their dominant red color tags indicating presence in bioactive extracts (Figure S1). The colors of the border (taxonomical origin mapping) suggested that the active nodes were mainly found in *B. monnieri*, while only a few were related to other species. The size of the nodes was based on the MS intensity, which was obtained from an average of the corresponding signal across all samples. In a MN, molecular families tend to cluster together, thus leading to similar ionization behaviours within clusters. Consequently, we hypothesized that the MS intensity of these molecules within a cluster was indicative of their relative abundance. According to this logic, five bioactive clusters (MN_1–MN_5, Figure 4B), were further prioritized based on the five largest nodes, leading to a selection of 25 potential bioactive features (Table 1). Among these, seventeen features corresponded to unique molecules, whereas the other neighboring nodes connected to these features were dimeric or adduct forms. Thus, seventeen compounds from MN_1-MN_5 were considered as bioactive candidates from MN (Table 1). An example of unprioritized cluster (MN_6), potentially linked to non-active metabolites, with dominant grey color tags is also shown in Figure 4C for comparison purposes.

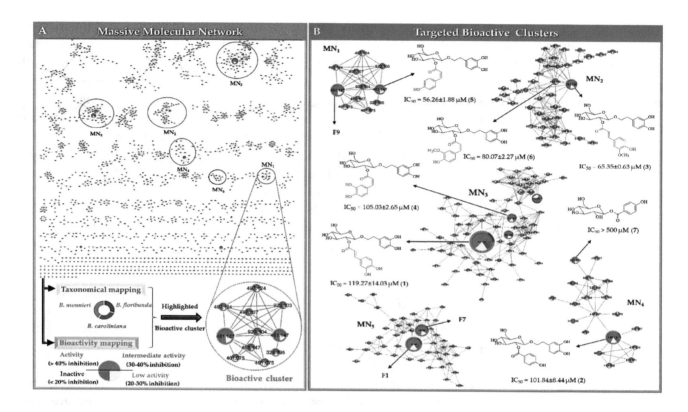

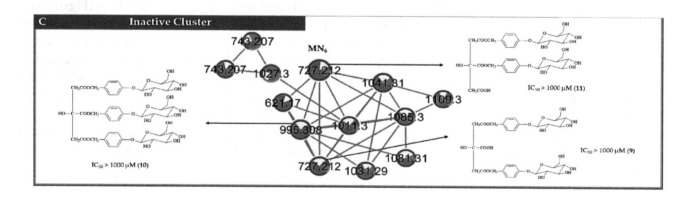

Figure 4. Multi-informational molecular map obtained from the analyses of 59 extracts of three *Bacopa* species mapping with taxonomy and anti-lipid peroxidation activity. Taxonomies of the samples are shown in different colors on the border of each node. Green, blue and purple represent BM, BC and BF, respectively. Bioactivities of the samples are shown in different colors inside each node. The active extracts with an inhibition higher than 40% are represented in red and inactive extracts with less than 40% inhibition are represented in gray. The size of each node is based on the peak height intensity. (**A**) A multi-informative massive molecular network created from MS^2 datasets. (**B**) Five selected bioactive clusters, MN_1-MN_5 with two potential candidates in each cluster, (**C**) an inactive cluster, MN_6. Chemical structures of the active compounds in Figure 4B,C are expressed with IC$_{50}$ values of anti-lipid peroxidation activity.

Table 1. The nineteen bioactive candidate features (**F1–F19**) ranked by p[1] value from S-plot of MVA and twenty-five bioactive candidates selected from prioritized clusters of MN (MN_1–MN_5). Ten potential bioactive compounds prioritized from the merging of MVA and MN approach are highlighted (one color per cluster). IC_{50} values of the compounds on anti-lipid peroxidation activity are expressed in µM and as an average from triplicate experiments ± standard deviation.

ID	m/z	RT (min)	p[1] Value*	Selected Bioactive Cluster	Chemical Formula	Δ ppm	Dereplicated Compounds (MSMS Based Identification)**	Isolated Compounds (NMR Identification)	Anti-Lipid Peroxidation Activity (IC_{50} (µM))
F1	191.0197[M – H]⁻	0.25	0.239	MN_5	$C_6H_8O_7$	0.14	Idaric acid-1,4-lactone		
F2	217.0487[M + Cl]⁻	0.23	0.207	NS	$C_6H_{14}O_6$	-1.20	Adduct of F18		
F3	477.1420[M – H]⁻	1.38	0.204	MN_3	$C_{23}H_{26}O_{11}$	-3.91	Plantainoside B[b]	Plantainoside B (1)	119.27 ± 14.03
F4	377.0873[M – H]⁻	0.24	0.183	NS	$C_{18}H_{18}O_9$	1.08	4,8-Dihydroxy-1,2,3,6,7-pentamethoxy-9H-xanthen-9-one		
F5	315.1099[M – H]⁻	0.60	0.166	NS	$C_{14}H_{20}O_8$	-4.31	2-(3,5-Dihydroxyphenyl)ethanol-3'-O-β-D-glucopyranoside	3,4-dihydroxyphenethyl glucoside (8)	>500
F6	435.1313[M – H]⁻	1.28	0.165	MN_4	$C_{21}H_{24}O_{10}$	-3.74	Monnieraside III[a]	Monnieraside III (2)	101.84 ± 8.44
F7	191.0197[M – H]⁻	0.31	0.163	MN_5	$C_6H_8O_7$	0.14	Idaric acid-1,4-lactone isomer		
F8	955.2917[2M – H]⁻	1.38	0.156	MN_3	$C_{23}H_{26}O_{11}$	-4.91	Dimer of F3		
F9	461.1473[M – H]⁻	1.60	0.154	MN_1	$C_{23}H_{26}O_{10}$	-4.29	8-O-(6'-O-trans-Coumaroyl-β-D-glucopyranosyl)-3,4-dihydroxyphenylethanol		
F10	491.1580[M – H]⁻	1.67	0.152	MN_2	$C_{24}H_{28}O_{11}$	-4.51	Monnieraside II[a]	Monnieraside II (3)	65.35 ± 0.63
F11	1063.4467[M – H]⁻	3.07	0.128	NS	$C_{49}H_{76}O_{23}S$	-3.92	Unidentified[c]		
F12	477.1420[M – H]⁻	1.53	0.119	MN_3	$C_{23}H_{26}O_{11}$	-3.91	Plantainoside B[b]	Monnieraside IV[e] (4)	105.03 ± 2.65
F13	219.0458[M – H]⁻	0.23	0.118	NS	$C_{15}H_8O_2$	-3.41	Unidentified[c]		
F14	461.1473[M – H]⁻	1.71	0.115	MN_1	$C_{23}H_{26}O_{10}$	-4.29	8-O-(6'-O-trans-Coumaroyl-β-D-glucopyranosyl)-3,4-dihydroxyphenylethanol	Monnieraside V[e] (5)	56.26 ± 1.88
F15	491.1579[M – H]⁻	1.78	0.113	MN_2	$C_{24}H_{28}O_{11}$	-4.31	Monnieraside II[a]	Monnieraside VI[e] (6)	80.07 ± 2.27
F16	977.4458[M – H]⁻	3.00	0.112	NS	$C_{46}H_{74}O_{20}S$	-3.75	Bacopaside I[a]		>1000[f]
F17	299.0786[M – H]⁻	0.78	0.110	MN_4	$C_{13}H_{16}O_8$	-4.54	4-Hydroxybenzoyl glucose[b]	4-hydroxybenzoyl glucose (7)	>500
F18	181.0717[M – H]⁻	0.23	0.107	NS	$C_6H_{14}O_6$	-0.21	Mannitol[d]		
F19	631.2274[M – H]⁻	0.60	0.104	NS	$C_{46}H_{32}O_3$	0.74	Unidentified[c]		
F20	497.1243[M + Cl]⁻	1.58	0.033	MN_1	$C_{23}H_{26}O_{10}$	-4.63	Adduct of F9		
F21	461.0749[M – H]⁻	1.56	0.003	MN_1	$C_{21}H_{18}O_{12}$	-5.09	3',4',5,7-Tetrahydroxyflavone5-O-β-D-glucurono-pyranoside		
F22	497.1243[M + Cl]⁻	1.71	0.029	MN_1	$C_{23}H_{26}O_{10}$	-4.63	Adduct of F14		
F23	521.1685[M – H]⁻	1.66	0.053	MN_2	$C_{25}H_{30}O_{12}$	-3.93	Aucubigenin-10-O-(4-hydroxy-3- methoxy-cinnamoyl), 1-O-β-D-glucopyranoside[b]		
F24	983.3235[2M – H]⁻	1.67	0.084	MN_2	$C_{24}H_{28}O_{11}$	-4.53	Dimer of F10		
F25	527.1347[M + Cl]⁻	1.67	0.030	MN_2	$C_{24}H_{28}O_{11}$	-4.05	Adduct of F10		
F26	341.0893[M – H]⁻	0.66	0.064	MN_3	$C_{15}H_{18}O_9$	-4.37	Chaenorrhinoside[b]		
F27	477.1421[M – H]⁻	1.62	0.043	MN_3	$C_{23}H_{26}O_{11}$	-3.90	Plantainoside B[b]		
F28	871.2706[2M – H]⁻	1.29	0.077	MN_4	$C_{21}H_{24}O_{10}$	-4.57	Dimer of F6		
F29	471.1084[M + Cl]⁻	1.29	0.033	MN_4	$C_{21}H_{24}O_{10}$	-4.36	Adduct of F6		
F30	599.1642[2M – H]⁻	0.79	0.068	MN_4	$C_{13}H_{16}O_8$	-4.07	Dimer of F17		
F31	421.0046[M – H]⁻	0.31	0.008	MN_5	$C_{17}H_{10}O_{13}$	0.63	Unidentified[c]		
F32	405.0308[M – H]⁻	0.31	0.057	MN_5	$C_{14}H_{14}O_{14}$	0.69	Unidentified[c]		
F33	191.0198[M – H]⁻	0.38	0.027	MN_5	$C_6H_8O_7$	-0.38	Idaric acid-1,4-lactone		
Three isolated inactive compounds selected from inactive cluster (MN_6) of the MN and in S-plot of MVA									
F34	727.2125[M – H]⁻	1.20	-0.026	MN_6	$C_{32}H_{40}O_{19}$	-4.67	Unidentified[c]	Parishin C (9)	>1000
F35	995.3078[M – H]⁻	1.40	-0.037	MN_6	$C_{45}H_{56}O_{25}$	-4.03	Parishin A[d]	Parishin A (10)	>1000
F36	727.2123[M – H]⁻	1.12	-0.060	MN_6	$C_{32}H_{40}O_{19}$	-4.40	Unidentified[c]	Parishin B (11)	>1000

* The values obtained from S-plot of OPLS and ** DNP-ISDB in silico fragmented results unless specified (Top 1 result only are reported). [a,b] The compound has been previously reported in *B. monnieri* and Plantaginaceae family, respectively; [c] No matching with DNP-ISDB or GNPS libraries, [d] Annotated compound from GNPS libraries, [e] New compound and [f] Standard compound. NS: not selected from bioactive clusters (MN_1–MN_5) but from other clusters in MN.

2.2.4. Merging MVA and MN for Bioactive Candidate Prioritization

The S-plot of MVA brings statistical correlation between features and bioactivity but can however be biased by scaling and normalization processes. On the other side, the bioactivity-informed MN approach allows to highlight structural relations between putative bioactive compounds and thus, despite the lack of statistics, allows to indirectly discriminate possible MS artefacts from specialized metabolites features. In order to prioritize unique bioactive molecules from the merging of MVA and MN, common features found in both approaches were highlighted with color tags (see in Table 1) and prioritized as potential bioactive candidates. The two largest nodes found in each five selected clusters (MN$_1$-MN$_5$, Figure 4B) represented features also found in the list of putative bioactive candidates in MVA. Therefore, these ten features (**F1, F3, F6, F7, F9, F10, F12, F14, F15** and **F17**) were prioritized as potential bioactive compounds for this study (Table 1).

2.3. DNP-ISDB Dereplication and Purification of Bioactive Candidates

In the MN, the acquired MS^2 spectra of each node from the whole MN were matched automatically against GNPS spectral libraries and then annotated against an in silico spectral database build from the Dictionary of Natural Products (DNP-ISDB) as previously described [1] thus providing an identification of level 2 [52]. These spectra were subsequently matched against with a subset of the DNP-ISDB restricted to Plantaginaceae specialized metabolites in order to refine the dereplication results. The top five candidate structures with highest spectral similarity scores were retrieved and the chemical structures for each node was directly visualized within the network using Cytoscape and the ChemViz plugin. The candidate structures for each node were ranked according to their spectral similarity score and the structure with the highest score was reported (Table 1).

Compounds **F1** and **F7** (m/z 191.0197 [M − H]$^-$) were isomers, which were both annotated as idaric acid-1,4-lactone. The other three pairs of isomers i.e., **F3** and **F12** (m/z 477.1421 [M − H]$^-$), **F9** and **F14** (m/z 461.1473 [M − H]$^-$) and **F10** and **F15** (m/z 491.1581 [M − H]$^-$), were proposed to be plantainoside B, 8-O-(6'-O-trans-coumaroyl-β-D-glucopyranosyl)-3,4-dihydroxyphenylethanol and monnieraside II, respectively. The **F6** was predicted to be monnieraside III. The unprioritized features, **F34–36**, did not match with MS^2 spectra libraries from DNP–ISDB, however **F35** was matched against the GNPS spectral library entry parishin A. From these dereplication results, the four pairs of isomers could not be differentiated and two inactive features were given no annotation. Therefore, they may have been new compounds. To establish their structures and evaluate their bioactivity potential, targeted purification of these potential bioactive and inactive compounds was carried out. In order to isolate these compounds, the active extract of *B. monnieri* was fractionated by medium pressure liquid chromatography coupled to an ultraviolet detector (MPLC-UV). The conditions of this separation were first developed by HPLC–UV using a column with identic stationary phase. After this, the analytical HPLC conditions were geometrically transferred to semi–preparative MPLC-UV [53]. All of the MPLC fractions obtained were systematically analyzed by LC-MS. Using the retention time and molecular weight, it was possible to localize the ten potential bioactive candidates (**F1, F3, F6, F7, F9, F10, F12, F14, F15** and **F17**) and three unprioritized features (**F34–36**). MPLC fractions were further purified by semi–preparative HPLC. As for the separation using MPLC, the conditions of the semi–preparative HPLC were first developed in an analytical method using a column with a similar stationary phase chemistry. After this step, the condition was successfully transferred to the semi–preparative HPLC [54] (Figure S2). In order to avoid loss of resolution, the sample was introduced into the semi–preparative HPLC column by dry load according to a recently developed protocol [55]. Thanks to this approach, it was possible to obtain a high–resolution separation of the majority of the polar compounds, allowing them to be obtained in a high degree of purity. Using this system, seven bioactive candidates prioritized by MVA and MN (compounds **1–7**, corresponding to features **F3, F6, F10, F12, F14, F15** and **F17**, respectively) and one compound highlighted MVA only (compound **8**, corresponding to feature **F5**) were isolated. In addition, compounds **9–11** (features **F34–36**), which were all found in a non–prioritized cluster (MN_6, Figure 4C) and in an area of the S-plot indicative of potential inactive compounds (lower left corner, Figure 3E), were also isolated.

2.4. Identification and Structure Elucidation of Compounds 1–11

After purification, all isolated compounds were fully characterized by extensive 2D NMR experiments, which complemented the $HRMS^2$ results. Compounds 1–3 and 7–11, were identified as plantainoside B (1), monnieraside III (2), monnieraside II (3) [48], 4-hydroxybenzoyl glucose (7) [56], 3,4-dihydroxyphenethyl glucoside (8) [57], parishin C (9), parishin A (10) and parishin B (11) [58], respectively, by comparing their spectral data with literature. Compounds 4–6 were isolated for the first time and identified as new phenylethanoid glycosides: monnieraside IV (4), monnieraside V (5), and monnieraside VI (6). The ^1H and ^{13}C-NMR of 4–6 are provided in Table 2 and their COSY, HMBC and ROESY correlations are shown in Figure 5.

Table 2. ^1H- and ^{13}C-NMR (600/151 MHz, in CD_3OD) of 4–6.

Position	Monnieraside IV (4)		Monnieraside V (5)		Monnieraside VI (6)	
	δ_C	δ_H (J in Hz)	δ_C	δ_H (J in Hz)	δ_C	δ_H (J in Hz)
1	131.5		131.3		131.2	
2	117.0	6.61, d (2.1)	116.8	6.62, d (2.1)	116.6	6.61, d (2.1)
3	146.0		145.8		145.8	
4	144.6		144.4		144.3	
5	116.3	6.61, d (8.1)	116.1	6.61, d (8.1)	116.2	6.60, d (8.1)
6	121.4	6.49, dd (8.1, 2.1)	121.1	6.50, dd (8.1, 2.1)	121.1	6.48, dd (8.1, 2.1)
7	36.5	2.68, t (7.2)	36.3	2.68, m	36.3	2.67, t (7.1)
8	71.9	3.64, dt (9.8, 7.2) 4.00, dt (9.8, 7.2)	71.5	3.63, dt (9.4, 7.3) 4.01, dt (9.4, 6.9)	71.6	3.63, dt (9.8, 7.1) 4.00, dt (9.8, 7.1)
1'	102.3	4.45, d (8.1)	102.0	4.44, d (8.1)	102.1	4.46, d (8.0)
2'	74.9	4.79, dd (9.3, 8.1)	74.6	4.79, dd (9.3, 8.1)	74.7	4.79, dd (9.3, 8.0)
3'	76.2	3.51, t (9.3)	75.9	3.50, t (9.3)	76.0	3.52, t (9.3)
4'	71.8	3.38, t (9.3)	71.5	3.38, t (9.3)	71.5	3.38, t (9.3)
5'	78.1	3.29 (overlapped)	77.9	3.28 (overlapped)	77.9	3.30 (overlapped)
6'	62.6	3.69, dd (12.0, 5.7) 3.88, dd (12.0, 2.3)	62.4	3.69, dd (11.9, 5.8) 3.88, dd (11.9, 1.8)	62.4	3.69, dd (12.0, 5.8) 3.88, dd (12.0, 2.3)
1"	128.2		127.6		127.9	
2"	118.7	7.38, d (2.1)	133.4	7.60, d (8.7)	114.8	7.72, d (2.0)
3"	145.7		115.5	6.74, d (8.7)	148.0	
4"	148.3		159.8		149.1	
5"	115.7	6.72, d (8.2)	115.5	6.74, d (8.7)	115.4	6.76, d (8.2)
6"	125.1	7.08, dd (8.2, 2.1)	133.4	7.60, d (8.7)	126.4	7.12, dd (8.2, 2.0)
7"	145.1	6.81, d (12.8)	144.6	6.88 d (12.7)	145.1	6.87, d (12.8)
8"	116.7	5.73, d (12.8)	116.6	5.76, d (12.7)	116.5	5.77, d (12.8)
9"	167.4		167.3		167.1	
OCH_3					56.2	3.85, s

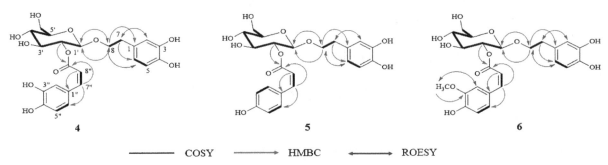

4   5   6

———— COSY   ———→ HMBC   ←——→ ROESY

Figure 5. The COSY, HMBC and ROESY correlations of new compounds 4–6.

The 2D NMR spectra and HRMS spectra are provided as supplementary data (Figures S3–S21). The structures of seven isolated bioactive candidates are displayed on the prioritized clusters in Figure 4B and structure of the three unprioritized compounds are provided in Figure 4C.

Compound **4** was obtained as a white amorphous powder. The HRESIMS of this compound exhibited a deprotonated molecular ion at m/z 477.1420 [M − H]⁻ corresponding to the molecular formula $C_{23}H_{26}O_{11}$ (calcd. 477.1402), indicating an isomer of plantainoside B (**1**). The NMR data of **4** showed close similarities to those of plantainoside B except that the value of the coupling constant between the two ethylenic protons at δ_H 5.73 (H-8″) and 6.81 (H-7″) of 12.8 Hz indicated a *cis*-form for the caffeoyl group in **4**. The structure of **4** was therefore established as 8-*O*-(2′-*O*-*cis*-caffeoyl-β-ᴅ-glucopyranosyl)-3,4-dihydroxyphenylethanol (monnieraside IV).

Compound **5** was obtained as a white amorphous powder and it showed a deprotonated molecular ion at m/z 461.1473 [M − H]⁻, which was consistent with the molecular formula $C_{23}H_{26}O_{10}$ (calcd. 461.1453). The NMR data of **5** exhibited a *para*-disubstituted moiety at δ_H 6.74 (2H, d, J = 8.7 Hz, H-3″, H-5″) and 7.60 (2H, d, J = 8.7 Hz, H-2″, H-6″) instead of the tri-substituted group of the *cis*-caffeoyl of **4**. The 16 Da mass difference between these two compounds was consistent with this NMR observation. The structure of **5** was established as 8-*O*-(2′-*O*-*cis*-coumaroyl-β-ᴅ-gluco-pyranosyl)-3,4-dihydroxyphenylethanol (monnieraside V).

The molecular formula of compound **6** (white amorphous powder) was calculated as $C_{24}H_{28}O_{11}$ by analysis of its HRESIMS (m/z 491.1580 [M − H]⁻, calcd. 491.1559). The NMR data of **6** showed similarities with those of compound **3** (monnieraside II) both of them being isomers. A *cis*-feruoyl group was present in **6**, as confirmed by the coupling constant value of 12.8 Hz between H-7″ and H-8″ protons. The structure of **6** was thus established as 8-*O*-(2′-*O*-*cis*-feruloyl-β-ᴅ-glucopyranosyl)-3,4-dihydroxyphenylethanol (monnieraside VI).

According to DNP-ISDB dereplication results for the eleven isolated compounds (**1-11**), four compounds; plantainoside B (**1**), monnieraside III (**2**), monnieraside II (**3**) and 4-hydroxybenzoyl glucose (**7**) were correctly annotated as confirmed by NMR results (Table 1). Compound **8** was attributed an incorrect structure (2-(3,5-dihydroxyphenyl)ethanol-3′-*O*-β-ᴅ-glucopyranoside) by MS² dereplication, however this annotation was related to the structure later established by NMR (3,4-dihydroxyphenethyl glucoside). In addition, DNP-ISDB dereplication proposed the structure of **F9** and **5** (m/z 461.1473 [M − H]⁻) as 8-*O*-(6′-*O*-*trans*-coumaroyl-β-ᴅ-glucopyranosyl)-3,4-dihydroxy-phenylethanol. However, NMR data of **5** suggested it as 8-*O*-(2′-*O*-*cis*-coumaroyl-β-ᴅ-glucopyranosyl)-3,4-dihydroxyphenylethanol. This indicated that the structure of **F9** could indeed be the dereplicated *trans*–isomer. Furthermore, previous observation showed that the *trans*-isomers of phenylpropanoid derivatives (compounds **1** and **3**) had shorter retention time than their *cis*-isomers counterpart (compounds **4** and **6**). The same phenomenon was also observed for **F9** and **5**. Consequently, **F9** could therefore correspond to as 8-*O*-(2′-*O*-*trans*-coumaroyl-β-ᴅ-glucopyranosyl)-3,4-dihydroxy-phenylethanol. In addition, we found that the annotation against GNPS spectral libraries of compound **10** (parishin A) was correct, as confirmed by NMR structural elucidation. In MN₆, the annotation of node m/z 995.3078 [M − H]⁻ with parishin A and the mass difference of 268.0950 with two neighboring nodes at m/z 727.2121 [M − H]⁻, RT 1.19 min and 727.2124 [M − H]⁻, RT 1.10 min indicated a possible loss of the 4-(β-ᴅ-glucopyranosyloxy)benzyl alcohol moiety (−$C_{13}H_{16}O_6$, calcd. 268.0946) present on parishin A. After isolation and NMR identification structural elucidation, **9** and **11** were indeed found to be parishin C and parishin B, respectively, illustrating the interest of MN for dereplication purposes.

2.5. Evaluation of the Anti-Lipid Peroxidation Activity of the Isolated Compounds

In order to verify the bioactivity potential of the compound prioritized by the combination of MVA and multi-informative MN, the seven isolated compounds were tested for their anti-lipid peroxidation activity with the TBAR assay. Six compounds, **1–6**, showed inhibitory activity with IC₅₀ values < 120 μM and one compound, **7**, had lower activity (IC₅₀ > 500 μM) (Table 1). The positive control (Trolox) showed an IC₅₀ value of 13.92 ± 0.32 μM. For this study, we defined compounds presenting IC₅₀ values not higher than 10-fold of the control's IC₅₀ value as active compounds.

Some prioritized features (**F1, F7** and **F9**) could not be isolated, their bioactivity potential is however discussed according to the following evidences. Features **F1** and **F7** were proposed to be idaric acid-1,4-lactone and its isomer by MS^2. The D enantiomer, D-glucaric-1,4-lactone, has been reported to exert anti-lipid peroxidation and anti-oxidant activities [59]. Compound **F9** was also likely to exhibit anti-lipid peroxidation activity similar to its isomer (**5**), in the same fashion as isomeric compounds **1/4** and **3/6** also shared the same range of anti-lipid peroxidation activity. Given the structure similarity of **1–6**, their inhibitory activities were compared. The activity of the compounds tends to decrease when C3'' was substituted with methoxy (**3, 6**) and hydroxy groups (**1, 4**), respectively (Figure 4B). Such substitutions might reduce the ability of the compounds to protect the oxidation of Fe^{2+} to Fe^{3+} in the lipid peroxidation process.

To verify that the proposed merging of MVA and MN decreased the numbers of false positive candidate compounds, two features **F5** and **F16** (identified to bacopaside I using standard comparison) highlighted by MVA only were assayed. Both showed low levels of activity with IC_{50} values > 500 μM and > 1000 μM, respectively. This indicated that the combination of both prioritization approaches could help to further refine the prioritization process and lower the rate of false positives isolation.

Additionally, three unprioritized compounds **9–11** were isolated and their anti-lipid peroxidation activity assayed. We found that these three compounds displayed very low inhibition of lipid peroxidation with the IC_{50} values > 1000 μM, indicating that the employed strategy was effective to highlight bioactive compounds from complex mixtures of NPs prior to isolation.

Further investigations of ten prioritized bioactive features **F1, F7, F9** and compounds **1–7** revealed that they were differently distributed (% of MS intensities) in the three *Bacopa* species (Figure 6). The highest mean distribution of these compounds was observed in *B. monnieri* (77%), followed by *B. floribunda* (21%). This result agreed with the finding that *B. monnieri* had higher anti-lipid peroxidation activity than *B. floribunda* (Figure 2), suggesting that these compounds are the bioactives responsible for the anti–lipid peroxidation effects observed in *B. monnieri* and *B. floribunda*. Even though *B. caroliniana* presented the lowest level of these active compounds (~2%), it still showed some inhibition of lipid peroxidation, which could indicate the presence of other bioactive compounds in the plant.

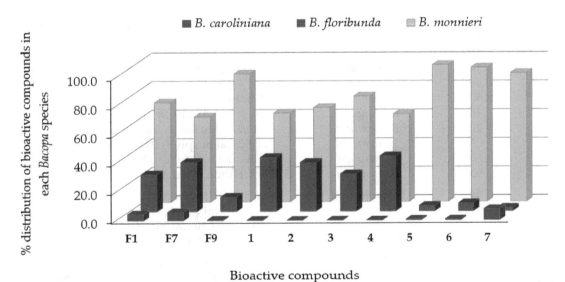

Figure 6. Percentage distribution of ten bioactive compounds in each *Bacopa* species, calculated by division of the average MS signal intensity of the compound in each species by a sum of signal intensities of the compound in three *Bacopa* species ×100.

The biological evaluation of the compounds prioritized by merging MVA and MN, indicated the validity of the approach. However, some bioactive compounds could be missed since the selection in MN was partly based on MS signal intensity, which is non–quantitative and highly dependent on the chemical structure of the analytes. The hyphenation of MS analytical platforms with universal detectors such as evaporative light scattering detector (ELSD) should offer a more accurate view of the precise quantitative repartition of metabolites within complex matrices, hence enhancing the power of MS–based prioritization approaches.

3. Materials and Methods

3.1. Chemicals and Plant Materials

All chemicals used were of analytical grade and obtained from Sigma-Aldrich (St. Louis, MO, USA). All solvents were HPLC and LC-MS grades. Acetonitrile (ACN), methanol (MeOH) and formic acid were purchased from Merck (Darmstadt, Germany). Water was purified by a Milli–Q purification system from Millipore (Bedford, MA, USA).

Three *Bacopa* species i.e., 36 samples of *B. monnieri* (BM1-12), 12 samples of *B. caroliniana* (BC1-4), and 11 samples of *B. floribunda* (BF1 from nature and BF2-11 from tissue culture) were collected from different regions and seasons. Only collected BM and BC samples were planted under the same growing conditions in the Faculty of Pharmaceutical Sciences, Naresuan University and subsequently harvested during different seasons in 2017: January (represented winter), April (summer), and July (rainy season) to enable an evaluation of the effect of these seasonal conditions. These plants species were identified by Dr. Pranee Nangngam and their voucher specimens (Saesong001-17) have been deposited at Department of Biology, Faculty of Science, Naresuan University. The codes and information regarding the samples are presented in Table 3.

Table 3. The geographical details of the *Bacopa* samples collected in this study. Samples 1–16 were collected in 3 seasons i.e., winter, summer, and rainy season (48 samples). Only sample 17 was collected in summer (1 sample). Plant tissue cultures of *B. floribunda* (samples 18–27) were collected in April, 2017 (10 samples).

No.	Code	*Bacopa* spp.	Sources
1	BM1	*B. monnieri*	Perth, Australia
2	BM2	*B. monnieri*	Wat Phra Sri Mahathat, Bangkok, Thailand
3	BM3	*B. monnieri*	Samphan garden, Nakhon Pathom, Thailnd
4	BM4	*B. monnieri*	Naresuan University, Phitsanulok, Thailand
5	BM5	*B. monnieri*	Kasetsart University, Bangkok, Thailand
6	BM6	*B. monnieri*	Nakhon Nayok, Thailand
7	BM7	*B. monnieri*	Chatuchak Market, Bangkok, Thailand
8	BM8	*B. monnieri*	Ayutthaya, Thailand
9	BM9	*B. monnieri*	Fukuoka, Japan (originated in India)
10	BM10	*B. monnieri*	Siriraj hospital, Bangkok, Thailand
11	BM11	*B. monnieri*	Chatuchak Market, Bangkok, Thailand
12	BM12	*B. monnieri*	Phetchabun, Thailand (originated in India)
13	BC1	*B. caroliniana*	Naresuan University, Phitsanulok, Thailand
14	BC2	*B. caroliniana*	Nakhon Nayok, Thailand
15	BC3	*B. caroliniana*	Chiang Mai, Thailand
16	BC4	*B. caroliniana*	Bangkok, Thailand
17	BF1	*B. floribunda*	Sakolnakorn, Thailand
18–27	BF2 to BF11	*B. floribunda*	Plant tissue cultures obtained from Department of Biology, Faculty of Science, Naresuan University

The shoot part (10 cm) of each *Bacopa* sample was collected based on a previous method [45]. Then it was cleaned and dried at 50 °C in a hot air oven for 24 h. The dried plants were crushed and passed through a 60 mesh sieve and stored in plastic containers under refrigeration at −20 °C until used.

3.2. Sample Preparation

Metabolites of *Bacopa* were extracted by adding 1 mL of 70%MeOH to a powdered sample (20 mg). The solution was then sonicated at room temperature for 15 min and filtered through a 0.45 µm nylon filter. Each extract solution was analyzed by UPHLC-HRMS^2 and tested for anti-lipid peroxidation activity in parallel.

3.3. TBAR Assay

Lipid peroxidation inhibitory activity was tested by TBARs assay, with minor modification to a previous study [50]. In this process, 20 µL of sample and 140 µL of homogenate rat brain (contained 5.72 mg/mL total protein) were mixed and incubated at 37 °C for 30 min. Then, 20 µL of 4 mM Fe_2SO_4 and 2 mM ascorbic acid were added to the mixture solution and incubated at 37 °C for 1 h. After incubation, 200 µL of TBARs reagent (40% trichloroacetic acid, 1.4% thiobarbituric acid, and 8% HCl) was added and incubated at 90 °C for 60 min. The mixture was then allowed to cool to room temperature and centrifuged at 10,000 rpm at 4 °C for 5 min to pelletize the precipitated protein. The absorbance of the supernatant was read at 530 nm by a microplate reader (BioTek Instruments, Winooski, Vermont, USA). The inhibition was calculated by comparison with the negative control. The homogenized rat brain in this assay was prepared in 1x PBS buffer (pH 7.4). The protein content in the homogenized rat brain was measured using a bicinchoninic acid (BCA) assay [60].

3.4. UHPLC-ESI-HRMS^2 Analysis

The UHPLC−HRMS^2 was carried out on a Waters Acquity UPLC IClass system system interfaced to a Q-Exactive Focus mass spectrometer (Thermo Scientific, Bremen, Germany), using a heated electrospray ionization (HESI-II) source. Chromatographic separation was performed on a Waters BEH C18 column (50 × 2.1 mm, 1.7 µm), the mobile phase consisted of 0.1% formic acid in water (A) and 0.1% formic acid in acetonitrile (B), the flow rate was 600 µL/min, the injection volume was 1 µL, and the linear gradient elution initially increased from 5–100% B for 7 min, followed by isocratic conditions at 100% B for 1 min, and then decreased to 5% B for the final step for 2 min. The negative ionization mode was applied in this study because the molecular ion peak of the most important metabolites could not be observed in positive ion mode. The optimized HESI-II parameters were set as follows: source voltage, 3.5 kV; sheath gas flow rate (N_2), 48 units; auxiliary gas flow rate, 11 units; spare gas flow rate, 2.0 units; capillary temperature, 300 °C, S-Lens RF Level, 55. The mass analyzer was calibrated using a mixture of caffeine, methionine-arginine-phenylalanine-alanine-acetate (MRFA), sodium dodecyl sulfate, sodium taurocholate, and Ultramark 1621 in an acetonitrile/methanol/water solution containing 1% formic acid by direct injection. The data-dependent MS/MS events were performed on the three most intense ions detected in full scan MS (Top3 experiment). The MS/MS isolation window width was 2 Da, and the normalized collision energy (NCE) was set to 35 units. In data-dependent MS/MS experiments, full scans were acquired at a resolution of 35,000 fwhm (at m/z 200) and MS/MS scans at 17,500 fwhm, both with a maximum injection time of 50 ms. After being acquired in a MS/MS scan, parent ions were placed in a dynamic exclusion list for 3.0 s. All samples were performed by UHPLC-HRMS^2 in one batch and a single pool of all samples was used as a quality control (QC). The QC sample was processed to monitor the reproducibility and stability of the system, which was injected at the beginning, then once every ten tested samples, and at the end of the batch analysis.

3.5. MZmine data preprocessing

The UHPLC−HRMS^2 raw data were converted to .mzXML format using MSConvert software, part of the ProteoWizard package and processed with MZmine version 2.32. Six main steps, consisting in mass detection, chromatogram building, deconvolution, isotopic peak grouping, alignment and gap filling, were carried. The mass detection was set in centroid mode and the noise level was kept at 1×10^6 for MS^1 and 0 for MS^2. The ADAP chromatogram builder was selected and run using a minimum group size in number of scans of 5, minimum height of 1×10^6, and m/z tolerance of 0.001 Da (or 5 ppm). The chromatogram deconvolution was set as follows: wavelets (ADAP) was used as the algorithm for peak recognition, m/z and RT range for MS^2 scan pairing were 0.3 Da and 0.1 min, S/N threshold was 20, minimum feature height was 1×10^6, coefficient/area threshold was 110, peak duration range was 0.01–1.0 min, and the RT wavelets range was 0.001–0.04. Chromatograms were then deisotoped by isotopic peaks a grouper algorithm with a m/z tolerance of 0.001 Da and an RT tolerance of 0.05 min. Peak alignment was carried out using a join aligner, with m/z tolerance set at 0.001 Da, absolute RT tolerance at 0.05 min, and weight for m/z and RT at 30. The missing peaklist after alignment was filled by gap filling of same RT and m/z range gap filler module with a m/z tolerance of 0.001 Da. After gap filling, all peaklists were done with identification of adduct search, complex search, and molecular formula prediction. This resulted in a peaklist of 6082 features which was further filtered to a peaklist of 4191 features having an associated data dependent MS^2 spectra. This resulting peaklist of 4191 features was exported as input for the MVA (MS^1 data only) and for MN generation (MS^1 and MS^2 data).

3.6. Multivariate Analysis

After data treatment with MZmine, a three-dimensional data matrix comprising of retention time, m/z value and peak height were analyzed by SIMCA-P software (version 13.0, Umerics, Umea, Sweden). Pareto-scaling was applied to normalize data for PCA and OPLS analysis. In addition, R^2 and Q^2 (cum) were used for model evaluation. Values of both parameters close to 1.0 indicated a good fitness for the created model. OPLS, a supervised multivariate statistical method, was completed with percent inhibition of lipid peroxidation activity as the Y input. The features with potential bioactivity from S-plot in OPLS model were selected based on their p[1] values.

3.7. Molecular Networking Analyses

The MN of MS^2 spectra of the *Bacopa* species was generated using the online workflow of the Global Natural Products Social Molecular Networking (GNPS). The MS^2 spectra were then clustered with MS-Cluster with a parent mass tolerance at 0.02 Da and a fragment ion mass tolerance at 0.02 Da to create consensus spectra, and consensus spectra containing less than two spectra were discarded. A network was then created, where edges were filtered to have a cosine score above 0.7 and more than 6 matching peaks. Furthermore, the edges between two nodes were kept in the network if each of the nodes appeared in each other's respective top 10 most similar nodes. The spectra in the network were automatically searched against GNPS spectral libraries and then against DNP-ISDB according to a previously described methodology [1]. ChemViz 1.3 plugin (freely available at [61]) was used to display the structure of the dereplication hits directly within Cytoscape 3.6.1. The generated MN in this study can be seen in [62] and the MASSIVE datasets contained all raw data was provided in the link of [63].

3.8. Purification of Candidate Bioactive Compounds

3.8.1. Extraction Procedure

The dried powder of BM4 (100 g) was macerated three times with MeOH and shaken for 24 h to give 24.2 g of MeOH extract. The polar substances (sugar) of the extract were removed using solid phase extraction prior to purification using the following protocol. The 200 g of C18 (ZEOprep® 60 C18, 40–63 μm) was packed in a column and activated by MeOH (1 L), followed by conditioning with water (1 L). Then, 2 g of Brahmi extract in 10 mL water was loaded and the column was washed with water (1 L) to remove polar substances. Remaining compounds were finally eluted with MeOH (1 L).

3.8.2. Purification Methods

The isolation steps of candidate compounds were performed by MPLC and followed by semi–preparative HPLC. A system of MPLC was carried out on an LC instrument conducted with a 681-pump module C-615, UV-Vis module C-640, and a fraction collector module C-660 (Buchi, Flawil, Switzerland). Fractionation was performed with an ZEOprep® C18 column (70 × 460 mm, 15–25 μm) with elution of 0.1% formic acid in water (A) and 0.1% formic acid in acetonitrile (B). The gradient elution started from 0-20 min of 35% B and then increased to 100% B for 284 min. The flow rate was 20 mL/min. This condition was first optimized on an analytical HPLC column (250 × 4.6 mm i.d., 15–25 μm, Zeochem, Uetikon am See, Switzerland) packed with the same stationary phase and then geometrically transferred to the preparative scale [53]. The extract was introduced into the MPLC column by dry injection by mixing 5.62 g of the extract with 18.30 g of the Zeoprep C18 stationary phase (40–63 μm, Zeochem). The mixture was conditioned in a dry-load cell (11.5 × 2.7 cm i.d.) and it was connected subsequently between the pumps and the MPLC column. Twenty-five fractions were collected by peak-based detection under UV at 205, 254 and 366 nm. When there were no peaks, 250 mL of each of the fractions was collected. The candidate compounds in the fractions were tracked down by LC-MS using the same conditions as mentioned in session 3.4.

The candidate bioactive compounds (**1–8**) and inactive compounds (**9–11**) were isolated from fraction 3 of MPLC using semi–preparative HPLC, which was performed on a HPLC-UV instrument with SPD-20A UV-Vis, a LC-20AP Pump, a FRC-10A fraction collector and a sample injector (Shimadzu, USA). The separation was carried out on an XBridge C18 OBD prep column (19 × 250 mm, 5 μm, Waters, Milford, MA, USA) with a guard column (4 × 20 mm, 5 μm), using an isocratic system of 0.1% formic acid in water and in acetonitrile at ratios of 86 and 14 as mobile phase. The separation time was 65 min with a post run of 10 min and the flow rate set at 17 mL/min. This semi–preparative HPLC condition was optimized on an analytical HPLC using a column with a similar stationary phase (XBridge C18, 4.6 × 250 mm, 5 μm) and then the optimum condition was geometrically transferred to the semi-preparative scale [54]. In order to avoid loss of resolution, the sample was loaded into the column by dry loading according to a recently developed protocol [55], which made it possible to obtain a high–resolution separation of the majority of the polar compounds to ensure a high degree of purity. Using this preparative system, eighty-four fractions were collected by peak-based detection under UV absorption of 205, 254 and scan 200–600 nm and volume based collection (8 mL of each fraction). All collected fractions were dried by speed vacuum (Genevac HT-4X, Genevac Ltd., North Carolina, USA). Isolation was achieved and afforded candidate bioactive compounds of **1** (8.5 mg), **2** (2.2 mg), **3** (0.9 mg), **4** (1.4 mg) **5** (0.1 mg) **6** (0.6 mg) and **7** (0.8 mg) and **8** (3.0 mg) and three inactive compounds of **9** (0.4 mg), **10** (3.0 mg) and **11** (1.2 mg). The purity and structure elucidation of each isolated compound was checked with HPLC, MS and NMR.

3.8.3. Identification Procedures

The NMR spectra of each isolated compound was recorded on a Bruker Avance Neo 600 MHz spectrometer equipped with a QCI 5mmCryoprobe and a SampleJet automated sample changer (Bruker BioSpin, Rheinstetten, Germany) (600). Chemical shifts (δ) were recorded in parts per million in methanol-d_4 using the residual solvent signal (δ_H 3.31; δ_C 49.0) as internal standards for ^{1}H and ^{13}C-NMR, respectively. Mass spectrometric data were obtained on a Waters Acquity UPLC IClass system system interfaced to a Q-Exactive Focus mass spectrometer (Thermo Scientific).

4. Conclusions

In this work, the integration of MVA and multi-informative MN based on LC–HRMS^2 metabolite profiling with bioactivity data was proven to be an efficient way to identify bioactive constituents in closely related plant extracts. The data generated allowed a rapid prioritization of bioactive compounds on a specific target from crude *Bacopa* extracts. Thanks to this approach the potential bioactivity for individual compounds could be anticipated prior to any physical separation process. This allowed the targeted isolation of six phenylethanoid glycosides **1–6** of *Bacopa* species with lipid-peroxidation inhibitory activity three of them being novel compounds i.e., monnieraside IV (**4**), monnieraside V (**5**) and monnieraside VI (**6**).

Additionally, the results in MVA and MN showed significant difference between Brahmi samples harvested in summer and other seasons in term of overall biological activity and amount of bioactive compounds. To our knowledge, Brahmi is collected throughout the year in Thailand and, based on our study, seasonal effects are important to consider and might affect the medicinal properties claimed for Brahmi. The described bioactive compounds could be used as biomarkers for quality control of this plant.

Author Contributions: T.S. performed whole experiments, data analysis, and prepared manuscript, P.-M.A. acquired UHPLC-HRMS^2 data and supervised data analysis, E.F.Q. helped for isolation, L.M. analyzed the NMR and structure elucidations, N.N. helped for data analysis, P.T. helped for data analysis, N.K. helped for data analysis, T.S., P.-M.A., J.-L.W. and K.I. conceived and designed the study. All authors reviewed the results and approved the final version of the manuscript.

Acknowledgments: We are gratefully to Pranee Nangngam for providing *Bacopa* samples and her help in plant identification. Additionally, we would like to thank the Bioactive Natural Products Unit, University of Geneva, Switzerland, who provided laboratory facilities.

References

1. Allard, P.-M.; Péresse, T.; Bisson, J.; Gindro, K.; Marcourt, L.; Pham, V.C.; Roussi, F.; Litaudon, M.; Wolfender, J.-L. Integration of molecular networking and In-Silico MS/MS fragmentation for natural products dereplication. *Anal. Chem.* **2016**, *88*, 3317–3323. [CrossRef] [PubMed]

2. Hubert, J.; Nuzillard, J.-M.; Renault, J.-H. Dereplication strategies in natural product research: How many tools and methodologies behind the same concept? *Phytochem. Rev.* **2017**, *16*, 55–95. [CrossRef]

3. Yuliana, N.D.; Khatib, A.; Choi, Y.H.; Verpoorte, R. Metabolomics for bioactivity assessment of natural products. *Phytother. Res.* **2011**, *25*, 157–169. [CrossRef] [PubMed]

4. Li, P.; AnandhiSenthilkumar, H.; Wu, S.-b.; Liu, B.; Guo, Z.-y.; Fata, J.E.; Kennelly, E.J.; Long, C.-l. Comparative UPLC-QTOF-MS-based metabolomics and bioactivities analyses of *Garcinia oblongifolia*. *J. Chromatogr. B* **2016**, *1011*, 179–195. [CrossRef] [PubMed]

5. D'Urso, G.; Pizza, C.; Piacente, S.; Montoro, P. Combination of LC–MS based metabolomics and antioxidant activity for evaluation of bioactive compounds in *Fragaria vesca* leaves from Italy. *J. Pharm. Biomed. Anal.* **2018**, *150*, 233–240. [CrossRef]

6. Ayouni, K.; Berboucha-Rahmani, M.; Kim, H.K.; Atmani, D.; Verpoorte, R.; Choi, Y.H. Metabolomic tool to identify antioxidant compounds of *Fraxinus angustifolia* leaf and stem bark extracts. *Ind. Crops. Prod.* **2016**, *88*, 65–77. [CrossRef]

7. Caesar, L.K.; Kellogg, J.J.; Kvalheim, O.M.; Cech, N.B. Opportunities and Limitations for Untargeted Mass Spectrometry Metabolomics to Identify Biologically Active Constituents in Complex Natural Product Mixtures. *J. Nat. Prod.* **2019**, *82*, 469–484. [CrossRef]

8. Patti, G.J.; Yanes, O.; Siuzdak, G. Innovation: Metabolomics: The apogee of the omics trilogy. *Nat. Rev. Mol. Cell Biol.* **2012**, *13*, 263–269. [CrossRef]

9. Kim, H.K.; Choi, Y.H.; Verpoorte, R. NMR-based plant metabolomics: Where do we stand, where do we go? *Trends Biotechnol.* **2011**, *29*, 267–275. [CrossRef]

10. Wolfender, J.-L.; Rudaz, S.; Hae Choi, Y.; Kyong Kim, H. Plant Metabolomics: From Holistic Data to Relevant Biomarkers. *Curr. Med. Chem.* **2013**, *20*, 1056–1090.

11. Wolfender, J.-L.; Nuzillard, J.-M.; van der Hooft, J.J.J.; Renault, J.-H.; Bertrand, S. Accelerating Metabolite Identification in Natural Product Research: Toward an Ideal Combination of Liquid Chromatography–High-Resolution Tandem Mass Spectrometry and NMR Profiling, in Silico Databases, and Chemometrics. *Anal. Chem.* **2019**, *91*, 704–742. [CrossRef]

12. Yang, J.Y.; Sanchez, L.M.; Rath, C.M.; Liu, X.; Boudreau, P.D.; Bruns, N.; Glukhov, E.; Wodtke, A.; de Felicio, R.; Fenner, A.; et al. Molecular networking as a dereplication strategy. *J. Nat. Prod.* **2013**, *76*, 1686–1699. [CrossRef]

13. Wang, M.; Carver, J.J.; Phelan, V.V.; Sanchez, L.M.; Garg, N.; Peng, Y.; Nguyen, D.D.; Watrous, J.; Kapono, C.A.; Luzzatto-Knaan, T.; et al. Sharing and community curation of mass spectrometry data with Global Natural Products Social Molecular Networking. *Nat. Biotechnol.* **2016**, *34*, 828. [CrossRef]

14. Olivon, F.; Allard, P.-M.; Koval, A.; Righi, D.; Genta-Jouve, G.; Neyts, J.; Apel, C.; Pannecouque, C.; Nothias, L.-F.; Cachet, X.; et al. Bioactive natural products prioritization using massive multi-informational molecular networks. *Acs Chem. Biol.* **2017**, *12*, 2644–2651. [CrossRef]

15. Naman, C.B.; Rattan, R.; Nikoulina, S.E.; Lee, J.; Miller, B.W.; Moss, N.A.; Armstrong, L.; Boudreau, P.D.; Debonsi, H.M.; Valeriote, F.A.; et al. Integrating molecular networking and biological assays to target the isolation of a cytotoxic cyclic octapeptide, samoamide A, from an American Samoan Marine Cyanobacterium. *J. Nat. Prod.* **2017**, *80*, 625–633. [CrossRef]

16. Nothias, L.-F.; Nothias-Esposito, M.; da Silva, R.; Wang, M.; Protsyuk, I.; Zhang, Z.; Sarvepalli, A.; Leyssen, P.; Touboul, D.; Costa, J.; et al. Bioactivity-based molecular networking for the discovery of drug leads in natural product bioassay-guided fractionation. *J. Nat. Prod.* **2018**, *81*, 758–767. [CrossRef]

17. Global Natural Product Social Molecular Networking. Available online: http://gnps.ucsd.edu (accessed on 10 Aprile 2018).

18. Olivon, F.; Elie, N.; Grelier, G.; Roussi, F.; Litaudon, M.; Touboul, D. MetGem Software for the Generation of Molecular Networks Based on the t-SNE Algorithm. *Anal. Chem.* **2018**, *90*, 13900–13908. [CrossRef]

19. Kind, T.; Tsugawa, H.; Cajka, T.; Ma, Y.; Lai, Z.; Mehta, S.S.; Wohlgemuth, G.; Barupal, D.K.; Showalter, M.R.; Arita, M.; et al. Identification of small molecules using accurate mass MS/MS search. *Mass Spectrom. Rev.* **2018**, *37*, 513–532. [CrossRef]

20. Tem, S. *Thai Plant Names*, 2014 ed.; The Forest Herbarium, Royal Forest Department: Bangkok, Thailand, 2014.

21. Mukherjee, G.D.; Dey, C.D. Clinical trial on Brahmi. I. *J. Exp. Med. Sci.* **1966**, *10*, 5–11.

22. Vollala, V.R.; Upadhya, S.; Nayak, S. Effect of *Bacopa monniera* Linn. (brahmi) extract on learning and memory in rats: A behavioral study. *J. Vet. Behav.* **2010**, *5*, 69–74. [CrossRef]

23. Saraf, M.K.; Prabhakar, S.; Khanduja, K.L.; Anand, A. *Bacopa monniera* attenuates scopolamine-induced impairment of spatial memory in mice. *Evid. Based Complement. Alternat. Med.* **2011**, *2011*, 10. [CrossRef]

24. Nathan, P.J.; Clarke, J.; Lloyd, J.; Hutchison, C.W.; Downey, L.; Stough, C. The acute effects of an extract of *Bacopa monniera* (Brahmi) on cognitive function in healthy normal subjects. *Hum. Psychopharmacol. Clin. Exp.* **2001**, *16*, 345–351. [CrossRef]

25. Stough, C.; Lloyd, J.; Clarke, J.; Downey, L.A.; Hutchison, C.W.; Rodgers, T.; Nathan, P.J. The chronic effects of an extract of *Bacopa monniera* (Brahmi) on cognitive function in healthy human subjects. *Psychopharmacology* **2001**, *156*, 481–484. [CrossRef]

26. Peth-Nui, T.; Wattanathorn, J.; Muchimapura, S.; Tong-Un, T.; Piyavhatkul, N.; Rangseekajee, P.; Ingkaninan, K.; Vittaya-areekul, S. Effects of 12-week *Bacopa monnieri* consumption on attention, cognitive processing, working memory, and functions of both cholinergic and monoaminergic systems in healthy elderly volunteers. *Evid. Based Complement. Alternat. Med.* **2012**, *2012*, 606424. [CrossRef]

27. Kongkeaw, C.; Dilokthornsakul, P.; Thanarangsarit, P.; Limpeanchob, N.; Norman Scholfield, C. Meta-analysis of randomized controlled trials on cognitive effects of *Bacopa monnieri* extract. *J. Ethnopharmacol.* **2014**, *151*, 528–535. [CrossRef]

28. Roodenrys, S.; Booth, D.; Bulzomi, S.; Phipps, A.; Micallef, C.; Smoker, J. Chronic effects of Brahmi (*Bacopa monnieri*) on human memory. *Neuropsychopharmacology* **2002**, *27*, 279–281. [CrossRef]

29. Morgan, A.; Stevens, J. Does Bacopa monnieri Improve Memory Performance in Older Persons? Results of a Randomized, Placebo-Controlled, Double-Blind Trial. *J. Altern. Complementary Med.* **2010**, *16*, 753–759. [CrossRef]

30. Gour, S.; Tembhre, M. Cholinergic inhibitory effects of bacopa monnieri and acephate in the kidney of rat. *Int. J. Curr. Adv. Res.* **2018**, *7*, 14136–14141.

31. Teschke, R.; Bahre, R. Severe hepatotoxicity by Indian Ayurvedic herbal products: A structured causality assessment. *Ann. Hepatol.* **2009**, *8*, 258–266. [CrossRef]

32. Sumathi, T.; Nongbri, A. Hepatoprotective effect of Bacoside-A, a major constituent of Bacopa monniera Linn. *Phytomedicine* **2008**, *15*, 901–905. [CrossRef]

33. Menon, B.R.; Rathi, M.A.; Thirumoorthi, L.; Gopalakrishnan, V.K. Potential Effect of Bacopa monnieri on Nitrobenzene Induced Liver Damage in Rats. *Indian J. Clin. Biochem.* **2010**, *25*, 401–404. [CrossRef]

34. Singh, H.; Dhawan, B.N. Neuropsychopharmacological effects of the ayurvedic nootropic *Bacopa monnieri* Linn. *Indian J. Pharmacol.* **1997**, *29*, 359–365.

35. Russo, A.; Borrelli, F. *Bacopa monniera*, a reputed nootropic plant: An overview. *Phytomedicine* **2005**, *12*, 305–317. [CrossRef]

36. Deepak, M.; Sangli, G.K.; Arun, P.C.; Amit, A. Quantitative determination of the major saponin mixture bacoside A in *Bacopa monnieri* by HPLC. *Phytochem. Anal.* **2005**, *16*, 24–29. [CrossRef]

37. Ganzera, M.; Gampenrieder, J.; Pawar, R.S.; Khan, I.A.; Stuppner, H. Separation of the major triterpenoid saponins in *Bacopa monnieri* by high-performance liquid chromatography. *Anal. Chim. Acta* **2004**, *516*, 149–154. [CrossRef]

38. Murthy, P.B.; Raju, V.R.; Ramakrisana, T.; Chakravarthy, M.S.; Kumar, K.V.; Kannababu, S.; Subbaraju, G.V. Estimation of twelve bacopa saponins in *Bacopa monnieri* extracts and formulations by high-performance liquid chromatography. *Chem. Pharm. Bull. (Tokyo)* **2006**, *54*, 907–911. [CrossRef]

39. Phrompittayarat, W.; Wittaya-Areekul, S.; Jetiyanon, K.; Putalun, W.; Tanaka, H.; Ingkaninan, K. Determination of saponin glycosides in *Bacopa monnieri* by reversed phase high performance liquid chromatography. *Thai Pharm. Health Sci. J.* **2007**, *2*, 26–32.

40. Bhandari, P.; Kumar, N.; Singh, B.; Singh, V.; Kaur, I. Silica-based monolithic column with evaporative light scattering detector for HPLC analysis of bacosides and apigenin in *Bacopa monnieri*. *J. Sep. Sci.* **2009**, *32*, 2812–2818. [CrossRef]

41. British Pharmacopoeia Commission. *The British Pharmacopoeia 2016*; The Stationery Office: London, UK, 2016; Volume 1.

42. Mathur, S.; Sharma, S.; Gupta, P.M.; Kumar, S. Evaluation of an Indian germplasm collection of the medicinal plant Bacopa monnieri (L.) Pennell by use of multivariate approaches. *Euphytica* **2003**, *133*, 255–265. [CrossRef]

43. Bansal, M. Diversity among wild accessions of Bacopa monnieri (L.) Wettst. and their morphogenetic potential. *Acta Physiol. Plant.* **2014**, *36*, 1177–1186. [CrossRef]

44. Bansal, M.; Reddy, M.S.; Kumar, A. Seasonal variations in harvest index and bacoside A contents amongst accessions of Bacopa monnieri (L.) Wettst. collected from wild populations. *Physiol. Mol. Biol. Plants* **2016**, *22*, 407–413. [CrossRef]

45. Phrompittayarat, W.; Jetiyanon, K.; Wittaya-Areekul, S.; Putalun, W.; Tanaka, H.; Khan, I.; Ingkaninan, K. Influence of seasons, different plant parts, and plant growth stages on saponin quantity and distribution in *Bacopa monnieri*. *SJST* **2011**, *33*, 193–199.

46. Bhandari, P.; Kumar, N.; Singh, B.; Kaul, V.K. Bacosterol Glycoside, a New 13,14-Seco-steroid Glycoside from *Bacopa monnieri*. *Chem. Pharm. Bull. (Tokyo)* **2006**, *54*, 240–241. [CrossRef]

47. Bhandari, P.; Kumar, N.; Gupta, A.P.; Singh, B.; Kaul, V.K. A rapid RP-HPTLC densitometry method for simultaneous determination of major flavonoids in important medicinal plants. *J. Sep. Sci.* **2007**, *30*, 2092–2096. [CrossRef]

48. Chakravarty, A.K.; Sarkar, T.; Nakane, T.; Kawahara, N.; Masuda, K. New Phenylethanoid Glycosides from *Bacopa monniera*. *Chem. Pharm. Bull. (Tokyo)* **2002**, *50*, 1616–1618. [CrossRef]

49. Ohta, T.; Nakamura, S.; Nakashima, S.; Oda, Y.; Matsumoto, T.; Fukaya, M.; Yano, M.; Yoshikawa, M.; Matsuda, H. Chemical structures of constituents from the whole plant of Bacopa monniera. *J. Nat. Med.* **2016**, *70*, 404–411. [CrossRef]

50. Limpeanchob, N.; Jaipan, S.; Rattanakaruna, S.; Phrompittayarat, W.; Ingkaninan, K. Neuroprotective effect of *Bacopa monnieri* on beta-amyloid-induced cell death in primary cortical culture. *J. Ethnopharmacol.* **2008**, *120*, 112–117. [CrossRef]

51. Katajamaa, M.; Miettinen, J.; Orešič, M. MZmine: Toolbox for processing and visualization of mass spectrometry based molecular profile data. *Bioinformatics* **2006**, *22*, 634–636. [CrossRef]

52. Schymanski, E.L.; Jeon, J.; Gulde, R.; Fenner, K.; Ruff, M.; Singer, H.P.; Hollender, J. Identifying Small Molecules via High Resolution Mass Spectrometry: Communicating Confidence. *Environ. Sci. Technol.* **2014**, *48*, 2097–2098. [CrossRef]

53. Challal, S.; Queiroz, E.F.; Debrus, B.; Kloeti, W.; Guillarme, D.; Gupta, M.P.; Wolfender, J.L. Rational and Efficient Preparative Isolation of Natural Products by MPLC-UV-ELSD based on HPLC to MPLC Gradient Transfer. *Planta Med.* **2015**, *81*, 1636–1643. [CrossRef]

54. Guillarme, D.; Nguyen, D.T.T.; Rudaz, S.; Veuthey, J.-L. Method transfer for fast liquid chromatography in pharmaceutical analysis: Application to short columns packed with small particle. Part I: Isocratic separation. *Eur. J. Pharm. Biopharm.* **2007**, *66*, 475–482. [CrossRef]

55. Queiroz, E.F.; Alfattani, A.; Afzan, A.; Marcourt, L.; Guillarme, D.; Wolfender, J.-L. Utility of dry load injection for an efficient natural products isolation at the semi-preparative chromatographic scale. *J. Chromatogr. A* **2019**, *1598*, 85–91. [CrossRef]

56. Tabata, M.; Umetani, Y.; Ooya, M.; Tanaka, S. Glucosylation of phenolic compounds by plant cell cultures. *Phytochemistry* **1988**, *27*, 809–813. [CrossRef]

57. Bianco, A.; Mazzei, R.A.; Melchioni, C.; Romeo, G.; Scarpati, M.L.; Soriero, A.; Uccella, N. Microcomponents of olive oil—III. Glucosides of 2(3,4-dihydroxy-phenyl)ethanol. *Food Chem.* **1998**, *63*, 461–464. [CrossRef]

58. Jer-Huei, L.; Yi-Chu, L.; Jiing-Ping, H.; Kuo-Ching, W. Parishins B and C from rhizomes of Gastrodia elata. *Phytochemistry* **1996**, *42*, 549–551. [CrossRef]

59. Saluk-Juszczak, J.; Olas, B.; Nowak, P.; Staroń, A.; Wachowicz, B. Protective effects of D-glucaro-1,4-lactone against oxidative modifications in blood platelets. *Nutr. Metab. Cardiovasc. Dis.* **2008**, *18*, 422–428. [CrossRef]

60. Smith, P.K.; Krohn, R.I.; Hermanson, G.T.; Mallia, A.K.; Gartner, F.H.; Provenzano, M.D.; Fujimoto, E.K.; Goeke, N.M.; Olson, B.J.; Klenk, D.C. Measurement of protein using bicinchoninic acid. *Anal. Biochem.* **1985**, *150*, 76–85. [CrossRef]

61. ChemViz: Cheminformatics Plugin for Cytoscape. Available online: http://www.cgl.ucsf.edu/cytoscape/chemViz/ (accessed on 10 July 2018).

62. Global Natural Product Social Molecular Networking. Available online: https://gnps.ucsd.edu/ProteoSAFe/status.jsp? (accessed on 19 June 2018).

63. MASSIVE datasets. Available online: ftp://massive.ucsd.edu/MSV000083989 (accessed on 18 June 2019).

9

Phytochemical and Analytical Characterization of Novel Sulfated Coumarins in the Marine Green Macroalga *Dasycladus vermicularis* (Scopoli) Krasser

Anja Hartmann [1,*]**, Markus Ganzera** [1]**, Ulf Karsten** [2]**, Alexsander Skhirtladze** [3] **and Hermann Stuppner** [1]

[1] Institute of Pharmacy, Pharmacognosy, CMBI, University of Innsbruck, Innrain 80-82, 6020 Innsbruck, Austria; markus.ganzera@uibk.ac.at (M.G.); hermann.stuppner@uibk.ac.at (H.S.)

[2] Institute of Biological Sciences, Applied Ecology & Phycology, University of Rostock, Albert-Einstein-Str. 3, 18059 Rostock, Germany; ulf.karsten@uni-rostock.de

[3] Department of Phytochemistry, Iovel Kutateladze Institute of Pharmacochemistry, Tbilisi State Medical University, 0159 Tbilisi, Georgia; aleksandre.skhirtladze@yahoo.com

* Correspondence: Anja.Hartmann@uibk.ac.at;

Academic Editor: Pinarosa Avato

Abstract: The siphonous green algae form a morphologically diverse group of marine macroalgae which include two sister orders (Bryopsidales and Dasycladales) which share a unique feature among other green algae as they are able to form large, differentiated thalli comprising of a single, giant tubular cell. Upon cell damage a cascade of protective mechanisms have evolved including the extrusion of sulfated metabolites which are involved in the formation of a rapid wound plug. In this study, we investigated the composition of sulfated metabolites in *Dasycladus vermicularis* (Dasycladales) which resulted in the isolation of two phenolic acids and four coumarins including two novel structures elucidated by nuclear magnetic resonance spectroscopy (NMR) as 5,8′-di-(6(6′),7(7′)-tetrahydroxy-3-sulfoxy-3′-sulfoxycoumarin), a novel coumarin called dascladin A and 7-hydroxycoumarin-3,6-disulfate, which was named dascladin B. In addition, an analytical assay for the chromatographic quantification of those compounds was developed and performed on a reversed phase C-18 column. Method validation confirmed that the new assay shows good linearity ($R^2 \geq 0.9986$), precision (intra-day R.S.D $\leq 3.71\%$, inter-day R.S.D $\leq 7.49\%$), and accuracy (recovery rates ranged from 104.06 to 97.45%). The analysis of several samples of *Dasycladus vermicularis* from different collection sites, water depths and seasons revealed differences in the coumarin contents, ranging between 0.26 to 1.61%.

Keywords: siphonous green algae; sulfated coumarins; *Dasycladus vermicularis*; isolation and quantification

1. Introduction

Dasycladus vermicularis (Scopoli) Krasser is an evolutionarily ancient, small siphonous green alga, which is widely distributed throughout tropical to temperate regions such as several Atlantic islands (Canary islands, Madeira, Antilles), many regions in the Mediterranean Sea, Central America (Belize), Caribbean islands, South America (Brazil), and Asia (Japan, South China Sea, Philippines) [1]. This chlorophyte inhabits well-illuminated shallow waters (0.3–20 m) with high light exposures in the upper littoral zone on rocky substrates and are often covered by a thin layer of sediment [2]. To thrive under enhanced doses of UV radiation, photo-protective mechanisms are needed. In 1983, Menzel et al. [3] isolated and identified 3,6,7-trihydroxycoumarin (thyc) as a UV absorbing compound from

D. vermicularis for the first time, which was also the first report of coumarins in algae. Subsequently, several studies have been carried out to investigate the relevance of thyc in *D. vermicularis*. They indicated an elevated excretion of thyc due to increasing UV exposure and temperatures suggesting that this compound is a natural sunscreen/UV protectant [4–6]. Another very remarkable characteristic of *D. vermicularis* is its morphology. *D. vermicularis* is a member of the so-called siphonous green macro algae comprising unique giant single cells without cross walls. These thalli can grow up to 10 cm long, gaining stability by surrounding themselves with a calcareous coating which supports the long unicellular algae with sufficient stability to grow upright. Siphonous algae typically contain a huge central vacuole and a thin layer of cytoplasm, the latter inhabiting multiple nuclei (Bryopsidales) or just one nucleus (Dasycladales) [7]. After cell damage, for example due to herbivory, a rapid wound closure is essential for the survival of such organisms. Therefore, immediately upon injury a cascade of biochemical reactions is induced to assimilate cellular contents into an insoluble wound plug initially formed by gelling, followed by a slower hardening process (1–2 h) [8,9]. This mechanism is indispensable to avoid cytoplasmic loss and limits the intrusion of extracellular components, herbivore attack or pathogenic invasion, which could otherwise result in high mortality rates [8,10]. A few years ago Welling et al. [8] investigated both the intact and wounded alga to monitor changes in chemical composition, which may be involved in the wound plug formation. This study surprisingly revealed the dominant secondary metabolite to be 6,7-dihydroxycoumarin-3-sulfate (dhycs) in the methanolic extracts of intact *D. vermicularis*, while the previously reported major compound 3,6,7-trihydroxycoumarin was only found in the methanolic extracts after wounding. Thus, the dhycs is supposed to act as a precursor and is transformed into the more active thyc in the presence of sulfatases. According to Welling et al. [9] thyc acts as an intermediate which is rapidly oxidized and serves as a protein cross-linker for the formation of a wound sealing co-polymer in combination with amino acid side chains from the alga. Such polymerization processes are known from other marine organisms, which are usually involved in bioadhesive processes that are needed for sessile marine organisms such as tubeworms and mussels to attach themselves to surfaces. For example, the common blue mussel *Mytilus edulis* uses a metal centered chelate that initiates the biopolymerisation process which includes secondary metabolites such as protein-bound-dopamine [11]. Sulfated secondary metabolites are widely distributed among marine species and are stored therein in a dormant state. They are then transformed enzymatically into more active metabolites, for example, psammaplin A sulfate from the sponge *Aplysinella rhax* or zosteric acid, an antifouling metabolite in the seagrass *Zostera marina*. Both metabolites are converted upon tissue disruption to their desulfated form thereby increasing activity as a defensive metabolite [12,13]. Kurth et al. [14] just recently revealed the presence of two sulfated phenolic acids in *D. vermicularis* namely 4-(sulfooxy)benzoic acid (SBA) and 4-(sulfooxy)phenylacetic acid (SPA), which are also proposed to exist in a dormant state prior to transformation to more active desulfated metabolites. However, these two sulfated phenolic acids are most likely not involved in the wound plug formation, but could be serving as biofilm inhibitor. In this study we investigated the phytochemical composition of *D. vermicularis* extracts of different polarities. The coumarin composition of this alga seems to be more complex than previously described, and hence we report on two novel coumarins from *D. vermicularis* and their analysis via HPLC-MS and NMR. Coumarins are natural benzopyrone derivatives with a variety of desirable pharmacological properties which are commonly found in higher plants [15], however sulfated molecules are rather uncommon and beyond that *D. vermicularis* is the first alga known to contain these secondary metabolites. Therefore, we report on the first validated HPLC assay for the separation and quantification of sulfated coumarins in algae which has been applied to samples from three different sampling sites across the Mediterranean Sea to compare their coumarin content.

2. Results

2.1. Isolation and Identification of the Coumarins

With the aim of isolating the major compounds present in *Dasycladus vermicularis* four coumarins and two phenolic acids were isolated from the methanol and the aqueous extract. A sample (2.5 g) of the aqueous extract was separated by means of repeated flash chromatography and semi-preparative HPLC, which resulted in the isolation of compounds **1**, **4** and **8**. Compounds **2**, **3** and **7** were obtained from 4.5 g of crude methanol extract by silica gel and Sephadex LH 20 column chromatography. ^{1}H- and ^{13}C-NMR shift values of all isolated coumarins are summarized in Table 1. The shift values for thyc were in good agreement with literature values [16]. Compounds **1** and **2** were identified as new natural products.

Table 1. NMR shift values of compounds isolated from the marine green alga *Dasycladus vermicularis*; spectra were recorded on a 600 MHz NMR instrument in deuterated water.

Position	Dasycladin A (1) in D₂O		HMBC C	Dasycladin B (2) in D₂O		HMBC C
	δ_H	δ_C, Type		δ_H	δ_C, Type	
2		163.3, C			161.0, C	
3		136.1, C			134.1, C	
4	7.40 (s)	134.4, CH	2, 3, 5, 9	7.94 (s)	133.3, CH	2, 3, 5, 9
5		118.3, C		7.64 (s)	122.4, CH	4, 6, 7, 9
6		144.1, C			137.6, C	
7		152.7, C			153.0, C	
8	7.10 (s)	106.8, CH	6, 7, 9, 10	7.05 (s)	105.1, CH	6, 7, 9, 10
9		150.2, C			151.1, C	
10		113.5, C			112.1, C	
2'		163.0, C				
3'		135.8, C				
4'	7.96 (s)	135.8, CH	2', 3', 5', 9'			
5'	7.28 (s)	115.8, CH	4', 6', 7', 9'			
6'		145.7, C				
7'		151.5, C				
8'		111.2, C				
9'		147.7, C				
10'		113.9, C				

Compound **1** was isolated as a yellowish amorphous powder. Its molecular formula was established as $C_{18}H_{10}O_{16}S_2$ by HR-ESI–MS (m/z 544.934, calcd. for $[C_{18}H_{10}O_{16}S_2$-H]$^-$, 544.936) indicating the presence of a sulfated dicoumarin. Fragments at m/z 464.9 [M-H-80]$^-$ and 385.0 [M-H-80-80]$^-$ could be attributed to the loss of sulfate groups, respectively. The melting point was measured to as 278–280 °C The IR spectra shows a strong and characteristic S=O stretching vibration at about 1038 cm^{-1} for the R-OSO₃H groups, 1689 and 1629 cm^{-1} for (C=O), 3059 and 3203 cm^{-1} (OH). In the ^{1}H-NMR (Table 1) spectrum, four singlet aromatic proton resonances at δ_H 7.96 (1H, s, H-4'), 7.40 (1H, s, H-4), 7.28 (1H, s, H-5'), 7.10 (1H, s, H-8) were observed. The ^{13}C-NMR (Table 1) spectrum showed eighteen carbon signals, which were assigned by DEPT experiments to four aromatic methines and fourteen quaternary carbons, two of which (δ_C 163. 3 and 163.0) could be attributed to intramolecular ester groups. The spectroscopic data suggested that **1** is composed of two identical coumarin moieties substituted in positions C-3(C-3'), C-6(C-6'), and C-7 (C-7'). The absence of corresponding signals in the ^{1}H-NMR spectrum and the low field-shifted C-5 and C-8' signals in the ^{13}C-NMR spectrum indicated that the two symmetric coumarin moieties were connected at 5–8' through a C-C bond. Localization of the two sulfate groups was established based on the low field-shifted signals of C-3 and C-3' as well as by comparison of NMR data with those of thyc (**4**) [16] and compound **3**. HSQC and HMBC experiments of **1** were useful to assign all signals in the ^{1}H and ^{13}C spectra. C-4 (δ 134.4) and C-8 (δ 106.8) were used to assign the H-4 (7.40, s) and H-8 (7.10, s) as well as C-4' (δ 135.8) and C-5' (δ 115.8) which were assigned to H-4' (7.96, s) and H-5' (7.28, s) by ^{1}H-^{13}C HSQC.

The HMBC spectrum showed key correlation peaks between the proton signal at δ_H 7.93 (1H, s, H-4') and carbon resonances at δ_C 163.0 (C-2'), 147.7 (C-9'), 135.8 (C-3'), 115.8 (C-5'); and between the proton signal at δ_H 7.38 (1H, s, H-4) and carbon resonances at δ_C 163.3 (C-2), 150.3 (C-9), 136.1 (C-3), 118.3 (C-5).   Thus, compound **1** was identified as 5,8'-di-(6(6'),7(7')-tetrahydroxy-3-sulfoxy-3'-sulfoxycoumarin), a new coumarin for which we propose the trivial name "dasycladin A".

Compound **2** was also isolated as a yellowish amorphous powder. The molecular formula of $C_9H_6O_{11}S_2$ was determined by HR-ESI–MS (negative mode) with a mass peak at m/z 352.928 (calcd. for $[C_9H_6O_{11}S_2\text{-}H]^-$, 352.926). The mass spectrum showed a fragment at m/z 272.8 $[\text{M-H-80}]^-$ corresponding to the loss of a sulfate moiety. The melting point was measured as 233–238 °C. The IR spectra shows a strong and characteristic S=O stretching vibration at about 1038 cm^{-1} for the R-OSO$_3$H groups, 1697 cm^{-1} for (C=O), 3217 cm^{-1} (OH). The ^{1}H-NMR spectrum (Table 1) of **2** showed signals for three aromatic protons at δ_H 7.94 (1H, s, H-4), 7.64 (1H, s, H-5), 7.05 (1H, s, H-8). In the ^{13}C-NMR (Table 1) spectrum nine carbon signals, including three aromatic methines and six quaternary carbons were observed. HSQC and HMBC experiments of Compound **2** were useful to assign all signals in the ^{1}H- and ^{13}C-NMR spectra. C-4 (δ 133.3), C-5 (δ 122.4) and C-8 (δ 105.2) were used to assign the protons H-4 (7.94, s), H-5 (7.64, s) and H-8 (7.05, s) by ^{1}H-^{13}C HSQC. The HMBC spectrum showed correlation peaks between the proton signal at δ_H 7.94 (1H, s, H-4) and carbon resonances at δ_C 161.1 (C-2), 151.1 (C-9), 134.2 (C-3), 122.4 (C-5); between the proton signal at δ_H 7.64 (1H, s, H-5) and carbon resonances at δ_C 152.9 (C-7), 151.1 (C-9), 137.7 (C-6), 133.3 (C-4); and between the proton signal at δ_H 7.04 (1H, s, H-8) and carbon resonances at δ_C 152.9 (C-7), 151.1 (C-9), 137.7 (C-6), 112.3 (C-10). These spectroscopic data suggested that compound **2** is 3,6,7-trisubstituted coumarin. The low field-shifted signal of C-3 and the up field-shifted of C-6 indicated that the sulfate groups were attached at these carbons. The structure of **2** was deduced as 7-hydroxycoumarin-3,6-disulfate. Compound **2** represents a new coumarin for which we propose the trivial name "dasycladin B".

NMR spectra and HR-ESI–MS data for the novel sulfated coumarins **1** and **2** are shown in Figures S1A–E and S2A–E in the Supplementary Material.

2.2. HPLC-Method Development

A HPLC method was developed for quantification of the coumarins. Four coumarins were isolated as described above and used as standards in addition to the two synthetized sulfated phenolic acids and their educts (see Figure 1). Several different stationary phases were screened for the separation of the coumarins and phenolic acids in *D. vermicularis*, such as Zorbax SB-C18 3.5 μm, Hyperclone ODS 3 μm, YMC-triart C-18, 3.5 μm and Kinetex C-18 2.6 μm. However, the best separation was achieved on the Gemini C 18 110 Å, 3 μm (150 mm × 4.6 mm). The latter column yielded the best results concerning separation efficiency and peak shape, resulting in an optimum separation within less than 25 min (Figure 2).

5,8'-Di-(6(6'),7(7')-tetrahydroxy-3-sulfoxy-3'-sulfoxycoumarin) (**1**) eluted first (13.12 min), followed by 7-hydroxycoumarin-3,6-disulfate (**2**; 16.58 min), the sulfated phenolic acids 4-(sulfooxy)benzoic acid and 4-(sulfooxy)phenylacetic acid (**5**; 17.73 min, **6**; 18.3 min), then 6,7-dihydroxycoumarin-3-sulfate (**3**; 18.81 min), 3,6,7-trihydroxycoumarin (**4**; 20.63 min), 4-(hydroxyl)phenylacetic acid (**7**; 21.62 min), and finally 4-(hydroxyl)-benzoic acid (**8**; 22.07 min).

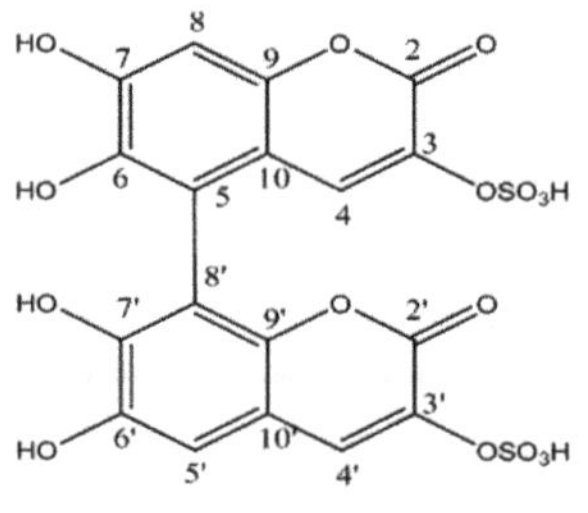

5,8′-di-(6(6′),7(7′)-tetrahydroxy-3-sulfoxy-3′-sulfoxycoumarin (**1**)

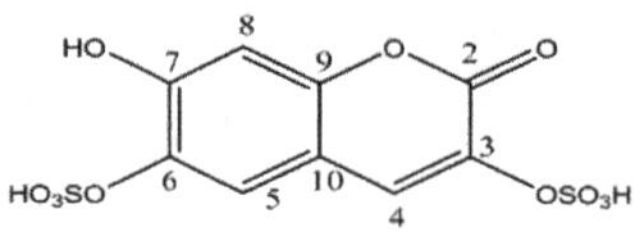

7-hydroxycoumarin-3,6-disulfate (**2**)

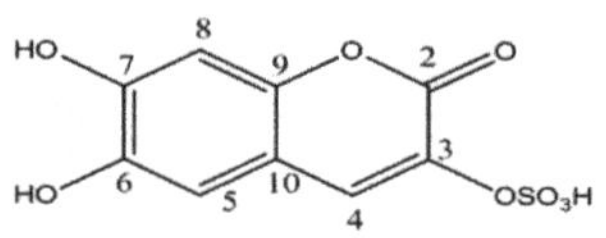

6,7-dihydroxycoumarin-3-sulfate (**3**)

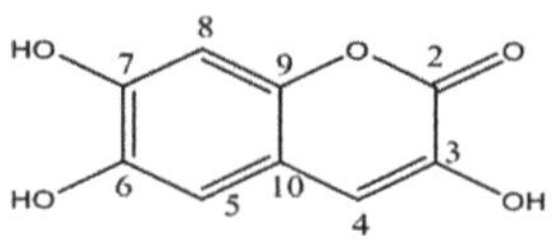

3,6,7-trihydroxycoumarin (**4**)

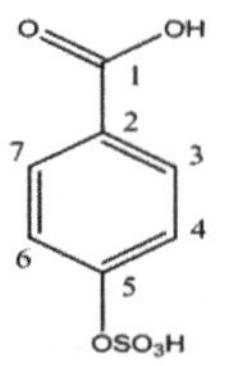

4-(sulfooxy)benzoic acid (**5**)

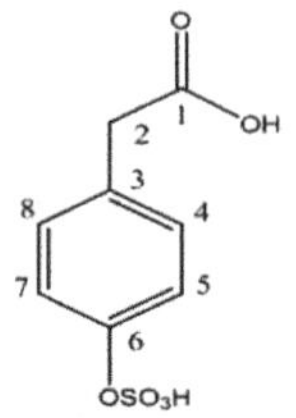

4-(sulfooxy)phenylacetic acid (**6**)

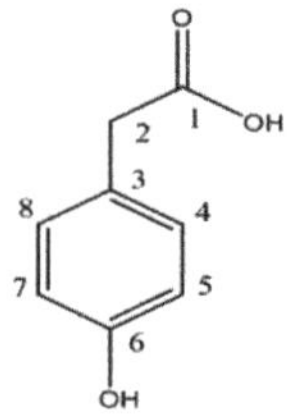

4-(hydroxy)phenylacetic acid (**7**)

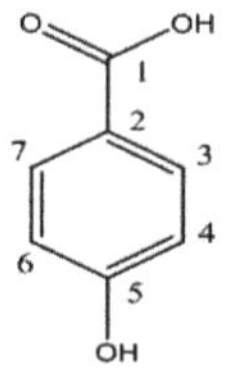

4-(hydroxy)benzoic acid (**8**)

Figure 1. Chemical structure of the isolated coumarins from the marine green alga *Dasycladus vermicularis*, the sulfated phenolic acids and their educts.

2.3. Method Validation

The new analytical method was validated according to the ICH guidelines [17] by establishing calibration curves of the two coumarin standards **1** and **4**, as well as the phenolic acids 4-hydroxy-benzoic acid and 4-hydroxyphenylacetic acid and their sulfated products 4-(sulfooxy)benzoic acid (SBA) and 4-(sulfooxy)phenylacetic acid (SPA) **5–8**. Sufficient material was not available for **2** and **3**. Excellent determination coefficients ($R^2 \geq 0.9986$) were obtained within a concentration range of 0.859–1154 µg/mL. Individual calibration levels were obtained by serial dilution, and each solution was analyzed under optimum HPLC conditions in triplicate. Limit of detection (LOD) and limit of quantification (LOQ) were calculated using defined concentration equivalents to S/N ratios of 3 (LOD) and 10 (LOQ). LOD and LOQ values ranged from 0.014–1.939 µg/mL, and from 0.044–5.876 µg/mL, respectively (Table 2). Selectivity of the method was assured by no visible co-elution (shoulders) in the relevant signals, LC-MS data, and by very consistent UV-spectra (as confirmed by the peak purity option in the operating software). The methods precision was confirmed by its repeatability, as well as inter- and intra-day variation which were determined in *D. vermicularis* sample (DV-2). For this purpose five individual samples at 250 mg/25 mL were extracted and analyzed on each of three consecutive days (Table 3). Intra-day (RSD $\leq$ 5.99%) and inter-day precision (RSD $\leq$ 7.49%) were within accepted limits. Accuracy was assured by spiking accurately weighed samples of DV-2 with three different concentrations of the standard substances. For all compounds the observed recovery rates were acceptable and ranged from 95.6 to 104.6%. Only for 3,6,7-trihydroxcoumarin the value for the low spike was at 91.3% (Table 3). This compound appeared to be stable in solution for at least several h, however when added to the extract it degrades rapidly and therefore the recovery rates are poor, especially at the lower concentrations.

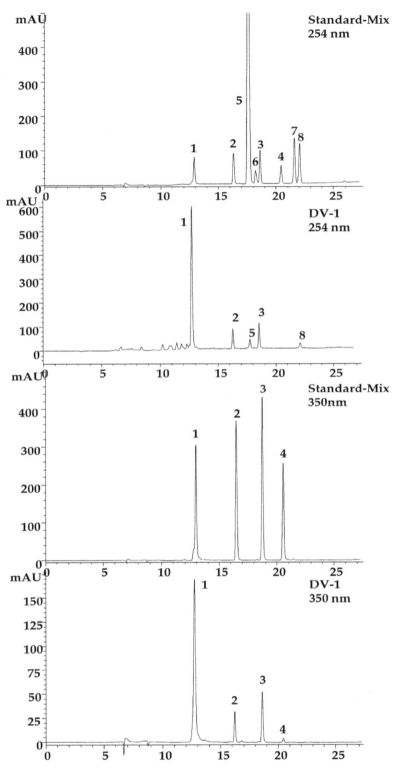

Figure 2. HPLC separation of all standards **1** to **8** at 254 nm and all coumarins **1** to **4** isolated from the marine green alga *Dasycladus vermicularis* at 350 nm, and the sample DV-1 from the marine green alga *Dasycladus vermicularis* at 254 nm and 350 nm under optimized conditions (column: Gemini C18, 110 Å column (150 × 4.6 mm, 3 μm); mobile phase (A) aqueous 20 mM ammonium acetate solution with 1.5% acetic acid and (B) methanol/water (9:1) with 20 mM ammonium acetate and 1.5% acetic acid. Gradient: 2% B to 15% B from 0 to 5 min and 15% B to 60% B from 5–20 min and 60% B to 98% B from 20–25 min; detection at 254 nm and 350 nm, flow rate 0.3 mL/min, injection volume 5 μL and 40 °C oven temperature. Peak assignment is according to Figure 1.

Table 2. Calibration data for the coumarins isolated from the marine green alga *Dasycladus vermicularis* and the respective phenolic acids.

Parameter	1 (Dasycladin A)	4 (thyc)	5 (SBA)	6 (SPA)	7 (4-OH-PAA)	8 (4-OH-BA)
Regr. Equation	Y = 22.953x – 7.904	Y = 67.354x – 296.52	Y = 19.684x + 22.158	Y = 0.652x – 1.475	Y = 97.057x + 14.771	Y = 2.110x + 2.757
σ rel of the slope	0.09	0.683	0.116	0.175	0.049	0.339
R	0.9999	0.9986	0.9999	1.000	1.000	1.000
Range (µg/mL)	440–0.859	445–6.953	629–1.229	1154–18.031	124.75–0.975	483–3.770
LOD [1]	0.192	0.589	0.039	1.939	0.014	1.045
LOQ [2]	0.581	1.784	0.117	5.876	0.044	3.168

[1] LOD: limit of detection determined with purified standards (in µg/mL). [2] LOQ: limit of quantification determined with purified standards (in µg/mL).

Table 3. Accuracy and precision of the new coumarin assay.

Substance	Accuracy [1]			Precision [2]			
	High Spike	Medium Spike	Low Spike	Day 1	Day 2	Day 3	Intra-Day
1	99.49	95.63	101.89	7.49	1.57	1.38	1.86
2	-	-	-	2.22	4.43	6.65	3.71
3	-	-	-	6.39	4.37	2.81	5.99
4	97.49	97.87	91.34	-	-	-	-
5	102.62	99.58	99.40	-	-	-	-
6	98.70	103.23	100.72	-	-	-	-
7	97.45	104.06	103.77	-	-	-	-
8	102.10	99.50	98.85	-	-	-	-

[1] Expressed as recovery rates in percent (sample DV-2 Alonissos). [2] maximum relative standard deviation (peak area) within one and three consecutive days (n = 5; sample: DV-2).

2.4. Analysis of Samples

Four different samples of *D. vermicularis*, all originating from the Mediterranean Sea, were analyzed for their coumarin content. For further details on collection sites, seasons and water depths see Supplementary Material Table S1. As expected, the total amount of coumarins in sample DV-2 (1.60–1.80 m depth) was much lower (3.66 mg/g DW) compared to sample DV-3 (0.30–0.80 m depth; 10.17 mg/g DW). The quantity of the monomeric sulfated coumarins **2** and **3** was the same, while the content of the dimeric compound **1** was about three times higher in the sample that was collected from shallow waters. The two samples that were collected from the same spot in Volos, Greece (DV-3 and DV-4) indicated that there might be seasonal changes in the coumarin content of *D. vermicularis* as well. In November (sample DV-4; 4.27 mg/g DW), the total coumarin content was only half the amount as in August (sample DV-3; 10.17 mg/g DW). The sample that was harvested from Malaga, Spain (DV-1) showed the highest amount of coumarins with 16.09 mg/g DW. The dimeric coumarin **1** was the most abundant compound in all samples, followed by **3**, the 6,7-dihydroxycoumarin-3-sulfate, and 7-hydroxycoumarin-3,6-disulfate (**2**). Thyc, which is reported to be the sole metabolite of compound **3**, only occurred in traces in the highest concentrated samples DV-1 and DV-3. Phenolic acids were also present in all samples, however, in much lower content. All samples contained 4-hydroxybenzoic acid and at a higher concentration its sulfated precursor 4-(sulfooxy)benzoic acid. All quantitative results are summarized in Figure 3. 4-(Sulfooxy)phenylacetic acid which was reported to be present in *D. vermicularis* in a previous publication by Kurth et al. [14] could not be detected in the samples by DAD; however, LC-MS revealed the presence of this compound in all samples. In addition to the standard compounds, three other signals were tentatively identified as coumarins based on the typical UV and MS-spectra; they are marked with a star (Figure 4). The compounds a* and b* both have UV absorption maxima of 346 nm and m/z of 465 [M-H$^-$]. These two compounds may be monosulfated dicoumarins. The assignment of other signals was easily possible by comparison to standards. For example, the determination of coumarins in sample DV-1 is shown in Figure S5 in the Supplementary Material. Chromatograms were recorded at 254 nm and 350 nm, the other traces show the identification of individual compounds by LC-MS in EIC mode.

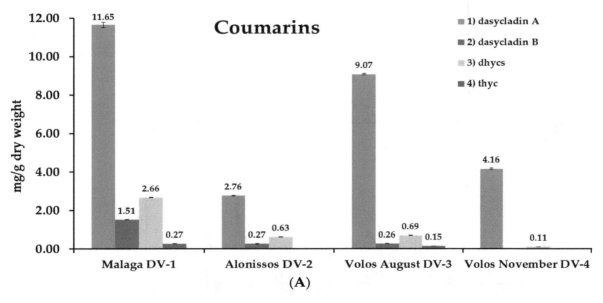

Figure 3. *Cont.*

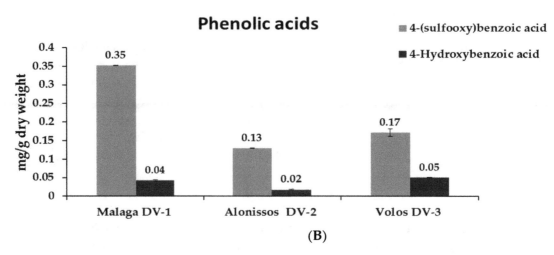

Figure 3. Quantification of the coumarins (**1**) dasycladin A, (**2**) dasycladin B, (extbf3) 6,7-dihydroxycoumarin-3-sulfate, (**4**) 3,6,7-trihydroxycoumarin. Concentrations are given as mg coumarins/g dry weight (**A**) and as mg/g phenolic acids as dry weight (**B**) (n = 3) in the green alga *Dasycladus vermicularis* collected at different sampling sites and dates in the Mediterranean Sea.

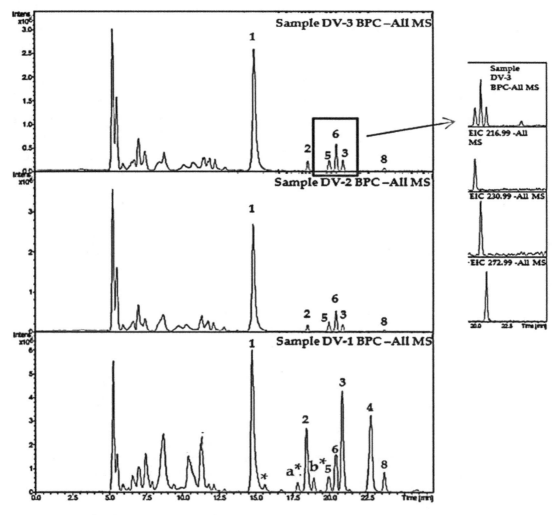

Figure 4. Base peak chromatograms of all extracts DV1-DV3 prepared from the marine green alga *Dasycladus vermicularis*. The red area is enlarged and shows the extracted ion chromatograms (EIC) for the sulfated phenolic acids SBA (**5**) and SPA (**6**). Tentatively identified minor coumarins are marked with a star (similar UV spectra) and with **a***** and **b***** (similar UV spectra and molecular weight).

3. Discussion

The chemical composition of coumarins and phenolic acids in the marine green alga *D. vermicularis* was investigated in detail in this study, revealing that the coumarin composition is more complex than previously reported [8]. Dasycladin A is the major compound, which probably degrades to the previously reported 6,7 dihydroxycoumarin-3 sulfate. Similarly, it can be speculated that dasycladin B is metabolized to the corresponding monosulfated coumarin first and afterwards to the more active metabolite 3,6,7-trihydroxycoumarin, since the sulfated compounds have been reported as dormant forms which are enzymatically transferred into active metabolites through sulfatases [9]. The sulfated phenolic acids SPA and SBA were both present in the extract, however at very low concentrations. These findings are highlighted with red in Figure 4 and are in good agreement with the LC-MS data published by Kurth et al. [14]. Coumarins in general show a wide range of different pharmacological activities, including anti-HIV, anti-tumor, anti-hypertensive, anti-coagulant, anti-inflammatory just to name a few. They have become important lead compounds in drug research due to their high bioavailability, low molecular weight, and low toxicity [15,18]. For simple coumarins anti-oxidative activity has been reported especially for compounds with free hydroxyl groups. Likewise, the C-7 free hydroxyl group is important for anti-bacterial activity and is also important for an anti-inflammatory activity [19]. The C-6 free hydroxyl group is important for both anti-bacterial and anti-fungal activity. A free hydroxyl group in position 3 (e.g., Compound **4** in this study) is especially important for a strongly enhanced inhibition of 5-Lipoxygenase and α-D-glucosidase [20]. Sulfated coumarins are rather uncommon but due to their negative charge they could bind to heparin receptors or inhibit platelet aggregation [21].

Besides recently developed HPLC-DAD, LC-MS and SFC methods for the separation of furo-pyrano- and monocoumarins on reversed phase columns [22–24], this study presents the first method for the separation of the definitive more polar sulfated coumarins. Their content was found to be quite variable in the different samples suggesting that water depth and seasonal changes including fluctuations in the visible and ultraviolet part of solar radiation might have a strong influence. *D. vermicularis* has been reported to excrete UV-absorbing brown-green substances under in-situ conditions staining the nearby seawater and thus being beneficial as photo-protective compounds for other macroalgae living in the vicinity [6]. The responsible compounds were later identified as coumarins and since they are accumulated in the outer parts of the siphonous cell walls, particularly after UV exposure, they are considered to act as UV-sunscreens [6]. 3,6,7-trihydroxycoumarin (thyc) was found to be preferentially localized in the apical part of the *D. vermicularis* thallus, which usually experiences highest natural insolation, particularly in the internal part of the cell wall and around the tonoplast. The percentage of UVR absorbed by both thyc layers could be measured from the in-vitro total thallus concentration of thyc and histological measurements of these layers. While the cell wall thyc layer absorbed 88% of the incident UVR irradiance, the one close to the vacuole membrane absorbed a similar fraction with 87.5% [6]. These data strongly support the hypothesis of coumarins/phenolics as natural sunscreen compounds reducing biologically harmful UVR from reaching sensitive biomolecules in the cell such as DNA and proteins. Phenolic compounds also play an important role in the interaction of macroalgae with their environment. They are relevant for different supporting or protective tissues, for example in cell wall formation, they can be involved in defense mechanisms, for example in anti-herbivory or having antibacterial effects, and signaling properties, for example in allelopathy [25].

The conspicuous decrease of coumarin content in November could make *D. vermicularis* more susceptible to abiotic and biotic stressors, but UVR and biotic interactions are less strong in late autumn compared to summer in the Mediterranean Sea. However, a larger number of samples from different origins, seasons and water depths is definitely needed to examine the qualitative and quantitative metabolic composition of *D. vermicularis* and its chemical reaction after wounding or other stress situations.

4. Materials and Methods

4.1. Reagents and Chemicals

All solvents used for isolation, synthesis and analytical studies were of analytical grade and purchased from Merck (Darmstadt, Germany). HPLC grade water was produced by a Sartorius arium 611 UV water purification system (Sartorius Göttingen, Germany). Reagents for the synthesis of 4-(sulfooxy)benzoic acid and 4-(sulfooxy)phenylacetic acid (4-hydroxybenzoic acid, sulphur trioxide pyridine complex (Pyr*SO$_3$), and 4-hydroxyphenylacetic acid) were purchased from Sigma Aldrich (Taufkirchen, Germany). Deuterated water for NMR experiments was obtained from Euriso-top (Saint-Aubin Cedex, France).

4.2. Algal Material

Four samples of *Dasycladus vermicularis* were analyzed. DV-1(330 g dry weight) was collected in September 1998 from the upper part of the infralittoral zone (0.5 m depth) in the Cabo de Gata-Nijar Natural Park (36° 52′ N, 2° 12′ W, Almeria, Southern Spain) and identified by Prof. Felix Figueroa (University of Malaga), freeze-dried and sent to Ulf Karsten, who stored the material under cool, dry and dark conditions prior to further processing in Innsbruck. Sample DV-2 was harvested in August 2017 in Alonissos, Greece (39°08′23.8″ N, 23°50′43.3″ E) at 1.80 m depth; Sample DV-3 and DV-4 were both harvested in Volos, Greece (39°1900.0″ N, 23°01′11.5″ E), DV-3 in August 2017 and DV-4 in November 2017 at 30–80 cm depth. All samples from Greece were collected and identified by the author (A. Hartmann). All samples were air-dried and voucher specimen of all samples are stored at the Institute of Pharmacy, Pharmacognosy, University of Innsbruck.

4.3. Instrumentation

NMR experiments were conducted on an Avance II 600 spectrometer (Bruker, Karlsruhe, Germany) operating at 600.19 (^{1}H) and 150.91 MHz (^{13}C). Spectra of the respective compounds were recorded in deuterated solvents from Euriso-Top adding 3-(trimethylsilyl)-propionic acid sodium salt (TMSP) as an internal standard. Infrared (IR) spectra were recorded on an ALPHA Fourier transform (FT)-IR apparatus (Bruker, Billerica, MA, USA) equipped with a platinum attenuated total reflection module. Analytical HPLC experiments were carried out on an Agilent 1100 system (Agilent, Waldbronn, Germany) equipped with a binary pump, autosampler, diode array detector and column oven. For the purification of the compounds a semi-preparative HPLC from Dionex (ThermoFisher, Waltham, MA, USA), comprising of a HPG-3200 pump, a VWD-3100 detector, column oven and a fraction collector was utilized. Additionally, the exact mass of the novel compounds **1** and **2** were determined in negative ESI mode on a micrOTOF-Q II MS (Bruker, Bremen, Germany). The settings were: nebulizer gas: 4.4 psi, dry gas: 4 L/min, dry temperature: 180 °C, capillary voltage: 2.5 kV, set capillary V 3500, set endplate offset V-500.

4.4. Isolation and Structural Analysis of Coumarins

Dried algal material of *Dasycladus vermicularis* (300 g, DV-1, Malaga), were finely ground to powder and subsequently extracted five times with 100% dichloromethane (p.a.) for 15 min in an ultrasonic bath. After centrifugation at 1537× *g*, the combined solutions were evaporated to dryness at 40 °C under reduced pressure to yield 1.13 g of crude dichloromethane extract (DV-1D). The plant material was subsequently extracted with 100% methanol (p.a.) using the same procedure to yield 4.71 g of crude methanol extract (DV-1M). The algal residue was extracted for a third time using the same procedure with a 1:1 mixture of water and methanol to yield 7.9 g crude aqueous extract. The crude methanol extract (4.5 g) was separated into 10 fractions (DV-M-S1-10) on silica gel (40–63 μm particle size) using a dichloromethane/ethyl acetate/methanol/water gradient. Fraction DasyM-S7 was further purified using size-exclusion chromatography on Sephadex LH-20 material with methanol:water (1:1) as eluent to obtain 16 subfractions (DV-M 7.1-16). This resulted in the isolation of compounds **2** (5.24 mg) and **3**

(4.04 mg). A portion (2.5 g) of the crude aqueous extract was first separated using flash chromatography (on RP-18 material (80 g Reveleris cartridge, 40 μm) and a water/methanol gradient, containing 0.25% formic acid in each solvent. 20 subfractions were obtained (DV-W-R1-20). Fraction 18 resulted in the pure compound 4. DV-W-R6 (39.56 mg) was purified by semi-preparative HPLC on a Lichrosorb RP-18 (250 × 10 mm, 7 μm) column with a gradient of 2–50 % methanol in water within 25 min at a flow of 1 mL/min. The oven temperature was set to 20 °C and the UV-detector signal to 350 nm, resulting in 7.91 mg of compound 1. Fraction DV-W-R14 (123 mg) was re-chromatographed on a smaller C18 column using flash chromatography which resulted in 2.6 mg of compound 8. The samples were dissolved in deuterated water with sodium trimethylsilyl propionate (TSP) as internal standard and in case of 3,6,7-trihydroxycoumarin deuterated methanol was used. NMR data of the isolated coumarins are summarized in Table 1. The shift values for thyc were in good agreement to literature values [16]. NMR spectra for the novel sulfated coumarins 1 and 2 are shown in Figure 1A–D and Figure 2A–D in the Supplementary Material. Compounds 3 and 4 are known natural products. Their structures were identified by comparison of their reported spectroscopic data, including ESI-MS and NMR data:

6,7-Dihydroxycoumarin-3-sulfate (**3**, Figure 1): UV_{max} 268, 346 nm. It was assigned with a molecular formula $C_9H_5O_8S$ of ESI-MS, m/z 272.98 [M − H]⁻. ¹H-NMR (600 MHz, D_2O + 0.05% TSP) δ(ppm): 7.87 (s, 1H), 7.10 (s, 1H), 6.95 (s, 1H) ¹³C NMR δ(ppm): 163.6 (C-2), 135.9 (C-3), 135.8 (C-4), 115.7 (C-5), 145.1 (C-6), 151.8 (C-7), 106.0 (C-8), 149.7 (C-9), 114.2 (C-10) [9].

3,6,7-Trihydroxycoumarin (**4**, Figure 1): UV_{max} 268, 346 nm. It was assigned with a molecular formula $C_9H_6O_5$ of ESI-MS, m/z 193.14 [M − H]⁻. ¹H-NMR (600 MHz, D_2O + 0.05% TSP) δ(ppm): 6.94 (s, 1H), 6.79 (s, 1H), 6.73 (s, 1H) ¹³C-NMR δ (ppm): 161.7 (C-2), 140.3 (C-3), 117.6 (C-4), 111.6 (C-5), 144.5 (C-6), 148.0 (C-7), 103.5 (C-8), 145.3 (C-9), 113.9 (C-10) [16].

4.5. Sample Preparation

The powdered dried alga (200 mg) was extracted three times with 8 mL of water: methanol (1:1) each by 15 min of sonication (Sonorex 35 KHz, Bandelin, Berlin, Germany). After centrifugation (1000× g for 3 min), the supernatants were combined in a 25 mL volumetric flask. Samples were measured immediately after extraction.

4.6. Analytical Conditions

Experiments were performed on an Agilent 1100 HPLC system using a Gemini C18, 110 Å column (150 × 4.6 mm, 3 μm) from Phenomenex (Aschaffenburg, Germany). The mobile phase (A) contained water with 20 mM ammonium acetate and 1.5% acetic acid and (B) methanol/water (9:1) with 20 mM ammonium acetate and 1.5% acetic acid. Elution was performed in gradient mode starting with 2% B to 15% B from 0 to 5 min, 15% B to 60% B from 5–20 min and 60% B to 98% B from 20–25 min, followed by 10 min of re-equilibration with 98% A. The DAD was set to 254 nm and 350 nm, and flow rate, sample volume and column temperature were adjusted to 0.3 L/min, 5 μL and 40 °C, respectively. HPLC-MS experiments were carried out on an Agilent 1260 HPLC system coupled to an amaZon iontrap mass spectrometer (Bruker, Bremen, Germany). The chromatographic conditions were as described before; MS-spectra were recorded in negative ESI mode, with a drying gas temperature of 220 °C, the nebulizer gas (nitrogen) set to 23 psi, and a nebulizer flow (nitrogen) of 6 L/min. The scanned mass range was between m/z 70–1500, at a capillary voltage of 4.5 kV.

4.7. Synthesis of 4-(sulfooxy)benzoic Acid and Synthesis of 4-(sulfooxy)phenylacetic Acid

The synthesis of the two sulfated phenolic acids **5** and **6** was carried out as described recently by Kurth et al. [14], however using smaller quantities. 4-Hydroxybenzoic acid (1.5 g), sulfur trioxide pyridine complex (Pyr*SO₃, 1.72 g) were dissolved in water free pyridine (25 mL) and stirred in a 250 mL round bottomed flask at 25 °C for 48 h. For the synthesis of SPA, 4-hydroxyphenylacetic acid (0.75 g) and sulfur trioxide pyridine complex (Pyr*SO₃, 0.83 g) were used. Subsequently, the pyridine was removed by evaporation at 40 °C under reduced pressure. The remaining yellow-brown oil was dissolved in water (20 mL, HPLC grade) and the solution adjusted to pH 6–7 (pH-Meter, Mettler Toledo, Greifensee, Switzerland) using 25% potassium hydroxide. The aqueous solution was washed three times in a separatory funnel. A white precipitate was formed and filtered off after phase separation. Subsequently, the clear aqueous solution was evaporated at 45 °C under reduced pressure to give a white residue, which was re-dissolved in water and adjusted to pH 10 again using 25% KOH. To cleave the anhydride side products this solution was stirred at 60 °C for 1 h and subsequently neutralized using diluted sulfuric acid and afterwards evaporated again. The yellow-white residue was suspended in 10 mL water at 40 °C (5 mL for the synthesis of SPA). A white precipitate was formed by adding 20 mL (10 mL) of methanol, which was filtered off and subsequently washed with 10 mL (5 mL) of methanol. The methanol fractions were combined and left at 4 °C for 24 h in the fridge, so that a crystalline precipitate was formed; it was filtered off and the solution evaporated to dryness. The so obtained raw product was suspended in the ultrasonic bath using 2 mL (1 mL) methanol (HPLC-grade), which resulted in a white powder in a yellow solution. This step was repeated twice. Finally the product was washed with acetone and dried at 70 °C to give 660.93 mg (44% yield) SBA and 253.86 mg SPA (33.8% yield).

SBA: ^{1}H-NMR (600 MHz, D$_2$O + 0.05% TSP) δ(ppm): 7.91 (d, 2H; J = 8.4 Hz); 7.36 (d, 2H; J = 8.4 Hz), ^{13}C-NMR δ(ppm): 177.7(C, C-1), 123.9 (C, C-2), 136.8 (CH,C-3,C-7), 133.3 (CH, C-4,C-6), 156.4 (C, C-5) HPLC–MS m/z [M − H]$^-$: 216.99

SPA: ^{1}H-NMR (600 MHz, D$_2$O + 0.05% TSP) δ(ppm): 3.55 (s, 2H; J = 8.4 Hz), 7.26 (d, 2H; J = 8.5 Hz), 7.32 (d, 2H), ^{13}C-NMR δ(ppm): 183.5 (C, C-1), 46.5 (CH$_2$, C-2), 124.2 (C, C-3), 133.1 (CH,C5; CH, C7), 138.1 (CH,C4; CH,C8), 152.3 (C, C-6), HPLC–MS m/z [M − H]$^-$: 231.00.

4.8. Synthesis of 3,6,7-trihydroxycoumarin

The synthesis of thyc was performed as previously published by Cotelle et al. [26] Briefly, 2,4,5 trihydroxybenzaldehyde (2.31 g), acetylglycine (2.10 g) and sodium acetate (1.59 g) were weighted into a round bottomed flask (100 mL), acetic anhydride (7.5 g) was added and the mixture was heated under reflux for 4 h (130 °C). The solution was cooled to room temperature and ice water (10 mL) was added. The precipitate was filtered, washed with ethanol/water (50:50) and dried to give 3-acetamido-6,7-diacetoxycoumarin. A solution of this intermediate (1.59 g) in 3 M HCl (50 mL) plus acetic acid (2 mL) was refluxed for 1 h and subsequently cooled to room temperature. The obtained precipitate was washed again with water to give pure 3,6,7-trihydroxycoumarin (667.2 mg).

Author Contributions: A.H. did all analytical work, isolated/elucidated the coumarins and wrote the manuscript; M.G. aided in analytical questions and corrected the manuscript; U.K. supplied and identified the algae and edited the first draft. A.S. aided in the structure elucidation of the novel coumarins.

Acknowledgments: We thank Barbara Matuszczak for measuring the IR spectra.

References

1. Guiry, M.D.; Guiry, M.D.; Guiry, G.M. *AlgaeBase*; World-Wide Electronic Publication, National University of Ireland: Galway, Ireland. Available online: http://www.algaebase.org (accessed on 18 October 2018).
2. Carrillo, J.M.A. Algunas observaciones sobre la distribucion vertical de las algas en la Isla del Hierro (canarias). *Vieraea. Fol. Sci. Biol. Canar.* **1980**, *10*, 3–16.

3.	Menzel, D.; Kazlauskas, R.; Reichelt, J. Coumarins in the Siphonalean Green Algal Family Dasycladaceae Kutzing (Chlorophyceae). *Bot. Mar.* **1983**, *26*, 23–29. [CrossRef]

4.	Gomez, I.; Pérez-Rodríguez, E.; Viñegla, B.; Figueroa, F.L.; Karsten, U. Effects of solar radiation on photosynthesis, UV-absorbing compounds and enzyme activities of the green alga *Dasycladus vermicularis* from southern Spain. *J. Photochem. Photobiol. B* **1998**, *47*, 46–57. [CrossRef]

5.	Perez-Rodriguez, E.; Aguilera, J.; Gomez, I.; Figueroa, F.L. Excretion of coumarins by the Mediterranean green alga *Dasycladus vermicularis* in response to environmental stress. *Mar. Biol.* **2001**, *139*, 633–639. [CrossRef]

6.	Perez-Rodriguez, E.; Aguilera, J.; Figueroa, F.L. Tissular localization of coumarins in the green alga *Dasycladus vermicularis* (Scopoli) Krasser: A photoprotective role? *J. Exp. Bot.* **2003**, *54*, 1093–1100. [CrossRef] [PubMed]

7.	Coneva, V.; Chitwood, D.H. Plant architecture without multicellularity: Quandaries over patterning and the soma-germline divide in siphonous algae. *Front. Plant. Sci.* **2015**, *6*, 287. [CrossRef] [PubMed]

8.	Welling, M.; Pohnert, G.; Küppert, F.C.; Ross, C. Rapid Biopolymerisation During Wound Plug Formation in Green Algae. *J. Adhes.* **2009**, *85*, 825–838. [CrossRef]

9.	Welling, M.; Ross, C.; Pohnert, G.A. Desulfatation-Oxidation Cascade Activates Coumarin-Based Cross-Linkers in the Wound Reaction of the Giant Unicellular Alga *Dasycladus vermicularis*. *Angew. Chem.-Int. E* **2011**, *50*, 7691–7694. [CrossRef] [PubMed]

10.	Ross, C.; Vreeland, V.; Waite, J.H.; Jacobs, R.S. Rapid assembly of a wound plug: Stage one of a two-stage wound repair mechanism in the giant unicellular chlorophyte *Dasycladus vermicularis* (Chlorophyceae). *J. Phycol.* **2005**, *41*, 46–54. [CrossRef]

11.	Sever, M.J.; Weisser, J.T.; Monahan, J.; Srinivasan, S.; Wilker, J.J. Metal-mediated cross-linking in the generation of a marine-mussel adhesive. *Angew. Chem.-Int. E* **2004**, *43*, 448–450. [CrossRef] [PubMed]

12.	Thoms, C.; Schupp, P.J. Activated chemical defense in marine sponges—A case study on *Aplysinella rhax*. *J. Chem. Ecol.* **2008**, *34*, 1242–1252. [CrossRef] [PubMed]

13.	Kurth, C.; Cavas, L.; Pohnert, G. Sulfation mediates activity of zosteric acid against biofilm formation. *Biofouling* **2015**, *31*, 253–263. [CrossRef] [PubMed]

14.	Kurth, C.; Welling, M.; Pohnert, G. Sulfated phenolic acids from Dasycladales siphonous green algae. *Phytochemtry* **2015**, *117*, 417–423. [CrossRef] [PubMed]

15.	Haensel, R.; Sticher, O. *Pharmakognosie Phytopharmazie*, 9th ed.; Springer Medizin Verlag GmbH: Heidelberg, Germany, 2010; pp. 419–420.

16.	Bailly, F.; Maurin, C.; Teissier, E.; Vezin, H.; Cotelle, P. Antioxidant properties of 3-hydroxycoumarin derivatives. *Bioorg. Med. Chem.* **2004**, *12*, 5611–5618. [CrossRef] [PubMed]

17.	ICH Harmonization for Better Health. Available online: http://www.ich.org/products/guidelines.html (accessed on 6 August 2018).

18.	Zhu, J.J.; Jiang, J.G. Pharmacological and Nutritional Effects of Natural Coumarins and Their Structure-Activity Relationships. *Mol. Nutr. Food Res.* **2018**, *62*, 1701073. [CrossRef] [PubMed]

19.	Kayser, O.; Kolodziej, H. Antibacterial Activity of Simple Coumarins: Structural Requirements for Biological Activity. *Naturforschung C* **1999**, *54*, 169. [CrossRef]

20.	Aihara, K.; Higuchi, T.; Hirobe, M. 3-Hydroxycoumarins: First direct preparation from coumarins using a $Cu^{2(+)}$-ascorbic acid-O_2 system, and their potent bioactivities. *Biochem. Biophys. Res. Commun.* **1990**, *168*, 169–175. [CrossRef]

21.	Verespy, S.; Metha, A.Y.; Afosah, D.; Al-Horani, R.A.; Desai, U.R. Allosteric partial Inhibition of Monomeric Proteases. Sulfated Coumarins Induce Regulation, not just Inhibition of Thrombin. *Sci. Rep.* **2016**, *6*, 24043. [CrossRef] [PubMed]

22.	Li, B.; Zhang, X.; Wang, J.; Zhang, Z.; Gao, B.; Shi, S.; Wang, X.; Li, J.; Tu, P. Simultaneous characterization of fifty coumarins from the roots of *Angelica dahurica* by off-line two-dimensional high-performance liquid chromatography coupled with electrospray ionization tandem mass spectrometry. *Phytochem. Anal.* **2014**, *25*, 229–240. [CrossRef] [PubMed]

23.	Wu, Y.; Wang, F.; Ai, Y.; Ma, W.; Bian, Q.; Lee, D.; Dai, R. Simultaneous determination of seven coumarins by UPLC-MS/MS: Application to a comparative pharmacokinetic study in normal and arthritic rats after administration of Huo Luo Xiao Ling Dan or single herb. *J. Chromatogr. B* **2015**, *991*, 108–117. [CrossRef] [PubMed]

24.   Li, G.J.; Wu, H.J.; Wang, Y.; Hung, W.L.; Rouseff, R.L. Determination of citrus juice coumarins, furanocoumarins and methoxylated flavones using solid phase extraction and HPLC with photodiode array and fluorescence detection. *Food Chem.* **2019**, *15*, 29–38. [CrossRef] [PubMed]

25.   Schoenwaelder, M.E.A. The Biology of Phenolic Containing Vesicles. *Algae* **2008**, *23*, 163–175. [CrossRef]

26.   Cotelle, P.; Vezin, H. EPR of free radicals formed from 3-hydroxyesculetin and related derivatives. *Res. Chem. Intermed.* **2003**, *29*, 365–377. [CrossRef]

10

In Silico Studies on Compounds Derived from *Calceolaria*: Phenylethanoid Glycosides as Potential Multitarget Inhibitors for the Development of Pesticides

Marco A. Loza-Mejía *, Juan Rodrigo Salazar * and Juan Francisco Sánchez-Tejeda

Benjamín Franklin 45, Cuauhtémoc, Mexico City 06140, Mexico; juansanchez@lasallistas.org
* Correspondence: marcoantonio.loza@ulsa.mx (M.A.L.-M.); juan.salazar@ulsa.mx (J.R.S.);

Abstract: An increasing occurrence of resistance in insect pests and high mammal toxicity exhibited by common pesticides increase the need for new alternative molecules. Among these alternatives, bioinsecticides are considered to be environmentally friendly and safer than synthetic insecticides. Particularly, plant extracts have shown great potential in laboratory conditions. However, the lack of studies that confirm their mechanisms of action diminishes their potential applications on a large scale. Previously, we have reported the insect growth regulator and insecticidal activities of secondary metabolites isolated from plants of the *Calceolaria* genus. Herein, we report an in silico study of compounds isolated from *Calceolaria* against acetylcholinesterase, prophenoloxidase, and ecdysone receptor. The molecular docking results are consistent with the previously reported experimental results, which were obtained during the bioevaluation of *Calceolaria* extracts. Among the compounds, phenylethanoid glycosides, such as verbascoside, exhibited good theoretical affinity to all the analyzed targets. In light of these results, we developed an index to evaluate potential multitarget insecticides based on docking scores.

Keywords: molecular docking; bioinsecticides; structure–activity relationship; phenylethanoid glycosides; *Calceolaria*; multitarget

1. Introduction

The continuous growth of the world population has created an enormous pressure to satisfy the global demand for agricultural products. The challenges include the depletion of soil fertility, the constant depredation of natural soils to convert them into agricultural ecosystems, and the ability of the arthropods to obtain resistance against traditional insecticidal controls.

Insecticides have been used for combating insect pests, mainly to increase the yield of food production among other agricultural products. From ancient times, there are records that describe the use of different types of products to combat insect pests [1]. It is known that various nonspecific agents have been used, such as sulfur and poisonous natural extracts, then organochlorines, organophosphates, carbamates, pyrethroids, and rotenoids, among others, and finally compounds, which are specifically designed and synthesized against enzymatic systems of arthropods.

The increasing need for agricultural goods has resulted in misutilization of insecticides, and this has led to the use of a higher concentration of insecticides or to the need for more toxic products. This has resulted in increased toxic effects on other beneficial organisms that coexist with pests in agroecosystems and on the bioaccumulation of higher concentrations of toxic insecticides in the bodies of predators or the final consumers, including humans. Despite these problems, the use of insecticides is needed to satisfy global demand for products. Thus, we can say that insecticides are a necessary evil. However, research must be carried out to identify better alternatives.

Among these alternatives, bioinsecticides enjoy a good reputation and are generally regarded as environmentally friendly and safer than synthetic insecticides [2]. For some years, many groups have conducted studies for biodirected phytochemical screening on plants toward the isolation and characterization of extracts and compounds that are useful as biocides. In most of published reports, authors investigate the effect of extracts or compounds against specific pest organisms, or against one or more isolated molecular targets, such as acetylcholinesterase (AChE) [3]. We use the extraordinary ability of plants to respond dynamically to herbivory through several molecular mechanisms, including the biosynthesis of defensive compounds to identify those with potential to be used for pest control. Those compounds can affect feeding, growth, and survival of insects and are widely distributed in nature [4]. The organic extracts prepared from the botanical material are a rich source of many classes of secondary metabolites. Many of them have been isolated via traditional chromatographic techniques and even used as active components in botanical pest management products, mainly rotenone, nicotine, strychnine, neem extracts, and essential oils [5]. Thus, the traditional methodology to discover new insecticides includes phytochemical work for the screening of microbial metabolites, terrestrial plants, algae, marine organisms, and so forth. Several factors make harder or more complicated the transition from synthetic insecticides to bioinsecticides. Specifically, the use of an extract generally does not offer guarantees of success in combating pests, and often, the insecticidal mechanisms involved are unknown or are too difficult to elucidate due to the complexity of mixtures of natural extracts [6].

However, less emphasis is given to pesticide-discovery efforts based upon natural products as templates for new structures via semisynthesis. In recent years, a renewed interest in obtaining biologically active compounds from natural sources has emerged, not only as a source of new molecules but also with innovative methodologies, including fragment-based design, high-throughput screening, and genetic engineering, towards the development of new pest-management products with low or absent toxicity towards nontarget insects and mammal organisms, low final concentrations caused by ambient degradability, and a relatively low cost compared with those compounds obtained via complete chemical synthesis [7].

Our group has conducted studies on the *Calceolaria* genus for the identification, isolation, and characterization of new bioinsecticides. The extracts and several secondary metabolites isolated from *Calceolaria* exhibit insect growth regulator (IGR) or insecticidal activities. The insecticidal activity was assayed against the fruit fly (*Drosophila melanogaster*, Diptera), yellow meal worm (*Tenebrio molitor*, Coleoptera: Tenebrionidae), and fall armyworm (*Spodoptera frugiperda*, J. E. Smith, Lepidoptera: Noctuidae), which are important insect pests in fruits, stored grains, and corn [8]. The experimental results indicate that some extracts and compounds isolated from *Calceolaria* interfere with sclerotization and molting processes, suggesting interaction with an ecdysone receptor [9]. Several of these extracts and compounds also act as enzymatic inhibitors against tyrosinase and protease enzymes [10], suggesting potential multitarget activity. Few examples of multitarget insecticides have been reported in the literature [11,12].

On the other hand, among the strategies used to find bioactive candidates, structure-based virtual screening (SBVS) has played a critical role, especially in the identification of potential chemotypes [13]. Docking-based virtual screening (DBVS) is probably the most widely used of these strategies. It involves docking of a library of ligands into a biological target and estimating the probability that a ligand will bind to the protein target by the application of a scoring algorithm, aiding in the identification of the most promising lead compounds for biological assays [14]. However, DBVS has some limitations: (a) the content and quality of the compound library has a profound effect on the success of DBVS, thus it is important to filter the library using the rule-of-five or other physicochemical filters, and (b) with the actual scoring functions, the prediction of correct binding poses is feasible but high accuracy prediction of binding affinity is still a challenge, thus there is little confidence on docking scores to rank potential ligands, particularly on those of the same structural frame [14,15].

Despite these limitations, DBVS has been successfully used in the identification of potential templates for new drug development [16–18]. Recently, some examples of the use of virtual screening and other computational chemistry tools in natural products research have been described [19–22].

With this in mind, we wanted to determine the potential use of compounds isolated from *Calceloraia* as leads in the discovery of multitarget insecticides using DBVS on some proteins recognized as targets for pesticides [12,23,24] and that could be targets for compounds present in *Calceolaria* extracts based on experimental results [9,25,26]: acetylcholinesterase (AChE), prophenoloxidase (PPO), and ecdysone receptor (EcR). Construction of a ligand library was based on compounds isolated and present in organic extracts with experimentally demonstrated pesticide activity aiming to identify potential structural templates that could be used in the development of new pesticides.

2. Materials and Methods

2.1. Ligand Construction

All of the ligands were chosen from a previously published review [27], which includes several compounds from different chemical families, including diterpenes, triterpenes, and naphthoquinones with a potential pesticidal activity, and some bioactive flavonoids and phenylethanoid glycosides as well. All of the structures were constructed using Spartan '10 for Windows, and these geometries were optimized using the MMFF force field. Then, these structures were exported to Molegro Virtual Docker 6.0.1 [28]; assignments of charges and ionization were based on standard templates as part of the Molegro software. A complete list of all ligands and their structures are presented in Supplementary Information.

2.2. Molecular Docking Studies

The docking studies were carried out based on the crystal structures of *Drosophila melanogaster* acetylcholinesterase (*Dm*AchE, PDB codes: 1DX4 [29] and 1QON [29]), *Heliothis virescens* ecdysone receptor (EcR, PDB code: 3IXP [30] and 2R40 [31]), and *Manduca sexta* prophenoloxidase (PPO, PDB code: 3HHS [32]). Two different structures from the Protein Data Bank (PDB) were selected to analyze repeatability of results, independent of the PDB structure selected. This was not possible for PPO as no other PDB structure has been reported. In addition, docking studies were carried out in human acetylcholinesterase (*h*AChE, PDB code: 4EY7 [33] and 4M0E [34]) to determine whether some of the compounds exhibited theoretical preference to the *Drosophila*/human enzyme. All structures were retrieved from the Protein Data Bank [35]. Docking studies were carried out using a previously reported methodology [36,37]. Briefly, all of the solvent molecules and cocrystallized ligands were removed from the structures. Molecular docking calculations for all of the compounds with each of the proteins were performed using Molegro Virtual Docker v. 6.0.1 [28]. Active sites of each enzyme were chosen as the binding sites and delimited with a 15 Å radius sphere centered on the cocrystallized ligand, except for the PPO structure, which has no cocrystallized ligand, and the sphere was centered on the active Cu^{2+} ions. Standard software procedure was used. The assignments of charges on each protein were based on standard templates as part of the Molegro Virtual Docker program, and no other charges were necessary to be set. The Root Mean Square Deviation (RMSD) threshold for multiple cluster poses was set to <1.00 Å. The docking algorithm was set to 5000 maximum iterations with a simplex evolution population size of 50 and a minimum of 25 runs for each ligand. After docking, *MolDock Score* was calculated as the theoretical binding affinity. To assess the efficacy of this procedure, cocrystallized ligands were also docked to their respective receptors (except for PPO), the top-ranking score was recorded, and the RMSD of that pose from the corresponding crystal coordinates was computed. In all the cases, the RMSD was lower than 2 Å. For each enzyme, the 10 compounds with lower *MolDock scores* were selected for analyzing their docking poses to identify potential structural requirements for enzyme binding.

2.3. Molecular Dynamics Simulations

Molecular Dynamics (MD) simulations were carried out to observe differences that could account for potential selectivity of phenylpropanoids for *Dm*AChE over *h*AChE. Simulations were performed in YASARA Dynamics v.18.4.24 [38,39] using AMBER14 force field [40]. The initial structures for the MD simulation were obtained from the docking complexes of compound **87** with *Dm*AChE (PDB code: 1QON) and with *h*AChE (PDB code: 4M0E). Compound **87** (verbascoside) was selected, as it is the most studied compound of the phenylpropanoids derived from *Calceolaria*. Each complex was positioned into a water box with a size of 100 Å × 100 Å × 100 Å, with periodic boundary conditions. Temperature was set at 298 K, water density to 0.997 g/cm^3, and pH to 7.4. Sodium (Na$^+$) and chlorine (Cl$^-$) ions were included to provide conditions that simulate a physiological solution (NaCl 0.9%). Particle mesh Ewald algorithm was applied with a cut-off radius of 8 Å. A timestep of 2.5 fs was set. The simulation snapshots were recorded at intervals of 100 ps until a total simulation time of 30 ns. Results were analyzed with a script included as part of YASARA software and included RMSD, ligand binding energy variations (using MM-PBSA calculations), and distance of ligand 87 to Ser 283 (*Dm*AChE) or Ser 203 (*h*AChE), as these residues play a key role in acetylcholinesterase enzymatic activity. For *Dm*AChE, we considered the interaction between the primary alcohol group of the central glucopyranose ring with Ser 238, and for *h*AChE, the interaction between the hydroxyl group of the ferouyl residue with Ser 203. A similar procedure has been recently reported for the simulation of complexes of drugs with some proteins [41–43].

2.4. Construction of the Virtual Multitarget Index and the Weighed Multi-Target Index

The virtual Multitarget index of each compound was determined. To compare the multitarget index of the analyzed compounds, we propose a virtual multitarget index (*vMTi*), which was calculated for the three insect targets (EcR, PPO, and *Dm*AChE) using formula (1):

$$vMTi = \sum_{i=1}^{n} \frac{MD_i}{MDr} \tag{1}$$

where MDi corresponds to the *MolDock* score of the molecule in a specific target and MDr is the *MolDock* score of the reference ligand; we considered the compound with the lowest *MolDock* score (which has the highest theoretical affinity) for each target as the reference. Compounds with higher values have a higher multitarget index. However, binding to *h*AChE is an undesirable condition. To take this into consideration, we propose a weighed *MTi* (*wMTi*), which was calculated using formula 2, using an external coefficient *n*, which represents the desirability of binding to a specific target:

$$wMTi = \sum_{i=1}^{n} n \frac{MD_i}{MDr} \tag{2}$$

To calculate *wMTi*, we gave values of *n* = 0.3 to desirable targets (EcR, PPO, and *Dm*AChE) and *n* = −0.3 to *h*AChE.

In addition to these calculations, a contour plot was built with Minitab using PPO, *Dm*AChE, and EcR docking scores. This plot can help identify potential multitarget compounds because those compounds would appear in valleys since they would have lower *MolDock* scores.

3. Results

3.1. Docking Studies Results

Tables 1–3 show data for the 10 compounds with a lower average *MolDock score* in the ecdysone receptor (EcR), prophenoloxidase (PPO), and acetylcholinesterase (both *Dm*AchE and *h*AChE) docking study. A table with complete docking results is presented in Supplementary Information.

Table 1. *MolDock Scores* obtained in the ecdysone receptor (EcR) docking. Top 10 compounds with the better theoretical binding. PEG = Phenylethanoid glycosides.

Ligand	Skeleton Type	Compound Name	PDB: 3IXP	PDB: 2R40	Average *MolDock Scores*
88	PEG	Calceolarioside C	−214.0	−207.2	−210.6
90	PEG	Forsythoside A	−202.8	−213.5	−208.2
89	PEG	Calceolarioside E	−184.7	−212.5	−198.6
92	PEG	Isoarenarioside	−183.0	−205.5	−194.2
87	PEG	Verbascoside	−197.4	−184.1	−190.8
86	PEG	Calceolarioside A	−174.2	−183.6	−178.9
91	PEG	Calceolarioside B	−162.1	−176.7	−169.4
93	PEG	Calceolarioside D	−160.2	−169.3	−164.7
68	Scopadulane	3-Isovaleroyl-7-malonyloxy-thyrsiflorane	−147.2	−157.1	−152.2
45	Isopimarane	3-β-Isovaleroyl-18-hydroxy-7-α-malonyloxyent-isopimara-9(11), 15-diene	−150.2	−151.5	−150.8

Table 2. *MolDock Scores* obtained in the PPO docking. Top 10 compounds with the better theoretical binding. PEG = Phenylethanoid glycosides.

Ligand	Skeleton	Compound Name	*MolDock* Score
86	PEG	Calceolarioside A	−161.187
110	Flavonoid	Kaempferol-7-methyl ether	−142.825
93	PEG	Calceolarioside D	−142.017
109	Flavonoid	Gossypetin-7,8,3′-trimethyl ether	−140.618
108	Flavonoid	Herbacetin-8,4′-dimethyl ether	−138.595
88	PEG	Calceolarioside C	−137.969
111	Flavonoid	Kaempferol-4′-methyl ether	−137.519
104	Flavonoid	Naringenin-4′-methyl ether	−137.451
107	Flavonoid	Isoscutellarein-8,4′-dimethyl ether	−137.188

Table 3. *MolDock* scores obtained in the AChE docking study. Top 10 compounds with the better theoretical binding.

Ligand	Compound Name	*Dm*AChE *MolDock* Scores			*h*AChE *MolDock* Scores			SR [1]
		PDB: 1DX4	PDB: 1QON	Average Score	PDB: 4EY7	PDB: 4M0E	Average Score	
90	Forsythoside A	−171.3	−254.5	−212.9	−177.7	−247.6	−212.6	1.00
88	Calceolarioside C	−174.0	−251.6	−212.8	−145.7	−217.7	−181.7	1.17
87	Verbascoside	−178.8	−233.5	−206.1	−152.6	−200.8	−176.7	1.17
89	Calceolarioside E	−169.0	−239.1	−204.0	−116.7	−209.0	−162.8	1.25
93	Calceolarioside D	−162.3	−227.7	−195.0	−147.9	−188.4	−168.2	1.16
92	Isoarenarioside	−141.1	−244.8	−193.0	−165.1	−208.0	−186.6	1.03
86	Calceolarioside A	−156.2	−212.8	−184.5	−164.6	−189.6	−177.1	1.04
91	Calceolarioside B	−128.0	−210.5	−169.2	−137.9	−183.9	−160.9	1.05
44	Isopimarane	−119.9	−180.3	−150.1	−137.0	−159.7	−148.4	1.01
43	Isopimarane	−127.3	−164.5	−145.9	−150.2	−154.6	−152.4	0.96

[1] Selectivity ratio (SR) = Average docking score *Dm*AChE / Average docking score *h*AChE.

3.2. Molecular Dynamics Studies on Complexes of Verbascoside with DmAChE and hAChE

Figure 1a shows the comparison of the RMSD time profile for protein backbone atoms during the 30 ns simulation of the complexes of compound **87** and *Dm*AChE and *h*AChE. Both complexes have RMSD average values around 2 Å (RMSD = 2.13 Å for *Dm*AChE and RMSD = 1.88 Å for *h*AChE).

We also wanted to check if the distance of compound **87** (verbascoside) to the catalytic site of acetylcholinesterase variates during the simulation time. We selected the potential interactions to Ser 203 in *h*AChE or Ser 238 in *Dm*AChE predicted by molecular docking as described in Methodology. Figure 1b shows the variation of distances of compound **87** to these key serine residues along the simulation time. As seen in this figure, the distance to catalytic site diminished from 4.8 Å to 3.0 Å after 3 ns of simulation in the case of *Dm*AChE (average distance = 3.6 Å), while it maintained almost the same in *h*AChE (average distance = 5.21 Å).

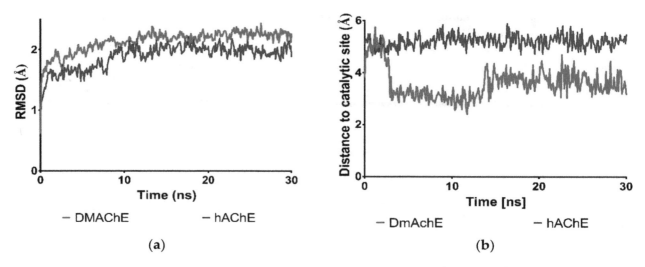

Figure 1. Plots of variations along time of Molecular Dynamics (MD) simulations of complexes of **87** with *Dm*AChE (red) and *h*AChE (blue). (**a**) The Root Mean Square Deviation (RMSD) of protein backbone; (**b**) distance of compound **87** to Ser 238 (*Dm*AChE) or Ser 203 (*h*AChE).

To estimate the difference in binding energy of compound **87** in its complex with *Dm*AChE and *h*AChE, MM-PBSA methods were applied. Ligand binding energy suggests better binding of compound **87** to *Dm*AChE (E = −131.5 kJ/mol) versus *h*AChE (E = −134.0 kJ/mol) as binding energy calculations implemented in YASARA Dynamics indicates that the higher the energy value, the better the binding.

3.3. Construction of the Virtual Multitarget Index and the Weighed Multitarget Index

Figure 2 shows a contour graphic that compares docking scores of the analyzed compounds on PPO, *Dm*AChE, and EcR. The zone in red corresponds to those molecules with high theoretical affinity against all the three molecular targets. Figure 3 shows the structure of the phenylpropanoids which resulted with the highest values of *vMTi* and *wMTi*. Table 4 shows a list of compounds with higher *vMti* and *wMTi* values; a full list is included in Supplementary Information.

Table 4. Compounds with higher *vMTi* and *wMTi* values. PEG = Phenylethanoid glycosides.

Ligand	Skeleton	Compound Name	*vMTi*	*wMTi*
88	PEG	Calceolarioside C	2.86	0.60
89	PEG	Calceolarioside E	2.67	0.57
86	PEG	Calceolarioside A	2.72	0.56
87	PEG	Verbascoside	2.67	0.55
93	PEG	Calceolarioside D	2.58	0.54
90	PEG	Forsythoside A	2.77	0.53
92	PEG	Isoarenarioside	2.64	0.53
91	PEG	Calceolarioside B	2.39	0.49
109	Flavonoid	Gossypetin-7,8,3′-trimethyl ether	2.05	0.43
110	Flavonoid	Kaempferol-7-methyl ether	2.03	0.43
77	Labdane	19-Malonyloxy-9-epi-ent-labda- 8(17), 12 Z, 14-triene	2.04	0.42
45	Isopimarane	3-β-Isovaleroyl-18-hydroxy-7-α-malonyloxyent-isopimara-9(11), 15-diene	2.13	0.42
3	Abietane	19-Malonyloxy-dehydroabietinol	1.99	0.42
57	Stemarane	17-Acetoxy-19-malonyloxy-ent-stemar-13(14)-ene	2.03	0.41
108	Flavonoid	Herbacetin-8,4′-dimethyl ether	1.92	0.40

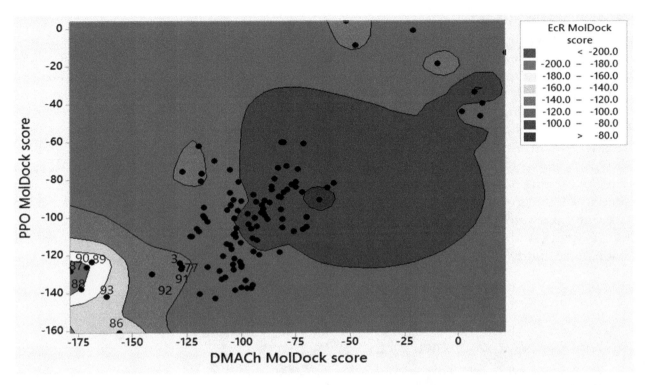

Figure 2. Contour plot correlating PPO, *Dm*AChE, and EcR docking scores. Zones in red-yellow indicate higher affinity to EcR than zones in purple or blue.

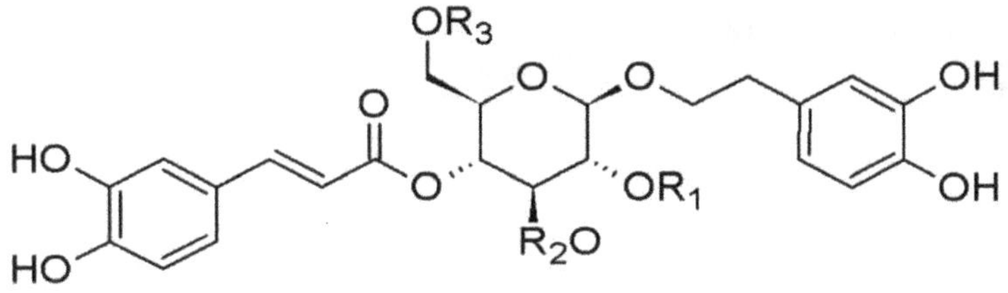

86 R_1= H, R_2= H, R_3=H   **87** R_1= H, R_2= Rhamnose, R_3=H
88 R_1= H, R_2= H, R_3=Xylose   **89** R_1= H, R_2= Apiose, R_3=H
90 R_1= H, R_2= H, R_3=Rhamnose

Figure 3. Structures of phenylethanoid glycosides (compounds **86–90**) which exhibited the highest *vMTi* and *wMTi* values.

4. Discussion

4.1. Docking Studies on Ecdysone Receptor

Induction of molting in Arthropods coincides with a release of 20-hydroxyecdysone (20-E), a steroidal-type hormone. Prior to each of the larval molts, at pupariation, at pupation, and during metamorphosis, the hormone is released in carefully timed spurts, coinciding with major morphological transitions. Ecdysone receptor (EcR) exists in three isoforms. Each requires a partner during the heterodimerization, a *Drosophila* homolog of vertebrate RXR protein named ultraspiracle (USP) protein. Although ecdysone can bind to EcR on its own, binding is significantly augmented by the participation of USP. The interaction between EcR and ecdysone is a crucial event for the development of insects, which is why it represents an interesting molecular target against pest insects [44].

Table 1 shows data for the 10 compounds with a lower average *MolDock score* in the ecdysone receptor docking study. Phenylethanoid glycoside derivatives have better theoretical binding to EcR among the evaluated compounds. Among them, the results indicate that binding to EcR occurs through hydroxyl groups of caffeoyl and phenyl ethyl residues in similar fashion to 20-E (Figure 4a). Analysis of Figure 4a,b reveals that compound **87** (verbascoside, which is a major phenylethanoid glycoside present in *Calceolaria* extracts) adopted a J-shaped conformation in the binding site of EcR, which is similar to the conformation adopted by natural ligand of EcR, 20-E [31] and the interaction pattern is very similar between these compounds: phenylethanoid residue interacts through hydrogen bonds with Arg383 and Glu309 (in magenta in Figure 4a,b) like 2β and 3β hydroxyl groups of ring-A in 20-E, rhamnose residue interacts with Ala398 (in blue in Figure 3a,b) like C-6 ketone moiety in ring-B in 20-E, feruoyl residue interacts with Thr 343 and rhamnose residue with Thr 346 (also in blue in set of Figure 4) like 14-α hydroxyl group, and additional interactions between feruoyl residue and central glucose ring of verbascoside with Tyr 408 and Asn 504 (shown in yellow) are seen in a similar fashion for 25-OH group of side chain of 20-E. This interaction is notable because 20-E interacts with this residue via a water linkage [31], hence the interaction of verbascoside with Asn504 could increase affinity, as some studies have demonstrated that ligands designed to displace the water molecules exhibit higher affinity [45].

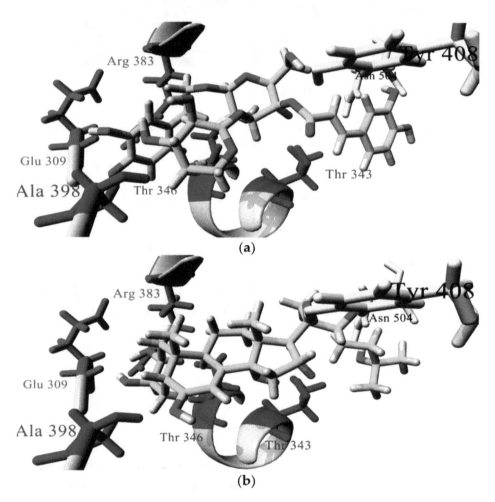

(a)

(b)

Figure 4. Comparison of (**a**) the docked pose of verbascoside (compound **87**) and (**b**) 20-E crystallized in the LBD of EcR (PDB:2R40).

Though there are no previous studies on phenylethanoid glycosides as EcR ligands, there is some experimental evidence that can support docking results. It has been previously reported that the ethyl acetate extract of *C. talcana*, of which verbascoside is its major component (compound **87**), caused a developmental disruption of *D. melanogaster* and *S. frugiperda* larvae. In addition, the authors of the study proposed verbascoside as a disruptor of ecdysteroid metabolism [26]. In another study, the incorporation of verbascoside in the artificial diet of the pest *Agrilus planipennis* caused a 100%

mortality at 45 mg/g of artificial diet [46] when testing the toxic effect of verbascoside against at least three different pest insect species. In addition, Harmatha and Dinan have reported that some polyhydroxylated stilbenoids have an antagonist EcR activity [47], and a previously reported pharmacophore model indicated that the presence of hydroxyl groups in an ecdysteroid template is important for EcR binding [48]. On the other hand, the presence of some other phenylethanoid glycosides, such as calceolarioside A, B, and C, in active extracts of *Calceolaria* as well as in *Fraxinus* spp. can be related to the strong larval molting disruption observed when the larvae of different species were exposed to extracts with high amounts of phenylethanoid glycosides or directly to different amounts of the isolated compounds [46]. All these experimental data strongly suggest that phenylpropanoid glycosides could be EcR ligands.

As described here, the effect of verbascoside and related phenylethanoid glycosides against the ecdysone receptor can explain only one of the multiple effects exerted by these compounds. The experimental evidence remarkably indicates that molting disruption exerted by phenylethanoid glycosides cannot be the only mechanism that explains the strong exerted insecticidal properties. The above information suggests a possible antagonist and multienzymatic inhibitory mechanism that phenylethanoid glycosides can exert, causing larvae disruption activity by acting as EcR antagonist in addition to other mechanisms.

4.2. Docking Studies on Prophenoloxidase

Melanization, a process performed by phenoloxidase (PO) and controlled by the prophenoloxidase (PPO) activation cascade, plays an important role in the invertebrate immune system in allowing a rapid response to pathogen infection. The activation of the PPO system, by the specific recognition of microorganisms by pattern-recognition proteins (PRPs), triggers a serine proteinase cascade, which eventually leads to the cleavage of the inactive PPO to the active PO that functions to produce melanin and toxic reactive intermediates. The importance of PPO–PO is due to cuticular sclerotization and defense against pathogens and parasites. PO catalyzes hydroxylation of monophenols to o-diphenols and oxidation of o-diphenols to quinones. Quinones take part in sclerotization and tanning of the cuticle and serve as precursors for synthesis of melanin [49,50]. Therefore, PPO is a very suitable molecular target for designing pesticide compounds.

Table 2 shows docking results from the PPO study. Among the compounds with better PPO binding, the best are flavonoids and phenylethanoid glycosides. The results are in agreement with several previous in vitro and in silico studies [10,51–55] in which most tyrosinase inhibitors possess a phenol moiety as the pharmacophore. Among them, flavonoids appear as effective competitive inhibitors of this enzyme. In addition, Karioti et al. [53] and Muñoz et al. [10] have reported tyrosinase inhibitory activities of some phenylethanoid glycosides, which have lower but comparable inhibitory activities compared with flavonols and flavones.

Hydroxyl groups of caffeoyl or phenylethyl residues have been proposed as essential structural requirements to display inhibitory activities against PPO because of their chelating properties. Figure 5 shows that phenylethanoid glycosides could bind to the PPO catalytic site through interaction with His residues, which are required to form a complex with copper ions. This is in agreement with the previously reported information that indicates verbascoside as a substrate for tyrosinase [10]. Among phenylethanoid glycosides, compounds **86** and **93** could bind better than other analogs. These compounds are monoglycosides, whereas other evaluated phenylethanoid glycosides are diglycosides, which is in agreement with previous reports that indicate the increase in the number of sugar units and the reduction of PPO inhibitory activity [53]. This observation could be explained in terms of the higher molecular volume of diglycosides that prevents them access to the active site as is shown Figure 5; the diglycoside compound **88** is shown in yellow and monoglycoside **86** is in cyan. From this figure, it can be concluded that it is possible that monoglycosides could bind closer to the catalytic site of PPO.

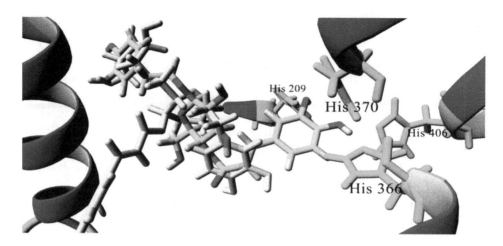

Figure 5. Overlap docking poses of compounds **86** (cyan) and **88** (yellow). Histidine residues of catalytic site are shown in green.

4.3. Docking Studies and Molecular Dynamics Simulations on Drosophila and Human Acetylcholinesterase

Acetylcholinesterase is a serine hydrolase that is vital for regulating the neurotransmitter acetylcholine in insects. This enzyme is an excellent molecular target for the development of insecticides [56,57]. The well-known active site has a deep and narrow gorge, with a catalytic site at the bottom and a peripheral site at the entrance. Acetylcholinesterase is a molecular target used to control insects that affect public health (e.g., mosquitoes, flies, cockroaches, among others) as well as those that affect agriculture and gardening (e.g., grasshoppers, aphids, caterpillars, among others) [58]. Current anticholinesterase insecticides work through phosphorylation of a serine residue at the AChE catalytic site, which disables the catalytic function and causes enzyme antagonism. Because this serine residue is also ubiquitous in AChEs of mammals and other species with cholinergic nerves, the use of anticholinesterase insecticides to target the serine residue causes serious off-target toxicity [59]. Therefore, it is necessary to evaluate in silico the affinity of molecules against the insect together with mammalian enzymes to determine whether there are some structural features that lead to design inhibitors specifically against insect enzymes.

Table 3 displays the *MolDock* scores of the top 10 compounds with better average docking scores for *Dm*AChE studies in PDB 1DX4 and 1QON structures. Data obtained during docking studies with *h*AChE (PDB structures 4EY7 and 4M0E) is also shown. Selectivity ratio versus *h*AChE was calculated with the average docking score obtained in both enzymes. Although some differences could be appreciated in docking scores values, the same tendency was observed in both *Dm*AChE structures and both *h*AChE structures as phenylethanoid glycosides are among the compounds with a better theoretical binding in the four docking studies. It has been reported that verbascoside and extracts containing other phenylethanoid glycosides are moderate inhibitors of AchE [25].

Figure 6a,b shows the predicted binding mode of verbascoside (compound **87**) in the active site of both *Dm*AchE and *h*AChE, respectively. In the case of the docking study carried out in *Dm*AChE, verbascoside and the rest of the analyzed PEGs adopted a Y-shaped conformation, with the central sugar core interacting with residues of the catalytic triad (colored in yellow in Figure 6a) and the phenylethoxy chain interacting with other residues within the bottom of the gorge. In the case of *h*AChE, the analyzed PEGs adopted a similar conformation, but the phenylethoxy chain did not reach the bottom of the gorge. An explanation to this is that PEGs interact with Asp74 through a hydrogen bond in *h*AChE, whereas this residue is absent in *Dm*AChE [60], limiting the access of PEGs to the catalytic triad, and this could explain the better theoretical affinity of PEGs to *Dm*AChE compared to *h*AChE.

To analyze additional differences that could account for potential selectivity of PGs to *Dm*AChE over *h*AChE, MD simulations were performed. The RMSD values could indicate the stability of the protein relative to its conformation. Figure 4 shows the comparison of the RMSD of the protein backbone profile during the 30 ns simulation of the complexes of compound **87** and *Dm*AChE and *h*AChE. Both complexes have RMSD values around 2Å (RMSD = 2.13 for *Dm*AChE and RMSD = 1.88 for *h*AChE), suggesting that both complexes are stable.

An important difference that was observed during visual analysis MD simulations was the variation of distance of verbascoside (compound **87**) to catalytic site in *Dm*AChE, as it appeared to move closer to key residues Glu 237 and Ser 238, while it seemed that compound **87** maintained a constant distance to equivalent residues Glu 202 and Ser 203 in *h*AChE complex. We confirmed this by measuring the distance of verbascoside to Ser 238 or Ser 203. As seen in Figure 2b, the distance to catalytic site diminished from 4.8 Å to 3.0 Å after 3 ns of simulation in the case of *Dm*AChE (average distance = 3.6 Å), while it maintained almost the same in *h*AChE (average distance = 5.21 Å). This could account for the better binding of **87** towards *Dm*AChE. This could be an important difference that could be useful to future design of selective inhibitors to *Dm*AChE based on the phenylethanoid glycoside template. Additionally, MM-PBSA calculations suggest that 87 binds better to *Dm*AChE (E = −131.5 kJ/mol) than to *h*AChE (E = −134.0 kJ/mol). Overall, we conclude that, based on molecular docking calculations and MD simulations, compound **87** is an interesting starting point for the design of selective *Dm*AchE inhibitors, an important factor to consider in terms of potential toxicity against human beings.

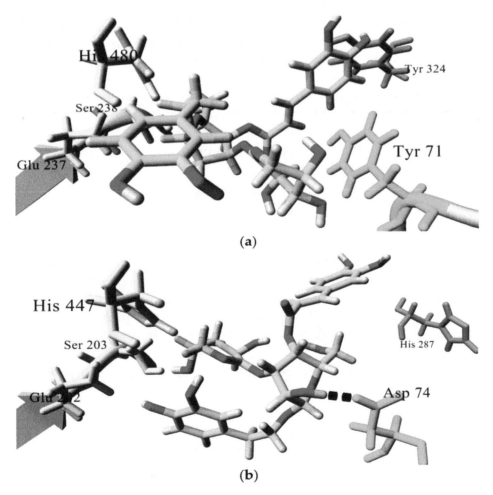

(a)

(b)

Figure 6. Comparison of the docking poses of compound **87** in *Dm*AChE (**a**) and *h*AChE (**b**). Catalytic residues are colored in yellow and residues at the entrance of the active site in orange. Tyr71/Asp 74 residues, which are different in each enzyme, are colored in green. Key hydrogen bond interaction of verbascoside to Asp 74 is shown in black.

4.4. Virtual Multitarget Index and Weighed Multitarget Index

A multitarget drug has been defined as the integration of multiple pharmacophores in one molecule with the purpose that it can have two or more simultaneous mechanisms of action [61]. Though the concept of multitarget drugs is an important research topic [62,63], there are few examples of the study of multitarget insecticides [12].

Computational tools like molecular docking and multitarget quantitative structure–activity relationship models (mt-QSAR) have been recently used for prediction and discovery of multitarget compounds [64–67]. However, the development of parameters to measure the multitarget index of a ligand is not an easy task. As described during the lapatinib discovery [68], the simple average of biological activity against several targets (or in our case, docking scores) can be misleading, because a compound with a promising average value of bioactivity on two or more targets could correspond to a multitarget compound or to a highly selective compound against only one target. Thus, a reference parameter and weighed coefficients for biological activities of interest should be included. Herein, we propose the use of contour graphics, such as the one shown in Figure 2, and a multitarget index (*vMTi*) to identify potential multitarget insecticides. In the contour plot of Figure 2, the docking scores in three targets of interest (EcR, PPO, and *Dm*AChE) are shown. Compounds that have shown greater theoretical affinity for the three targets will appear in the bottom left of the plot and inside the red and yellow contour areas. This would be a first criteria to identify potential multitarget compounds, because selective compounds would not appear in this area. As expected, the phenylethanoid glycosides appear in this area, but other compounds, such as abietane **3** and isopimarane **77**, can be considered to have potential multitarget properties.

Table 4 shows a list of compounds with higher *vMti* and *wMTi* values. In this table, phenylethanoid glycosides appear as compounds with a better multitarget profile. In addition, compounds **88**, **89**, and **87** (Figure 2) have not only high *vMTi* values, but also the highest *wMTi* due to their higher selectivity to *Dm*AChE than *h*AChE. Thus, these compounds are interesting candidates for the development and evaluation of safer multitarget insecticides.

5. Conclusions

Our results complement the experimental results obtained during *Calceolaria* extracts evaluation as biopesticides, and suggest that some of the compounds, such as the phenylethanoid family, can be used for the development of *multitarget* bioinsecticides. Based on the docking studies, it appears that verbascoside and other phenylethanoid glycosides could exert their bioactivity by modifying the activity of various receptors like EcR and enzymes like PPO and AChE, as was suggested and confirmed in previous experimental assays [25,26]. Theoretical affinity, together with *vMTi* and *wMTi*, can be useful for the rational design of *multitarget* bioinsecticides. Verbascoside appears as a good candidate for the development of a multitarget insecticide due to its prolific natural occurrence and its chemical and biological properties [69].

Author Contributions: Conceptualization, M.A.L.-M. and J.R.S.; methodology, M.A.L.-M. and J.F.S.-T.; formal analysis, M.A.L.-M., J.R.S., and J.F.S.-T.; investigation, M.A.L.-M., J.R.S., and J.F.S.-T.; writing—original draft preparation, M.A.L.-M., J.R.S., and J.F.S.-T.; writing—review and editing, M.A.L.-M., J.R.S., and J.F.S.-T.; supervision, M.A.L.-M.; project administration, M.A.L.-M. and J.R.S.; funding acquisition, M.A.L.-M.

Acknowledgments: The authors thank Dirección de Posgrado e Investigación of Universidad La Salle for access to additional computational resources.

References

1. Panagiotakopulu, E.; Buckland, P.C.; Day, P.M. Natural Insecticides and Insect Repellents in Antiquity: A Review of the Evidence. *J. Archeol. Sci.* **1995**, *22*, 705–710. [CrossRef]

2. Sporleder, M.; Lacey, L.A. Biopesticides. In *Insect Pests of Potato*; Elsevier: Amsterdam, The Netherlands, 2013; pp. 463–497. ISBN 9780123868954.

3. Isman, M.B. Bridging the gap: Moving botanical insecticides from the laboratory to the farm. *Ind. Crops Prod.* **2017**, *110*, 10–14. [CrossRef]

4. War, A.R.; Paulraj, M.G.; Ahmad, T.; Buhroo, A.A.; Hussain, B.; Ignacimuthu, S.; Sharma, H.C. Mechanisms of Plant Defense against Insect Herbivores. *Plant Signal. Behav.* **2012**, *7*, 1306–1320. [CrossRef] [PubMed]

5. Miresmailli, S.; Isman, M.B. Botanical insecticides inspired by plant-herbivore chemical interactions. *Trends Plant Sci.* **2014**, *19*, 29–35. [CrossRef] [PubMed]

6. Isman, M.B.; Grieneisen, M.L. Botanical insecticide research: Many publications, limited useful data. *Trends Plant Sci.* **2014**, *19*, 140–145. [CrossRef] [PubMed]

7. Schrader, K.K.; Andolfi, A.; Cantrell, C.L.; Cimmino, A.; Duke, S.O.; Osbrink, W.; Wedge, D.E.; Evidente, A. A survey of phytotoxic microbial and plant metabolites as potential natural products for pest management. *Chem. Biodivers.* **2010**, *7*, 2261–2280. [CrossRef] [PubMed]

8. Cespedes, C.L.; Aqueveque, P.M.; Avila, J.G.; Alarcon, J.; Kubo, I. New advances in chemical defenses of plants: Researches in calceolariaceae. *Phytochem. Rev.* **2015**, *14*, 367–380. [CrossRef]

9. Muñoz, E.; Escalona, D.; Salazar, J.R.; Alarcon, J.; Céspedes, C.L. Insect growth regulatory effects by diterpenes from *Calceolaria talcana* Grau & Ehrhart (Calceolariaceae: Scrophulariaceae) against *Spodoptera frugiperda* and *Drosophila melanogaster*. *Ind. Crops Prod.* **2013**, *45*, 283–292. [CrossRef]

10. Muñoz, E.; Avila, J.G.; Alarcón, J.; Kubo, I.; Werner, E.; Céspedes, C.L. Tyrosinase inhibitors from *Calceolaria integrifolia* s.l.: *Calceolaria talcana* aerial parts. *J. Agric. Food Chem.* **2013**, *61*, 4336–4343. [CrossRef] [PubMed]

11. Wang, Y.; Liu, T.; Yang, Q.; Li, Z.; Qian, X. A Modeling Study for Structure Features of β-*N*-acetyl-D-hexosaminidase from *Ostrinia furnacalis* and its Novel Inhibitor Allosamidin: Species Selectivity and Multi-Target Characteristics. *Chem. Biol. Drug Des.* **2012**, *79*, 572–582. [CrossRef] [PubMed]

12. Speck-Planche, A.; Kleandrova, V.V.; Scotti, M.T. Fragment-based approach for the in silico discovery of multi-target insecticides. *Chemom. Intell. Lab. Syst.* **2012**, *111*, 39–45. [CrossRef]

13. Cavasotto, C.N.; Orry, A.J.W. Ligand docking and structure-based virtual screening in drug discovery. *Curr. Top. Med. Chem.* **2007**, *7*, 1006–1014. [CrossRef] [PubMed]

14. Tuccinardi, T. Docking-based virtual screening: Recent developments. *Comb. Chem. High Throughput Screen.* **2009**, *12*, 303–314. [CrossRef] [PubMed]

15. Cheng, T.; Li, Q.; Zhou, Z.; Wang, Y.; Bryant, S.H. Structure-Based Virtual Screening for Drug Discovery: A Problem-Centric Review. *AAPS J.* **2012**, *14*, 133–141. [CrossRef] [PubMed]

16. Kontoyianni, M. Docking and Virtual Screening in Drug Discovery. *Methods Mol. Biol.* **2017**, *1647*, 255–266. [PubMed]

17. Toledo Warshaviak, D.; Golan, G.; Borrelli, K.W.; Zhu, K.; Kalid, O. Structure-Based Virtual Screening Approach for Discovery of Covalently Bound Ligands. *J. Chem. Inf. Model.* **2014**, *54*, 1941–1950. [CrossRef] [PubMed]

18. Wang, L.; Gu, Q.; Zheng, X.; Ye, J.; Liu, Z.; Li, J.; Hu, X.; Hagler, A.; Xu, J. Discovery of New Selective Human Aldose Reductase Inhibitors through Virtual Screening Multiple Binding Pocket Conformations. *J. Chem. Inf. Model.* **2013**, *53*, 2409–2422. [CrossRef] [PubMed]

19. Ribeiro, F.F.; Mendonca Junior, F.J.B.; Ghasemi, J.B.; Ishiki, H.M.; Scotti, M.T.; Scotti, L. Docking of Natural Products against Neurodegenerative Diseases: General Concepts. *Comb. Chem. High Throughput Screen.* **2018**, *21*, 152–160. [CrossRef] [PubMed]

20. Saldivar-Gonzalez, F.; Gómez-García, A.; Sánchez-Cruz, N.; Ruiz-Rios, J.; Pilón-Jiménez, B.; Medina-Franco, J. Computational Approaches to Identify Natural Products as Inhibitors of DNA Methyltransferases. *Preprints* **2018**. [CrossRef]

21. Singh, P.; Bast, F. Multitargeted molecular docking study of plant-derived natural products on phosphoinositide-3 kinase pathway components. *Med. Chem. Res.* **2013**, *23*. [CrossRef]

22. Ambure, P.; Bhat, J.; Puzyn, T.; Roy, K. Identifying natural compounds as multi-target-directed ligands against Alzheimer's disease: An in silico approach. *J. Biomol. Struct. Dyn.* **2018**, *23*, 1–25. [CrossRef] [PubMed]

23. Lee, S.-H.; Ha, K.B.; Park, D.H.; Fang, Y.; Kim, J.H.; Park, M.G.; Woo, R.M.; Kim, W.J.; Park, I.-K.; Choi, J.Y.; et al. Plant-derived compounds regulate formation of the insect juvenile hormone receptor complex. *Pestic. Biochem. Physiol.* **2018**, *150*, 27–32. [CrossRef] [PubMed]

24. Jankowska, M.; Rogalska, J.; Wyszkowska, J.; Stankiewicz, M.; Jankowska, M.; Rogalska, J.; Wyszkowska, J.; Stankiewicz, M. Molecular Targets for Components of Essential Oils in the Insect Nervous System—A Review. *Molecules* **2017**, *23*, 34. [CrossRef] [PubMed]

25. Cespedes, C.L.; Muñoz, E.; Salazar, J.R.; Yamaguchi, L.; Werner, E.; Alarcon, J.; Kubo, I. Inhibition of cholinesterase activity by extracts, fractions and compounds from *Calceolaria talcana* and *C. integrifolia* (Calceolariaceae: Scrophulariaceae). *Food Chem. Toxicol.* **2013**, *62*, 919–926. [CrossRef] [PubMed]

26. Muñoz, E.; Lamilla, C.; Marin, J.C.; Alarcon, J.; Cespedes, C.L. Antifeedant, insect growth regulatory and insecticidal effects of *Calceolaria talcana* (Calceolariaceae) on *Drosophila melanogaster* and *Spodoptera frugiperda*. *Ind. Crops Prod.* **2013**, *42*, 137–144. [CrossRef]

27. Céspedes, C.L.; Salazar, J.R.; Alarcon, J. Chemistry and biological activities of *Calceolaria* spp. (Calceolariaceae: Scrophulariaceae). *Phytochem. Rev.* **2013**, *12*, 733–749. [CrossRef]

28. Thomsen, R.; Christensen, M.H. MolDock: A New Technique for High-Accuracy Molecular Docking. *J. Med. Chem.* **2006**, *49*, 3315–3321. [CrossRef] [PubMed]

29. Harel, M.; Kryger, G.; Rosenberry, T.; Mallender, W.; Lewis, T.; Fletcher, R.; Guss, J.; Silman, I.; Sussman, J.L. Three-Dimensional Structures of *Drosophila melanogaster* Acetylcholinesterase and of its Complexes with Two Potent Inhibitors. *Protein Sci.* **2000**, *9*, 1063–1072. [CrossRef] [PubMed]

30. Moras, D.; Billas, I.M.; Browning, C. Adaptability of the ecdysone receptor bound to synthetic ligands. [CrossRef]

31. Browning, C.; Martin, E.; Loch, C.; Wurtz, J.-M.; Moras, D.; Stote, R.H.; Dejaegere, A.P.; Billas, I.M.L. Critical role of desolvation in the binding of 20-hydroxyecdysone to the ecdysone receptor. *J. Biol. Chem.* **2007**, *282*, 32924–32934. [CrossRef] [PubMed]

32. Li, Y.; Wang, Y.; Jiang, H.; Deng, J. Crystal structure of *Manduca sexta* prophenoloxidase provides insights into the mechanism of type 3 copper enzymes. *Proc. Natl. Acad. Sci. USA* **2009**, *106*, 17002–17006. [CrossRef] [PubMed]

33. Cheung, J.; Rudolph, M.J.; Burshteyn, F.; Cassidy, M.S.; Gary, E.N.; Love, J.; Franklin, M.C.; Height, J.J. Structures of human acetylcholinesterase in complex with pharmacologically important ligands. *J. Med. Chem.* **2012**, *55*, 10282–10286. [CrossRef] [PubMed]

34. Cheung, J.; Gary, E.N.; Shiomi, K.; Rosenberry, T.L. Structures of Human Acetylcholinesterase Bound to Dihydrotanshinone I and Territrem B Show Peripheral Site Flexibility. *ACS Med. Chem. Lett.* **2013**, *4*, 1091–1096. [CrossRef] [PubMed]

35. Berman, H.M.; Westbrook, J.; Feng, Z.; Gilliland, G.; Bhat, T.N.; Weissig, H.; Shindyalov, I.N.; Bourne, P.E. The protein data bank. *Nucleic Acids Res.* **2000**, *28*, 235–242. [CrossRef] [PubMed]

36. Ogungbe, I.V.; Erwin, W.R.; Setzer, W.N. Antileishmanial phytochemical phenolics: Molecular docking to potential protein targets. *J. Mol. Graph. Model.* **2014**, *48*, 105–117. [CrossRef] [PubMed]

37. Loza-Mejía, M.A.; Salazar, J.R. Sterols and triterpenoids as potential anti-inflammatories: Molecular docking studies for binding to some enzymes involved in inflammatory pathways. *J. Mol. Graph. Model.* **2015**, *62*, 18–25. [CrossRef] [PubMed]

38. Krieger, E.; Vriend, G. YASARA View—Molecular graphics for all devices—From smartphones to workstations. *Bioinformatics* **2014**, *30*, 2981–2982. [CrossRef] [PubMed]

39. Yasara Dynamics. Available online: www.yasara.org (accessed on 23 October 2018).

40. Duan, Y.; Wu, C.; Chowdhury, S.; Lee, M.C.; Xiong, G.; Zhang, W.; Yang, R.; Cieplak, P.; Luo, R.; Lee, T.; et al. A point-charge force field for molecular mechanics simulations of proteins based on condensed-phase quantum mechanical calculations. *J. Comput. Chem.* **2003**, *24*, 1999–2012. [CrossRef] [PubMed]

41. Gan, R.; Zhao, L.; Sun, Q.; Tang, P.; Zhang, S.; Yang, H.; He, J.; Li, H. Binding behavior of trelagliptin and human serum albumin: Molecular docking, dynamical simulation, and multi-spectroscopy. *Spectrochim. Acta Part A Mol. Biomol. Spectrosc.* **2018**, *202*, 187–195. [CrossRef] [PubMed]

42. Ding, X.; Suo, Z.; Sun, Q.; Gan, R.; Tang, P.; Hou, Q.; Wu, D.; Li, H. Study of the interaction of broad-spectrum antimicrobial drug sitafloxacin with human serum albumin using spectroscopic methods, molecular docking, and molecular dynamics simulation. *J. Pharm. Biomed. Anal.* **2018**, *160*, 397–403. [CrossRef] [PubMed]

43. Kumar, A.; Srivastava, G.; Negi, A.S.; Sharma, A. Docking, molecular dynamics, binding energy-MM-PBSA studies of naphthofuran derivatives to identify potential dual inhibitors against BACE-1 and GSK-3β. *J. Biomol. Struct. Dyn.* **2018**, 1–16. [CrossRef] [PubMed]

44. Schwedes, C.; Tulsiani, S.; Carney, G.E. Ecdysone receptor expression and activity in adult *Drosophila melanogaster*. *J. Insect Physiol.* **2011**, *57*, 899–907. [CrossRef] [PubMed]

45. Li, Z.; Lazaridis, T. The Effect of Water Displacement on Binding Thermodynamics: Concanavalin A. *J. Phys. Chem. B* **2005**, *109*, 662–670. [CrossRef] [PubMed]

46. Whitehill, J.; Rigsby, C.; Cipollini, D.; Herms, D.A.; Bonello, P. Decreased emergence of emerald ash borer from ash treated with methyl jasmonate is associated with induction of general defense traits and the toxic phenolic compound verbascoside. *Oecologia* **2014**, *176*, 1047–1059. [CrossRef] [PubMed]

47. Harmatha, J.; Dinan, L. Biological activities of lignans and stilbenoids associated with plant-insect chemical interactions. *Phytochem. Rev.* **2003**, *2*, 321–330. [CrossRef]

48. Dinan, L.; Hormann, R.E. *Comprehensive Molecular Insect Science*; Elsevier: Amsterdam, The Netherlands, 2005; ISBN 9780444519245.

49. Jiang, H.; Wang, Y.; Kanost, M.R. Pro-phenol oxidase activating proteinase from an insect, *Manduca sexta*: A bacteria-inducible protein similar to *Drosophila* easter. *Proc. Natl. Acad. Sci. USA* **1998**, *95*, 12220–12225. [CrossRef] [PubMed]

50. Sugumaran, M.; Barek, H. Critical Analysis of the Melanogenic Pathway in Insects and Higher Animals. *Int. J. Mol. Sci.* **2016**, *17*, 1–24. [CrossRef] [PubMed]

51. Aloui, S.; Raboudi, F.; Ghazouani, T.; Salghi, R.; Hamdaoui, M.H.; Fattouch, S. Use of molecular and in silico bioinformatic tools to investigate pesticide binding to insect (Lepidoptera) phenoloxidases (PO): Insights to toxicological aspects. *J. Environ. Sci. Health B* **2014**, *49*, 654–660. [CrossRef] [PubMed]

52. Kanteev, M.; Goldfeder, M.; Fishman, A. Structure–function correlations in tyrosinases. *Protein Sci.* **2015**, *24*, 1360–1369. [CrossRef] [PubMed]

53. Karioti, A.; Protopappa, A.; Megoulas, N.; Skaltsa, H. Identification of tyrosinase inhibitors from *Marrubium velutinum* and *Marrubium cylleneum*. *Bioorg. Med. Chem.* **2007**, *15*, 2708–2714. [CrossRef] [PubMed]

54. Yoshimori, A.; Oyama, T.; Takahashi, S.; Abe, H.; Kamiya, T.; Abe, T.; Tanuma, S.I. Structure-activity relationships of the thujaplicins for inhibition of human tyrosinase. *Bioorg. Med. Chem.* **2014**, *22*, 6193–6200. [CrossRef] [PubMed]

55. Tan, X.; Song, Y.H.; Park, C.; Lee, K.W.; Kim, J.Y.; Kim, D.W.; Kim, K.D.; Lee, K.W.; Curtis-Long, M.J.; Park, K.H. Highly potent tyrosinase inhibitor, neorauflavane from *Campylotropis hirtella* and inhibitory mechanism with molecular docking. *Bioorg. Med. Chem.* **2016**, *24*, 153–159. [CrossRef] [PubMed]

56. Houghton, P.J.; Ren, Y.; Howes, M.-J. Acetylcholinesterase inhibitors from plants and fungi. *Nat. Prod. Rep.* **2006**, *23*, 181–199. [CrossRef] [PubMed]

57. Thapa, S.L.; Xu, H. Acetylcholinesterase: A Primary Target for Drugs and Insecticides. *Mini Rev. Med. Chem.* **2017**, *17*, 1665–1676. [CrossRef] [PubMed]

58. Kobayashi, H.; Suzuki, T.; Akahori, F.; Satoh, T. Acetylcholinesterase and Acetylcholine Receptors: Brain Regional Heterogeneity. *Anticholinesterase Pestic. Metab. Neurotox. Epidemiol.* **2011**, 3–18. [CrossRef]

59. Pang, Y.; Brimijoin, S.; Ragsdale, D.W.; Zhu, K.Y.; Suranyi, R.; Gormley, M.; Company, K. Novel and Viable Acetylcholinesterase Target Site for Developing Effective and Environmentally Safe Insecticides. *Curr. Drug Targets* **2012**, *13*, 471–482. [CrossRef] [PubMed]

60. Wiesner, J.; Kříž, Z.; Kuča, K.; Jun, D.; Koča, J. Acetylcholinesterases—The structural similarities and differences. *J. Enzyme Inhib. Med. Chem.* **2007**, *22*, 417–424. [CrossRef] [PubMed]

61. Katselou, M.G.; Matralis, A.N.; Kourounakis, A.P. Multi-target drug design approaches for multifactorial diseases: From neurodegenerative to cardiovascular applications. *Curr. Med. Chem.* **2014**, *21*, 2743–2787. [CrossRef] [PubMed]

62. Lu, J.J.; Pan, W.; Hu, Y.J.; Wang, Y.T. Multi-target drugs: The trend of drug research and development. *PLoS ONE* **2012**, *7*, 1–9. [CrossRef] [PubMed]

63. Lavecchia, A.; Cerchia, C. In silico methods to address polypharmacology: Current status, applications and future perspectives. *Drug Discov. Today* **2016**, *21*, 288–298. [CrossRef] [PubMed]

64. Prado-Prado, F.; García-Mera, X.; Abeijón, P.; Alonso, N.; Caamaño, O.; Yáñez, M.; Gárate, T.; Mezo, M.; González-Warleta, M.; Muiño, L.; et al. Using entropy of drug and protein graphs to predict FDA drug-target network: Theoretic-experimental study of MAO inhibitors and hemoglobin peptides from *Fasciola hepatica*. *Eur. J. Med. Chem.* **2011**, *46*, 1074–1094. [CrossRef] [PubMed]

65. Prado-Prado, F.J.; García, I.; García-Mera, X.; González-Díaz, H. Entropy multi-target QSAR model for prediction of antiviral drug complex networks. *Chemom. Intell. Lab. Syst.* **2011**, *107*, 227–233. [CrossRef]

66. Speck-Planche, A.; Kleandrova, V.; Scotti, M.; Cordeiro, M. 3D-QSAR Methodologies and Molecular Modeling in Bioinformatics for the Search of Novel Anti-HIV Therapies: Rational Design of Entry Inhibitors. *Curr. Bioinform.* **2013**, *8*, 452–464. [CrossRef]

67. Speck-Planche, A.; Kleandrova, V.; Luan, F.; Natalia, D.S.; Cordeiro, M. Multi-Target Inhibitors for Proteins Associated with Alzheimer: In Silico Discovery using Fragment-Based Descriptors. *Curr. Alzheimer Res.* **2013**, *10*, 117–124. [CrossRef] [PubMed]

68. Lackey, K.E. The Discovery of Lapatinib. In *Designing Multi-Target Drugs*; Morphy, J.R., Harris, J.C., Eds.; Royal Society of Chemistry: Cambridge, UK, 2012; pp. 181–205.

69. Alipieva, K.; Korkina, L.; Orhan, I.E.; Georgiev, M.I. Verbascoside—A review of its occurrence, (bio)synthesis and pharmacological significance. *Biotechnol. Adv.* **2014**, *32*, 1065–1076. [CrossRef] [PubMed]

11

Identification and Growth Inhibitory Activity of the Chemical Constituents from *Imperata Cylindrica* Aerial Part Ethyl Acetate Extract

Yan Wang, James Zheng Shen, Yuk Wah Chan and Wing Shing Ho *

School of Life Sciences, Chinese University of Hong Kong, Shatin, Hong Kong, China;
1155070144@link.cuhk.edu.hk (Y.W.); james_shen_zheng@alumni.cuhk.net (J.Z.S.);
anthony.chan@link.cuhk.edu.hk (Y.W.C.)
* Correspondence: ws203ho@cuhk.edu.hk;

Abstract: *Imperata cylindrica* (L.) Raeusch. (IMP) aerial part ethyl acetate extract has anti-proliferative, pro-apoptotic, and pro-oxidative effects towards colorectal cancer in vitro. The chemical constituents of IMP aerial part ethyl acetate extract were isolated using high-performance liquid chromatography (HPLC) and identified with tandem mass spectrometry (ESI-MS/MS) in combination with ultraviolet-visible spectrophotometry and 400 MHz NMR. The growth inhibitory effects of each identified component on BT-549 (breast) and HT-29 (colon) cancer cell lines were evaluated after 48/72 h treatment by MTT assay. Four isolated compounds were identified as trans-p-Coumaric acid (**1**); 2-Methoxyestrone (**2**); 11, 16-Dihydroxypregn-4-ene-3, 20-dione (**3**); and Tricin (**4**). Compounds (**2**), (**3**), and (**4**) exhibited considerable growth inhibitory activities against BT-549 and HT-29 cancer cell lines. Compounds (**2**), (**3**), and (**4**) are potential candidates for novel anti-cancer agents against breast and colorectal cancers.

Keywords: *Imperata cylindrica*; HPLC; ESI-MS/MS; growth inhibitory activity; cancer

1. Introduction

Imperata cylindrica (L.) Raeusch. (IMP) is widely used for the treatment of hemorrhage, improvement of urination, and enhancement of the immune system [1]. Amounts of bio-active compounds isolated from IMP rhizomes and leaves were identified including benzoic acid and its derivatives [2], lignans [3], phenolic compounds [4], steroids [5], methoxylated flavonoids [6], and chromones [7].

Cancer is one of the leading causes of death worldwide. Herbal medicines are commonly used as both complementary ingredients and alternative therapies in cancer treatments. Potential bio-active components from herbal medicines can be isolated and purified using a high-performance liquid chromatography (HPLC) system. A tandem MS/MS detection system providing fragmentation information of the targets is one of the best choices adopted in chemical structural characterization and drug discovery [8,9].

Our previous study demonstrated that IMP aerial part ethyl acetate extract had growth-inhibiting, pro-apoptotic, and pro-oxidative effects on a colorectal cancer cell line HT-29 in vitro [10]. The present study aims to isolate the chemical constituents from IMP aerial part ethyl acetate extract and identify the bio-active compounds with considerable growth inhibitory activity against cancers.

2. Results

2.1. Isolation, Identification, and Quantification of Compounds (1)–(4)

Chemical structures of four compounds isolated from IMP aerial part ethyl acetate extract are shown in Figure 1.

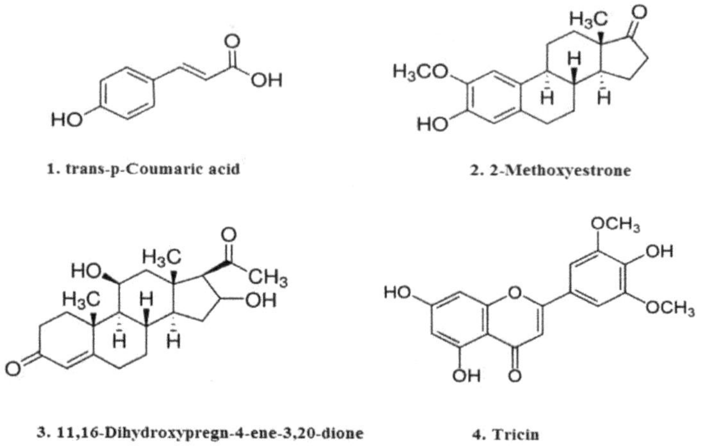

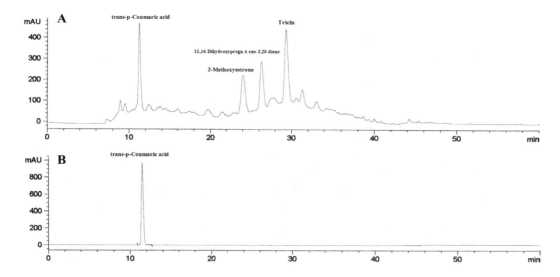

1. trans-p-Coumaric acid

2. 2-Methoxyestrone

3. 11,16-Dihydroxypregn-4-ene-3,20-dione

4. Tricin

Figure 1. Chemical structures of compounds (1)–(4) isolated from IMP aerial part ethyl acetate extract. These are trans-p-Coumaric acid (1); 2-Methoxyestrone (2); 11, 16-Dihydroxypregn-4-ene-3, 20-dione (3); and Tricin (4).

2.1.1. Compound (1): Trans-p-Coumaric Acid

The molecular formula of compound (1), $C_9H_8O_3$, was identified by comparing the liquid chromatographic retention time, UV absorption spectrum, and ESI-MS/MS spectrum with the trans-p-Coumaric acid standard (Sigma Aldrich, St. Louis, MO, USA). The HPLC chromatogram of compound (1) and trans-p-Coumaric acid standard (in methanol) possessed the same identical retention time (Figure 2A,B).

Figure 2. HPLC-DAD chromatogram of IMP aerial part ethyl acetate extract at 323 nm. IMP aerial part ethyl acetate extract solution (10 mg/mL in methanol, 20 µL) was analyzed in the 60 min HPLC gradient program. (**A**) The retention time of the trans-p-Coumaric acid standard (0.125 mg/mL in methanol, 20 µL) purchased from Sigma (**B**) was consistent with compound (1) in IMP aerial part ethyl acetate extract fingerprint.

The MS/MS fragmentation pattern of compound (1) accurately matched with the MS^2 spectrum from the NIST14 mass spectral database and the trans-p-Coumaric standard (Figure 3).

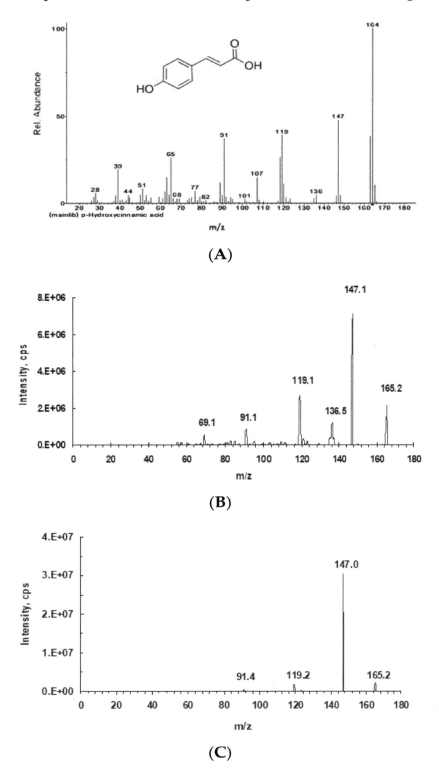

Figure 3. Relevant tandem mass (MS/MS) spectra. (**A**) trans-p-Coumaric acid spectrum (from NIST 14 mass spectral library); (**B**) isolated and purified compound (1); (**C**) trans-p-Coumaric acid standard (Sigma).

2.1.2. Compound (2): 2-Methoxyestrone

The molecular formula of compound (2), $C_{19}H_{24}O_3$, was identified with the MS/MS spectrum by searching the NIST14 mass spectral database (Figure 4).

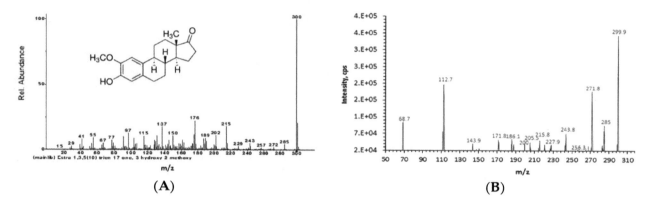

Figure 4. Relevant tandem mass (MS/MS) spectra. (**A**) 2-Methoxyestrone (from NIST 14 mass spectral library); (**B**) isolated and purified compound (2).

2.1.3. Compound (3): 11, 16-Dihydroxypregn-4-ene-3, 20-dione

The molecular formula of compound (3): $C_{21}H_{30}O_4$, was identified with the MS/MS spectrum by searching the NIST14 mass spectral database (Figure 5).

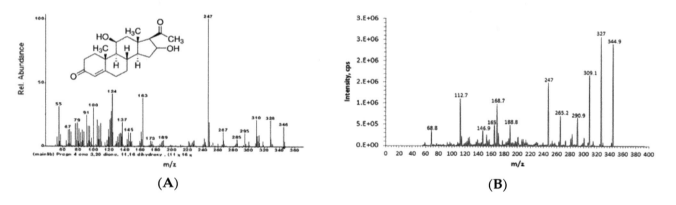

Figure 5. Relevant tandem mass (MS/MS) spectra. (**A**) 11, 16-Dihydroxypregn-4-ene-3, 20-dione (from NIST 14 mass spectral library); (**B**) isolated and purified compound (3).

2.1.4. Compound (4): Tricin

The molecular formula of compound (4), $C_{17}H_{14}O_7$, was identified by comparing the MS/MS spectrum with the published literature [11] (Figure 6A,B). The UV spectrum (Figure 6C), obtained using λ_{max} at 351 nm, was consistent with the previous description [12].

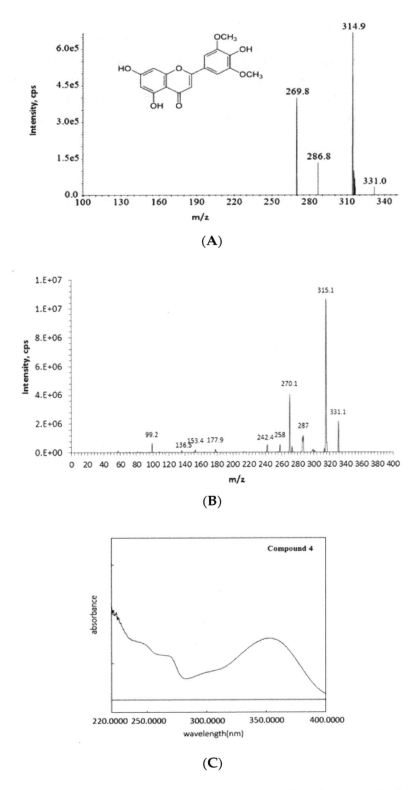

Figure 6. Relevant tandem mass (MS/MS) spectra. (**A**) Tricin (from literature [11]); (**B**) isolated and purified compound (**4**). (**C**) Compound (**4**) has absorption peaks (λ_{max}) at 351 nm. A control of 100% methanol was used and auto-zeroed automatically by the software.

1H-NMR (400 MHz, DMSO-d_6) δ (ppm): 12.964 (1H, s, 5-OH), 10.804 (s, 1H, 7-OH), 9.318 (s, 1H, 4-OH), 7.330 (2H, s, H-6′ and H-2′), 6.984 (1H, s, H-3), 6.564 (1H, d, J = 2.0 Hz, H-8), 6.209 (1H, d, J = 2.0 Hz, H-6), 3.887 (6H, s, 2OCH₃). 13C-NMR (100 MHz, DMSO-d_6) δ (ppm): 181.75 (C-4), 164.08 (C-2), 163.61 (C-7), 161.35 (C-5), 157.28 (C-9), 148.41 (C-3′ and C-5′), 139.81 (C-4′), 120.34 (C-1′), 104.35

(C-3), 103.68 (C-2′ and C-6′), 103.55 (C-10), 98.77 (C-6), 94.14 (C-8), 56.32 (2OCH$_3$). DEPT90-NMR (DMSO-d_6) δ (ppm): 94.12 (C-8), 98.75 (C-6), 103.53 (C-10), 104.31 (C-3). DEPT135-NMR (DMSO-d_6) δ (ppm): 56.31 (2OCH$_3$), 94.13 (C-8), 98.76 (C-6), 103.54 (C-10), 104.3 (C-3). DEPT spectra revealed that there were two primary carbons, five tertiary carbons, and ten quaternary carbons. A signal at δ3.887 (s, 6H) observed in the 1H-NMR spectrum and a signal at δ 56.32 observed in the 13C-NMR spectrum indicated that there were two equivalent methoxy groups. The NMR results (Figure 7) were consistent with the published data [13,14].

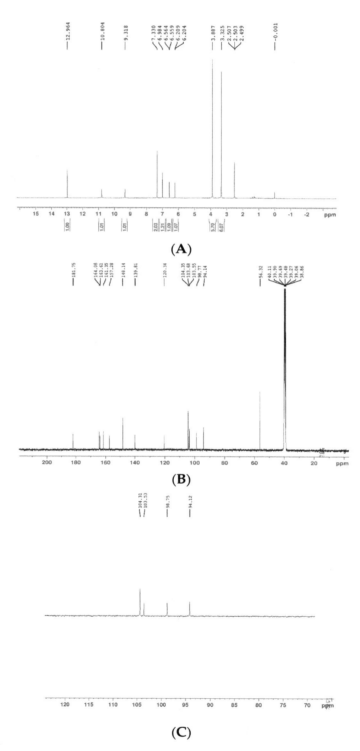

Figure 7. *Cont.*

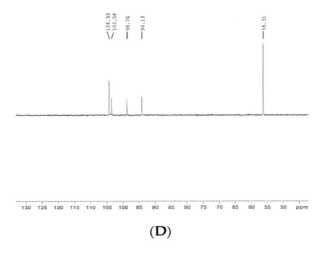

(D)

Figure 7. NMR spectra of Tricin. Purified Compound (**4**) in DMSO-d_6 solution was conducted NMR analysis. ^{1}H, ^{13}C, DEPT90, and DEPT135-NMR spectra are shown in (**A–D**), respectively.

Compounds (**1**)–(**4**) identified by tandem mass spectrometry (MS^2) are listed in Table 1.

Table 1. Characteristics of compound (**1**)–(**4**) identified by tandem mass spectrometry.

Analyte	Ion Mode	Molecular Formula	CAS No.	MS/MS Fragments (*m/z*)
trans-p-Coumaric acid	[M+H]$^+$	$C_9H_8O_3$	501-98-4	165.7, 147.4, 136.3, 118.9, 90.5
2-Methoxyestrone	[M-H]$^-$	$C_{19}H_{24}O_3$	362-08-3	299.9, 285.0, 271.8, 256.3, 243.8
11, 16-Dihydroxypregn-4-ene-3, 20-dione	[M-H]$^-$	$C_{21}H_{30}O_4$	55622-61-2	344.9, 327.0, 309.1, 290.9, 265.2, 247.0
Tricin	[M+H]$^+$	$C_{17}H_{14}O_7$	520-32-1	331.1, 315.0, 287.0, 270.1, 258.0, 242.4

2.1.5. Content of Analytes in IMP Aerial Part Ethyl Acetate Extract

Quantitative analysis of each isolated and purified compound in IMP aerial part ethyl acetate extract was determined by HPLC-DAD. The linearity of the calibration curve, limit of detection (LOD), and limit of quantification (LOQ) are listed in Table 2.

Table 2. Content of analytes in IMP aerial part ethyl acetate extract.

Analytes	Calibration Curves [a]	R^2 [b]	Linear Range (mg/mL)	LOD [c] (μg/mL)	LOQ [d] (μg/mL)	Contents of Analytes (mg/g Extract, n = 3)
trans-p-Coumaric acid	y = 114751x − 31.91	0.9999	0.0010–0.25	0.30	0.95	0.12 ± 0.010
2-Methoxyestrone	y = 13217x + 195.65	0.9992	0.031–1.00	7.28	24.84	0.86 ± 0.042
11,16-Dihydroxypregn-4-ene-3, 20-dione	y = 15063x + 1173.70	0.9995	0.12–2.50	6.71	22.91	0.65 ± 0.13
Tricin	y = 35025x − 126.29	0.9999	0.016–2.00	3.23	11.02	0.59 ± 0.041

[a] y, the value of peak area (by HPLC-DAD at 323 nm); x, the value of concentration (mg/mL); [b] R^2, correlation coefficient for six points on the calibration curves (n = 3); [c] LOD, limit of detection (S/N = 3); [d] LOQ, limit of quantification (S/N = 10).

2.2. Growth Inhibitory Evaluation of Compounds (1)–(4) on Breast Cancer and Colorectal Cancer In Vitro

The purified dried powder of each compound was dissolved in DMSO with a gradient of concentrations (μM). The growth inhibitory effects of compounds (**1**)–(**4**) on BT-549 (breast cancer cell line) were evaluated after 48/72 h treatment by MTT assay (Figure 8). Data are presented as mean values ±SD from three independent studies (*n* = 3).

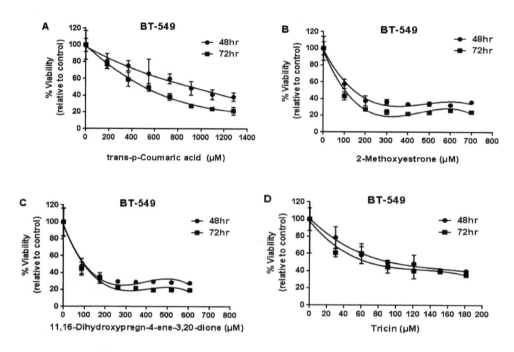

Figure 8. The growth inhibitory effects of compound (1)–(4) on BT-549 (breast cancer cell line) were evaluated after 48/72 h treatment by MTT assay.

The growth inhibitory effects of compounds (1)–(4) on HT-29 (colon cancer cell line) are shown in Figure 9.

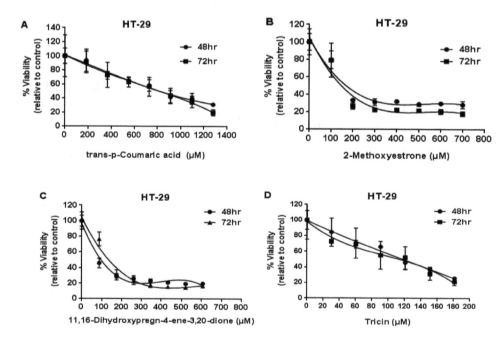

Figure 9. The growth inhibitory effects of compounds (1)–(4) on HT-29 (colon cancer cell line) were evaluated after 48/72 h treatment by MTT assay.

The half-maximal inhibitory concentration (IC50) of compounds (2), (3), and (4) on BT-549 breast cancer cell line (72 h) was 102, 97, and 68 µM, respectively. IC50 of compounds (2), (3), and (4) on a HT-29 colon cancer cell line (72 h) was 147, 134, and 114 µM, respectively. There were no statistically significant differences between 48 h and 72 h treatment groups ($p > 0.05$) (Table 3).

Table 3. IC50 of compounds (1)–(4) on BT-549 and HT-29 cancer cell lines.

Cancer Unit		Treatment Group (48/72 h)			
		Trans-p-Coumaric Acid	2-Methoxyestrone	11,16-Dihydroxypregn-4-ene-3, 20-dione	Tricin
BT-549	µg/mL	151/83	43/31	35/34	31/23
	µM	920/507	144/102 [a]	101/97 [a]	95/68 [a]
HT-29	µg/mL	135/135	51/44	33/46	39/38
	µM	821/821	169/147 [a]	96/134 [a]	118/114 [a]

[a] Numbers identified refer to the considerable growth inhibitory activity with half-maximal inhibitory concentration (IC50 < 150 µM).

3. Discussion

A previous study showed that the 50% growth inhibitory effect (GI50) of the IMP aerial part ethyl acetate extract against HT-29 was 14.5 µg/mL [10]. The three isolated compounds, including 2-Methoxyestrone (**2**), 11, 16-Dihydroxypregn-4-ene-3, 20-dione (**3**), and Tricin (**4**), have considerable growth inhibitory activities on BT-549 and HT-29 with the IC50 values among 23–51 µg/mL. Synergy and positive interactions between isolated constituents may contribute to the greater effect of the crude extract against cancers that can be further investigated.

Compound (**1**), trans-p-Coumaric acid, was able to induce apoptosis of HCT-15 colon cancer cells through a ROS-mitochondrial pathway with an IC 50 value of 1400 µM [15]. Natural trans-p-Coumaric acid exists in a wide variety of edible plants. The phenolic components from flaxseed oil was reported to have cytotoxic and pro-oxidant effects on MCF-7 human breast cancer cells [16]. The high gastric absorption efficiency of p-Coumaric acid was observed in rats, which makes it a potential bio-active compound in vivo [17]. Compound (**2**), 2-Methoxyestrone, is one kind of metabolite of estrone and estradiol. It is worth mentioning that 2-Methoxyestradiol was under a phase II clinical trial and expected to be a novel oral drug against multiple human melanoma, including breast cancer and ovarian cancer [18,19]. Metabolic inter-conversion between 2-Methoxyestrone and 2-Methoxyestradiol are based on the enzymatic catalyze reactions. Reductive activity promotes 2-Methoxyestrone conversion to 2-Methoxyestradiol. 2-Methoxyestrone can be formed by the enzymatic oxidation of 2-Methoxyestradiol [20]. Our study first reported the growth inhibitory activities of compound (**3**), 11, 16-Dihydroxypregn-4-ene-3, 20-dione, against BT-549 and HT-29 cancer cell lines. The structure of 11, 16-Dihydroxypregn-4-ene-3, 20-dione is similar to the well-known endogenous steroid (11α-Hydroxyprogesterone, $C_{21}H_{30}O_3$). Transformations of 11α-Hydroxyprogesterone generate a series of metabolites. Amounts of metabolites with different isoforms were identified as novel candidates of steroid drugs [21]. The molecular mechanisms of 11, 16-Dihydroxypregn-4-ene-3, 20-dione against cancers can be further investigated. Compound (**4**), Tricin, a well-studied bio-active flavonoid, is widely distributed in rice bran and bamboo leaves [22,23]. A previous study also isolated Tricin from the aerial part of *Imperata cylindrica* (L.) Beauv. [5]. Tricin was reported to have remarkable anti-cancer potential against SW-480 colon cancer cells and MDA-MB-468 breast cancer cells, and is safe for clinical development as a cancer preventive agent [24–28].

4. Materials and Methods

4.1. Cells, Chemicals and Reagents

BT-549 and HT-29 cell lines were obtained from ATCC (Manassas, VA, USA). BT-549 and HT-29 cells were cultured at 37 °C in a humidified atmosphere of 5% CO_2 in RPMI 1640 (Gibco, Carlsbad, CA, USA) supplemented with 10% fetal bovine serum (FBS) (Gibco, Carlsbad, CA, USA). Acetonitrile (ACN) (E. Merck, Darmstadt, Germany), Methanol (E. Merck, Darmstadt, Germany) and trifluoroacetic acid (TFA) (Sigma Aldrich, St. Louis, MO, USA) were of HPLC grade, and distilled and deionized water (ddH2O) was prepared using a Millipore water purification system (Millipore, Milford, MA, USA). All other reagents used in this study were of analytical reagent grade or higher and purchased from Sigma Aldrich.

4.2. Preparation of Powder Extract of IMP Aerial Part

The extraction method was described previously [10].

4.3. HPLC Analysis

The HPLC fingerprint was analyzed on a HP1100 series system (Santa Clara, CA, USA) equipped with a diode-array detector. An extract solution of 50 mg/mL (dissolved in methanol) was filtered with a 0.22 μm polytetrafluoroethylene (PTFE) membrane. A 15 μL sample was injected to a semi-preparative HPLC column (ALLTIMA C18, 5 μm, 250 mm × 10 mm i.d. Hichrom, Searle, UK) and detected at 323 nm. The initial mobile phase composed of solvent A (0.1% TFA in ddH$_2$O) and solvent B (100% methanol). The gradient for the HPLC analysis was programmed as follows: 0–5 min, 65% B; 5–15 min, 70% B; at a flow rate of 1.5 mL/min; 15–25 min, 80% B, at a flow rate of 1.0 mL/min; 25–40 min, 85% B, at a flow rate of 0.8 mL/min; 40–50 min, 100% B, at a flow rate of 2.0 mL/min, and then was held for additional 5 min.

4.4. Isolation and Purification of Compounds (1)–(4) by HPLC

Fractions were collected manually by observing the elution profile of the chromatography workstation. The elution profile was programmed with the gradient mobile phase composed of solvent A (0.1% TFA in ddH$_2$O), solvent B (100% methanol), and solvent C (100% ACN). Fractions were isolated and purified with the semi-preparative HPLC column (ALLTIMA C18, 5 μm, 250 mm × 10 mm i.d. Hichrom, Searle, UK). The gradients used for collecting each fraction were set as follows: Fraction (1), 0–14 min, 60% C; 14–19 min, 100%; at a flow rate of 1.5 mL/min; Fractions (2) and (3), 0–15 min, 85% B; 15–18 min, 100% B; at a flow rate of 2.0 mL/min; Fraction (4), 0–15 min, 85% B; at a flow rate of 2.0 mL/min; and 15–17 min, 100% B; at a flow rate of 2.5 mL/min. The purity of each HPLC fraction was calculated based on the proportion of the target peak area. The purified HPLC eluent was lyophilized and stored at −20 °C for further use.

4.5. Mass Spectrometry

The identification of each purified component was performed on a tandem mass spectrometer equipped with an electrospray ionization source. Each purified compound was dissolved in methanol at an appropriate concentration and was infused into the QTRAP 5500 mass spectrometer system (AB SCIEX, Framingham, MA, USA) equipped with a Turbo VTM Spray ion source. Multiple reaction monitoring (MRM) in both positive and negative mode was used to enhance the selectivity of detection. The source-dependent parameters for the mass spectrometer (MS) were set as follows: ion spray voltage (IS) = ±5500 V; curtain gas (CUR) = 20 psi; collision gas (CAD) = 10 psi; nebulizer gas (GS1) = 12 psi, heater gas (GS2) = 0 psi, and source temperature (TEM) = 0 °C. The fraction-dependent parameters were set as follows: declustering potential (DP) = +120.0 V/−130.0 V; entrance potential (EP) = ±10.0 V; collision cell exit potential (CXP) = ±13.0 V. The MS/MS optimized collision energy applied to compounds (1)–(4) was given as follows: 25 V in positive mode, 25 V in negative mode, 25 V in negative mode, and 40 V in positive mode, respectively. For trans-p-Coumaric acid standard, the collision energy applied was 10 V in positive mode. Raw data and images of spectra were generated by Analyst® Software (Redwood, CA, USA) and modified using Excel® (Redmond, WA, USA).

4.6. Ultraviolet-Visible Spectrophotometry

The UV spectrum of compound (4) was measured using a Shimadzu UV-3600 spectrophotometer (Shimadzu Corporation, Kyoto, Japan). Each absorption spectrum was recorded from 200.00 nm to 400.00 nm. Profiles were generated by UVProbe 2.21 Software (Shimadzu Corporation, Kyoto, Japan). A control of 100% methanol was set and auto-zeroed automatically by software.

4.7. NMR Analysis

A 5 mg sample of purified compound (4) was dissolved in DMSO-d_6, and 1H NMR (400 MHz), 13C NMR (100 MHz), DEPT 90, DEPT 135 spectra were recorded using the Bruker Avance III 400 MHz NMR spectrometer spectroscopy (Bruker Corporation, Solna, Sweden). All chemical shifts were reported in δ (ppm) relative to tetramethylsilane (TMS).

4.8. Quantitative Analysis

The content of each identified compound in IMP aerial part ethyl acetate extract was determined using a HPLC-DAD system. The linearity and range was evaluated by constructing a calibration curve (peak area vs concentration). Quantification was performed upon six levels of external standards. The limit of detection (LOD) was determined as the concentration with a signal-to-noise ratio of three, and the limit of quantification (LOQ) was determined as the concentration with a signal-to-noise ratio of ten.

4.9. MTT Assay

The growth inhibitory effects of compounds (1)–(4) on HT-29 (colon) and BT-549 (breast) cancer cell lines were evaluated. Cells were seeded at 4×10^3 cells per 96-well and incubated for 24 h. The cells were then treated by 0.5% DMSO (as solvent control) or various concentrations of compounds (as treatment group) and incubated at 37 °C for 48 and 72 h. The MTT assay and data analysis were performed as previously described [29].

4.10. Data Analysis

All statistics were calculated with SPSS 17.0 software and data were expressed as mean ± standard deviation (SD) for each analyte. For MS/MS spectrometry analysis, each mass spectrum shown was the average spectra of each sample detected with ten repetitions in each analysis. Compounds were identified by comparing the tandem mass (MS/MS) fragmentation patterns with those in the literatures, NIST14 mass spectral database, and the MS Search Program v.2.2 (National Institute of Standards and Technology, Gaithersburg, MD, USA). For the viability assay, a nonlinear regression test was applied to obtain a fit curve ($R^2 > 0.98$). Analysis of the differences between the 48/72 h treatment groups was carried out by one-way ANOVA (coupled with a post-test, Dunnett's test) with * $p < 0.05$.

5. Conclusions

In this study, it is the first time that trans-p-Coumaric acid (1); 2-Methoxyestrone (2); 11, 16-Dihydroxypregn-4-ene-3, 20-dione (3), and Tricin (4) were isolated and identified from IMP aerial part ethyl acetate extract. 2-Methoxyestrone, 11, 16-Dihydroxypregn-4-ene-3, 20-dione and Tricin possess considerable growth inhibitory activities against BT-549 breast and HT-29 colon cancer cell lines. The data provided important information about the bio-active components from IMP aerial part ethyl acetate extract. *Imperata cylindrica* (L.) Raeusch., one kind of traditional herbal medicine, has rational medical application potentials with respect to breast and colorectal cancer prevention.

Author Contributions: Y.W. and W.S.H. designed the experiments and wrote the paper; Y.W. and J.Z.S. purified each compound by HPLC system; Y.W.C. conducted the tandem MS analysis and analyzed the data; Y.W. identified each compound; J.Z.S. performed the MTT assay and evaluated the growth inhibitory activities of each purified compound against breast cancer and colon cancer cell lines. All authors approved the final manuscript.

Acknowledgments: We are grateful to the Biomedical Technology Support Center of Hong Kong Science and Technology Parks Corporation for their help with the mass spectrometry analysis and the generous support from Keenway Industries Ltd. (grant No. 6903088) to W.S.H.

Abbreviations

HPLC-DAD, high-performance liquid chromatography–diode array detector (HPLC-DAD); ESI-MS/MS, electrospray ionization tandem mass spectrometry; NMR, nuclear magnetic resonance; IMP, Imperata cylindrica; MTT, 3-(4,5-Dimethylthiazol-2-yl)-2,5-Diphenyltetrazolium Bromide; ACN, acetonitrile; TFA, trifluoroacetic acid; λmax, wavelength of maximum absorption; LOD, limit of detection; LOQ, limit of quantification; IC50, half-maximal inhibitory concentration; TMS, tetramethylsilane; SD, standard deviation.

References

1.   Pinilla, V.; Luu, B. Isolation and partial characterization of immunostimulating polysaccharides from *Imperata cylindrica*. *Planta Med.* **1999**, *65*, 549–552. [CrossRef] [PubMed]

2.   Eussen, J.H.H.; Niemann, G.J. Growth inhibiting substances from leaves of *Imperata cylindrica* (L.) Beauv. *Z. Pflanzenphysiol.* **1981**, *102*, 263–266. [CrossRef]

3.   Matsunaga, K.; Shibuya, M.; Ohizumi, Y. Graminone B, a novel lignan with vasodilative activity from *Imperata cylindrica*. *J. Nat. Prod.* **1994**, *57*, 1734–1736. [CrossRef] [PubMed]

4.   Matsunaga, K.; Shibuya, M.; Ohizumi, Y. Imperanene, a novel phenolic compound with platelet aggregation inhibitory activity from *Imperata cylindrica*. *J. Nat. Prod.* **1995**, *58*, 138–139. [CrossRef] [PubMed]

5.   Mohamed, G.A.; Abdel-Lateff, A.; Fouad, M.A.; Ibrahim, S.R.; Elkhayat, E.S.; Okino, T. Chemical composition and hepato-protective activity of *Imperata cylindrica* Beauv. *Pharmacogn. Mag.* **2009**, *5*, 28–36.

6.   Liu, R.H.; Chen, S.S.; Ren, G.; Shao, F.; Huang, H.L. Phenolic compounds from roots of *Imperata cylindrica* var. major. *Chin. Herb. Med.* **2013**, *5*, 240–243. [CrossRef]

7.   An, H.J.; Nugroho, A.; Song, B.M.; Park, H.J. Isoeugenin, a novel nitric oxide synthase inhibitor isolated from the rhizomes of *Imperata cylindrica*. *Molecules* **2015**, *20*, 21336–21345. [CrossRef] [PubMed]

8.   Tine, Y.; Renucci, F.; Costa, J.; Wélé, A.; Paolini, J. A Method for LC-MS/MS profiling of coumarins in *Zanthoxylum zanthoxyloides* (Lam.) B. Zepernich and Timler extracts and essential oils. *Molecules* **2017**, *22*, 174. [CrossRef] [PubMed]

9.   Chen, G.; Pramanik, B.N.; Liu, Y.H.; Mirza, U.A. Applications of LC/MS in structure identifications of small molecules and proteins in drug discovery. *J. Mass Spectrom.* **2007**, *42*, 279–287. [CrossRef] [PubMed]

10.   Kwok, A.H.Y.; Wang, Y.; Ho, W.S. Cytotoxic and pro-oxidative effects of *Imperata cylindrica* aerial part ethyl acetate extract in colorectal cancer in vitro. *Phytomedicine* **2016**, *23*, 558–565. [CrossRef] [PubMed]

11.   Lam, P.Y.; Zhu, F.Y.; Chan, W.L.; Liu, H.; Lo, C. Cytochrome P450 93G1 is a flavone synthase II that channels flavanones to the biosynthesis of Tricin O-linked conjugates in rice. *Plant Physiol.* **2014**, *165*, 1315–1327. [CrossRef] [PubMed]

12.   Li, M.; Pu, Y.; Yoo, C.G.; Ragauskas, A.J. The occurrence of Tricin and its derivatives in plants. *Green Chem.* **2016**, *18*, 1439–1454. [CrossRef]

13.   Kwon, Y.S.; Kim, C.M. Antioxidant constituents from the stem of Sorghum bicolor. *Arch. Pharm. Res.* **2003**, *26*, 535–539. [CrossRef] [PubMed]

14.   Kong, C.; Xu, X.; Zhou, B.; Hu, F.; Zhang, C.; Zhang, M. Two compounds from allelopathic rice accession and their inhibitory activity on weeds and fungal pathogens. *Phytochemistry* **2004**, *65*, 1123–1128. [CrossRef] [PubMed]

15.   Jaganathan, S.K.; Supriyanto, E.; Mandal, M. Events associated with apoptotic effect of p-Coumaric acid in HCT-15 colon cancer cells. *World J. Gastroenterol.* **2013**, *19*, 7726–7734. [CrossRef] [PubMed]

16.   Sorice, A.; Guerriero, E.; Volpe, M.G.; Capone, F.; La Cara, F.; Ciliberto, G.; Colonna, G.; Costantini, S. Differential response of two human breast cancer cell lines to the phenolic extract from flaxseed oil. *Molecules* **2016**, *21*, 319. [CrossRef] [PubMed]

17.   Konishi, Y.; Zhao, Z.; Shimizu, M. Phenolic acids are absorbed from the rat stomach with different absorption rates. *J. Agric. Food Chem.* **2006**, *54*, 7539–7543. [CrossRef] [PubMed]

18.   Dobos, J.; Tímár, J.; Bocsi, J.; Burián, Z.; Nagy, K.; Barna, G.; Peták, I.; Ladányi, A. In vitro and in vivo anti-tumor effect of 2-methoxyestradiol on human melanoma. *Int. J. Cancer* **2004**, *112*, 771–776. [CrossRef] [PubMed]

19.   Lakhani, N.J.; Sparreboom, A.; Xu, X. Characterization of in vitro and in vivo metabolic pathways of the investigational anticancer agent, 2-methoxyestradiol. *J. Pharm. Sci.* **2007**, *96*, 1821–1831. [CrossRef] [PubMed]

20.   Zhu, B.T.; Conney, A.H. Is 2-Methoxyestradiol an endogenous estrogen metabolite that inhibitsmammary carcinogenesis? *Cancer. Res.* **1998**, *58*, 2269–2277. [PubMed]

21. Choudhary, M.I.; Nasir, M.; Khan, S.N.; Atif, M.; Ali, R.A.; Khalil, S.M.; Rahman, A. Microbial hydroxylation of hydroxyprogesterones and α-glucosidase inhibition activity of their metabolites. *Z. Naturforsch.* **2007**, *62*, 593–599. [CrossRef]

22. Lee, D.E.; Lee, S.; Jang, E.S.; Shin, H.W.; Moon, B.S.; Lee, C.H. Metabolomic profiles of Aspergillus oryzae and Bacillus amyloliquefaciens during rice koji fermentation. *Molecules* **2016**, *21*, 773. [CrossRef] [PubMed]

23. Jiao, J.J.; Zhang, Y.; Liu, C.M.; Liu, J.E.; Wu, X.Q.; Zhang, Y. Separation and purification of Tricin from an antioxidant product derived from bamboo leaves. *J. Agric. Food Chem.* **2007**, *55*, 10086–10092. [CrossRef] [PubMed]

24. Hudson, E.A.; Dinh, P.A.; Kokubun, T.; Simmonds, M.S.; Gescher, A. Characterization of potentially chemopreventive phenols in extracts of brown rice that inhibit the growth of human breast and colon cancer cells. *Cancer Epidemiol. Biomarkers. Prev.* **2000**, *9*, 1163–1170. [PubMed]

25. Cai, H.; Hudson, E.A.; Mann, P.; Verschoyle, R.D.; Greaves, P.; Manson, M.M.; Steward, W.P.; Gescher, A.J. Growth-inhibitory and cell cycle-arresting properties of the rice bran constituent Tricin in human-derived breast cancer cells in vitro and in nude mice in vivo. *Br. J. Cancer* **2004**, *91*, 1364–1371. [CrossRef] [PubMed]

26. Verschoyle, R.D.; Greaves, P.; Cai, H.; Borkhardt, A.; Broggini, M.; D'Incalci, M.; Riccio, E.; Doppalapudi, R.; Kapetanovic, I.M.; Steward, W.P.; et al. Preliminary safety evaluation of the putative cancer chemopreventive agent Tricin, a naturally occurring flavone. *Cancer Chemother. Pharmacol.* **2006**, *57*, 1–6. [CrossRef] [PubMed]

27. Zhou, J.M.; Ibrahim, R.K. Tricin-a potential multifunctional nutraceutical. *Phytochem. Rev.* **2010**, *9*, 413–424. [CrossRef]

28. Jang, M.H.; Ho, J.K.; Hye, J.J. Tricin, 4',5',7'-trihydroxy-3',5'-dimethoxyflavone, exhibits potent antiangiogenic activity in vitro. *Int. J. Oncol.* **2016**, *49*, 1497–1504. [CrossRef]

29. Zheng, Y.M.; Shen, J.Z.; Wang, Y.; Lu, A.X.; Ho, W.S. Anti-oxidant and anti-cancer activities of Angelica dahurica extract via induction of apoptosis in colon cancer cells. *Phytomedicine* **2016**, *15*, 1267–1274. [CrossRef] [PubMed]

12

NP-Scout: Machine Learning Approach for the Quantification and Visualization of the Natural Product-Likeness of Small Molecules

Ya Chen [1], Conrad Stork [1], Steffen Hirte [1] and Johannes Kirchmair [1,2,3,*]

[1] Center for Bioinformatics (ZBH), Department of Informatics, Faculty of Mathematics, Informatics and Natural Sciences, Universität Hamburg, 20146 Hamburg, Germany; chen@zbh.uni-hamburg.de (Y.C.); stork@zbh.uni-hamburg.de (C.S.); steffen.hirte@studium.uni-hamburg.de (S.H.)

[2] Department of Chemistry, University of Bergen, 5007 Bergen, Norway

[3] Computational Biology Unit (CBU), Department of Informatics, University of Bergen, 5008 Bergen, Norway

[*] Correspondence: johannes.kirchmair@uib.no or kirchmair@zbh.uni-hamburg.de;

Abstract: Natural products (NPs) remain the most prolific resource for the development of small-molecule drugs. Here we report a new machine learning approach that allows the identification of natural products with high accuracy. The method also generates similarity maps, which highlight atoms that contribute significantly to the classification of small molecules as a natural product or synthetic molecule. The method can hence be utilized to (i) identify natural products in large molecular libraries, (ii) quantify the natural product-likeness of small molecules, and (iii) visualize atoms in small molecules that are characteristic of natural products or synthetic molecules. The models are based on random forest classifiers trained on data sets consisting of more than 265,000 to 322,000 natural products and synthetic molecules. Two-dimensional molecular descriptors, MACCS keys and Morgan2 fingerprints were explored. On an independent test set the models reached areas under the receiver operating characteristic curve (AUC) of 0.997 and Matthews correlation coefficients (MCCs) of 0.954 and higher. The method was further tested on data from the Dictionary of Natural Products, ChEMBL and other resources. The best-performing models are accessible as a free web service at http://npscout.zbh.uni-hamburg.de/npscout.

Keywords: natural products; natural product-likeness; machine learning; random forest; classification; similarity maps; visualization; molecular fingerprints; web service

1. Introduction

Natural products (NPs) continue to be the most prolific resource for drug leads [1–4]. A recent analysis found that over 60% of all small-molecule drugs approved between 1981 and 2014 are genuine NPs, NP analogs or their derivatives, or compounds containing an NP pharmacophore [5]. NPs are characterized by enormous structural and physicochemical diversity [6–8]. Some of the regions in chemical space covered by NPs are not, or only rarely, populated by synthetic molecules (SMs) [7,9]. The structural complexity of many NPs exceeds that of compounds found in conventional synthetic libraries for screening, in particular with respect to stereochemical aspects, molecular shape, and ring systems [10–18].

The primary bottleneck of NP research is the scarcity of materials for testing. In a recent study, we showed that the molecular structures of more than 250,000 NPs have been deposited in public databases, and that only approximately 10% of these are readily obtainable from commercial providers and other sources [19].

Given the fact that NPs exhibit a wide range of biological activities that are of immediate relevance to human health, new avenues that would make NP research more effective are being explored, in particular, research involving computational approaches [2]. For example, computational methods have been employed successfully for the identification of bioactive NPs [20–22] and their bio-macromolecular targets [23–26]. They have also been successfully utilized for the design of simple synthetic, bioactive mimetics of NPs [27–29]. In this context, computational methods for quantifying the NP-likeness of compounds can be valuable tools to guide the de novo generation of NP mimetics and optimize the NP-likeness of lead compounds. Such methods may also be useful for identifying genuine NPs in commercial compound libraries, which often also contain SMs [19]. This can be valuable in the context of library design and for the prioritization of compounds for experimental testing.

The best-known in-silico approach for identifying NPs is the NP-likeness score developed by Ertl et al. [30]. The NP-likeness score is a Bayesian measure that quantifies a compound's similarity with the structural space of NPs based on structural fragments. As such, the model can identify sub-structures characteristic to NPs. The method has been re-implemented, with some modifications, in various platforms (e.g., [31–33]). Among them is the Natural-Product-Likeness Scoring System [31], which allows the calculation of the NP-likeness score (with some modifications). The Natural-Product-Likeness Scoring System also allows the use of customized data sets for training. An alternative approach for quantifying NP-Likeness, following a similar modeling strategy, but based on extended connectivity fingerprints (ECFPs), was reported by Yu [34]. Also a rule-based approach has been reported [35].

In this work, we present the development and validation of new machine learning models for the discrimination of NPs and SMs. To the best of our knowledge, these models are trained on the largest collection of known NPs that have been employed for the development of such classifiers. Among further developments, we present the utilization of similarity maps [36] for the visualization of atoms of a molecule, which are characteristic for NPs or SMs, according to the models.

2. Materials and Methods

2.1. Data Preparation

NPs were compiled from several physical and virtual NP databases (see Results for details). The chemical structures were parsed directly from SMILES notation, where available. Alternatively, chemical structures stored in chemical table files (e.g., SDF) were parsed with RDKit [37] and converted into SMILES. Minor components of salts were removed by the method described in ref. [38]. Any compounds with a molecular weight below 150 Da or above 1500 Da, and any compounds consisting of elements other than H, B, C, N, O, F, Si, P, S, Cl, Se, Br, or I were filtered. The "canonicalize" method, which was implemented in the "tautomer" class of MolVS [39], was used for neutralizing the molecular structures and merging tautomers. After the removal of duplicate SMILES (ignoring stereochemistry), the processed NP reference data set consisted of a total of 201,761 NPs.

SMs were compiled from the "in-stock" subset of ZINC [40,41]. In a first step, 500,000 compounds of ZINC were picked by random selection from the complete "in-stock" subset and pre-processed following the identical protocol used for the NP databases. After generating unique, canonicalized SMILES, any molecules present in the NP reference data set were removed from the SM data set (as determined by the comparison of canonicalized SMILES). Then, random sampling was used to compile a reference data set of SMs of identical size as the NP reference data set (i.e., 201,761 compounds).

The Dictionary of Natural Products (DNP) [42] and the ChEMBL database [43,44] were pre-processed following the identical protocol outlined for the NP and SM data sets. The ChEMBL sub-set of molecules, published in the Journal of Natural Products, was retrieved directly from ChEMBL [43,45]. The natural products subset of ZINC was downloaded from the ZINC website [46].

2.2. Principal Component Analysis

Fifteen two-dimensional molecular descriptors calculated with the Molecular Operating Environment (MOE) [47] were used for principle component analysis (PCA): MW (Weight), log

P (log P (o/w)), topological polar surface area (TPSA), number of hydrogen bond acceptors (a_acc), number of hydrogen bond donors (a_don), number of heavy atoms (a_heavy), fraction of rotatable bonds (b_rotR), number of nitrogen atoms (a_nN), number of oxygen atoms (a_nO), number of acidic atoms (a_acid), number of basic atoms (a_base), sum of formal charges (FCharge), number of aromatic atoms (a_aro) and number of chiral centers (chiral), and number of rings (rings).

2.3. Model Building

Prior to model building, the preprocessed NP and SM reference data sets were merged, resulting in a total of 403,522 data records. The merged data set was then randomly split into a training set of 322,817 and a test set of 80,705 compounds (ratio of 4:1). In fingerprint space, structurally distinct molecules may have identical fingerprints. For this reason, de-duplication, based on fingerprints, was separately performed for all NPs and all SMs in the training data. Any fingerprints present in both the NP and SM subsets were removed, in order to avoid conflicting class labels. This procedure resulted in a training set of 156,119 NPs and 161,378 SMs represented by Morgan2 fingerprints, and in a training set of 108,393 NPs and 157,162 SMs represented by MACCS keys.

Morgan2 fingerprints (1024 bits) [48,49] and MACCS keys (166 bits) were calculated with RDKit, and 206 two-dimensional physicochemical property descriptors were calculated with MOE. Random forest classifiers (RFCs) were generated with scikit-learn [50,51] using default settings, except for "n_estimators", which was set to "100", and "class_weight", which was set to "balanced".

The NP-likeness calculator [30,31,52] was trained on atom signatures derived from the identical NP and SM data sets, used for training the RFCs. Subsequently, the NP-likeness score was calculated for each molecule in the test set, according to the atom signatures. All calculations used a signature height of 3, resulting in scores ranging from −3 to 3. Molecules with a score greater than 0.0 were labeled as NPs, and molecules with a score lower, or equal to 0.0 were labeled as SMs. NP class probabilities (and AUCs) were derived by normalizing these scores to a range from 0.0 to 1.0.

2.4. Similarity Maps

Similarity maps were computed with the RDKit [37] Chem.Draw.SimilarityMaps module based on RFCs derived from Morgan2 fingerprints (1024 bits).

3. Results

3.1. Compilation of Data Sets for Model Development

An NP reference data set of 201,761 unique NPs was compiled from 18 virtual NP libraries and nine physical NP databases. The reference data set is identical to that compiled as part of our previous work [8], with two amendments: First, the compounds of the DNP [42] were not included in the data set, as they serve as an external test set in this work, and second, the recently published Natural Products Atlas database [53] was added as a new data source. An overview of the NP data sources utilized in this work is provided in Table 1. The table also reports the number of molecules that are contained in the individual databases prior to, and after, data preprocessing. This is a procedure that includes the removal of salt components and stereochemical information, the filtering of molecules composed of uncommon elements, and with a molecular weight (MW) below 150 Da or above 1500 Da, and the removal of duplicate molecules (see Methods for details). An equal amount (i.e., 201,761) of synthetic organic molecules (SMs) was collected from the "in-stock" subset of ZINC [41] by random selection.

Table 1. Size of the individual data sets prior to and after data preprocessing.

Name [1]	Number of Molecules in SMILES Notation Successfully Parsed with RDKit	Number of Unique Molecules After Data Preprocessing	Scientific Literature and/or Online Presence
UNPD	229,140	161,228	[54,55]
TCM Database@Taiwan	56,325	45,422	[56,57]
NP Atlas	20,018	18,358	[53]
TCMID	13,188	10,918	[58,59]
TIPdb	8838	7620	[60–62]
Ambinter and Greenpharma NPs	7905	6680	[63,64]
AnalytiCon Discovery MEGx	4315	4063	[65]
NANPDB	6841	3734	[66,67]
StreptomeDB	3990	3353	[68,69]
NPs of PubChem Substance Database	3533	2638	[70,71]
NuBBE	1856	1637	[72,73]
Pi Chemicals NPs	1783	1511	[74]
NPCARE	1613	1479	[75,76]
NPACT	1516	1376	[77,78]
InterBioScreen NPs	1359	1116	[79]
AfroDb	954	865	[80,81]
TargetMol Natural Compound Library	850	745	[82]
HIM	1284	641	[83,84]
SANCDB	623	588	[85,86]
UEFS Natural Products	493	469	via ZINC [40,87]
p-ANAPL	538	456	[88]
NCI/NIH DTP NP set IV	419	394	[89]
HIT	707	362	[90,91]
AfroCancer	388	352	[92,93]
AfroMalariaDB	265	250	[94,95]
AK Scientific NPs	242	177	[96]
Selleck Chemicals NPs	173	163	[97]
NP data set TOTAL	-	**201761**	

[1] UNPD: the Universal Natural Products Database; TCM Database@Taiwan: the Traditional Chinese Medicine Database@Taiwan; NP Atlas: the Natural Products Atlas; TCMID: the Traditional Chinese Medicine Integrated Database; TIPdb: the Taiwan Indigenous Plant Database; NANPDB: the Northern African Natural Products Database; StreptomeDB: Streptome Database; NuBBE: Nuclei of Bioassays, Ecophysiology and Biosynthesis of Natural Products Database; NPCARE: Database of Natural Products for Cancer Gene Regulation; NPACT: the Naturally Occurring Plant-based Anti-Cancer Compound-Activity-Target Database; AfroDb: NPs from African medicinal plants; HIM: the Herbal Ingredients in-vivo Metabolism Database; UEFS Natural Products: the natural products database of the State University of Feira De Santana; p-ANAPL: the Pan-African Natural Products Library; NCI/NIH DTP NP set IV: the NP (plated) set IV of the Developmental Therapeutic Program of the National Cancer Institute/National Institutes of Health; HIT, the Herbal Ingredients' Targets Database; AfroCancer, the African Anticancer Natural Products Library; AfroMalariaDB, the African Antimalarial Natural Products Library.

3.2. Analysis of the Physicochemical Properties of Natural Products and Synthetic Molecules

Prior to model development, we compared the chemical space covered by the 201,761 unique NPs, and the equal number of unique SMs, using principal component analysis (PCA), based on 15 relevant physicochemical properties (see Methods for details). The score plot in Figure 1 shows that the chemical space of SMs is essentially a sub-space of NPs.

NPs have on average a higher MW than SMs (506 Da vs 384 Da) and a larger proportion of heavy compounds (38% vs. 10% of all molecules have a MW greater than 500 Da; Figure 2a). SMs have a narrower distribution of calculated log P values as compared to NPs (Figure 2b) but their averages are comparable (3.31 versus 3.25). SMs and NPs show clear differences in the entropy of element distributions in molecules, with NPs having, on average, a lower entropy than SMs (1.39 versus 1.63; Figure 2c). NPs tend to have more chiral centers (mean 6.66 vs. 0.75; Figure 2d), substantially fewer nitrogen atoms than SMs (mean 0.76 vs. 2.94; Figure 2e), and more oxygen atoms (mean 7.39 vs. 2.88; Figure 2f) [7,10,12–15,17].

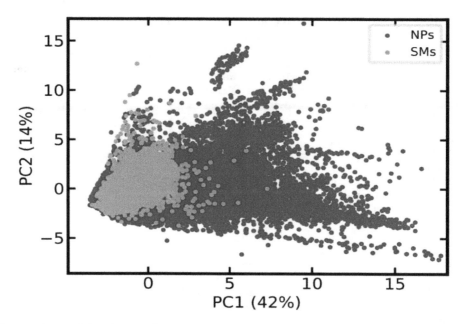

Figure 1. Comparison of the chemical space covered by natural products (NPs) and synthetic organic molecules (SMs). The score plot is based on the principle component analysis (PCA) of all molecules in the data set, characterized by 15 calculated physicochemical properties. PCA was performed on the full data sets. For the sake of clarity, only a randomly selected 10% of all data points are reported in the score plot. The percentage of the total variance explained by the first two principal components is reported in the respective axis labels.

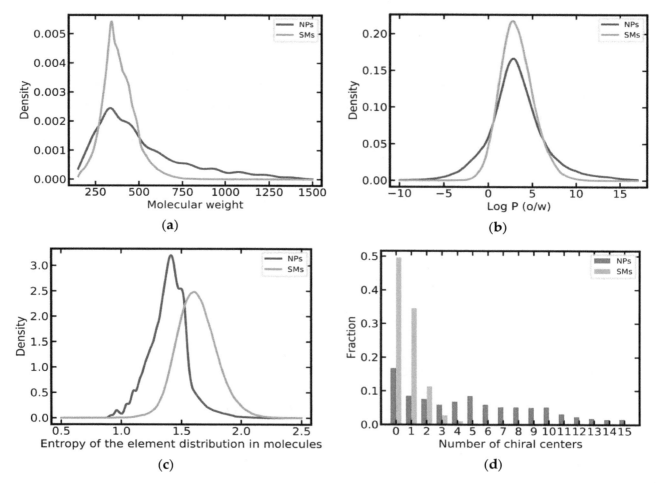

Figure 2. *Cont.*

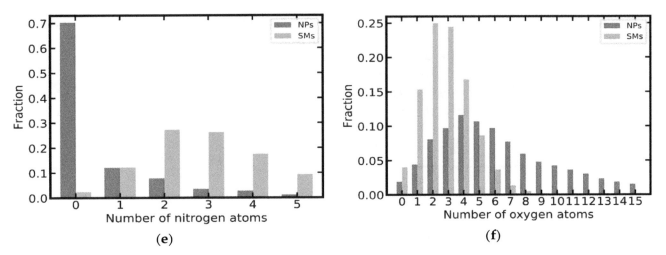

Figure 2. Distributions of key physicochemical properties among NPs and SMs: (**a**) Molecular weight; (**b**) log P (o/w); (**c**) entropy of the element distribution in molecules; (**d**) number of chiral centers; (**e**) number of nitrogen atoms; (**f**) number of oxygen atoms.

3.3. Model Development and Selection

Random forest classifiers [98] were trained on three different descriptor sets: 206 two-dimensional physicochemical property descriptors calculated with MOE [47], Morgan2 fingerprints (1024 bits) [48,49] calculated with RDKit [37], and MACCS keys (166 bits), also calculated with RDKit. Model performance was characterized utilizing the Matthews correlation coefficient (MCC) [99] and area under the receiver operating characteristic curve (AUC). The MCC is one of the most robust measures for evaluating the performance of binary classifiers, as it considers the proportion of all classes in the confusion matrix (i.e., true positives, false positives, true negatives, and false negatives). The AUC was used to measure how well the models are able to rank NPs early in a list.

As reported in Table 2, the models derived from any of the three descriptor sets performed very well. The AUC values, that were obtained during 10-fold cross-validation, were between 0.996 and 0.997; the MCC values were 0.950 or higher. No noticeable increase in performance was obtained by the further increase in the number of estimators (n_estimators) and the optimization of the maximum fraction of features considered per split (max_features; data not shown). Therefore, we chose to use 100 estimators, and the square root of the number of features, as the most suitable setup for model generation.

Table 2. Performance of models derived from different descriptors or fingerprints.

Test Method	Metric [1]	MOE Two-Dimensional Descriptors	Morgan2 Fingerprints (1024 Bits)	MACCS Keys	NP-Likeness Calculator
10-fold cross-validation	AUC	0.997	0.997	0.996	/
	MCC	0.953	0.958	0.950	/
Independent test set	AUC	0.997	0.997	0.997	0.997
	MCC	0.954	0.960	0.960	0.959

[1] AUC: area under the receiver operating characteristic curve: MCC: Matthews correlation coefficient.

3.4. Model Validation

In a first step, the performance of the selected models was tested on an independent test set. The AUC and MCC values, that were obtained for the selected models on this independent test set, are comparable with those obtained for the 10-fold cross-validation: AUC values were 0.997 for models based on any of the three types of descriptors and MCC values were 0.954 or higher.

Given the fact that the type of descriptor, used for model generation, did not have a substantial impact on model performance, we opted to select the model based on MACCS keys as the primary model for further experiments, because of its low complexity and good interpretability. This model achieved a very good separation of NPs and SMs for the independent test set, as shown in Figure 3a. Approximately 63% of all NPs were assigned an NP class probability of 1.0, whereas 51% SMs were assigned an NP class probability of 0.0. Only approximately 1% of all compounds were assigned values close to the decision threshold of 0.5 (i.e., between 0.4 and 0.6).

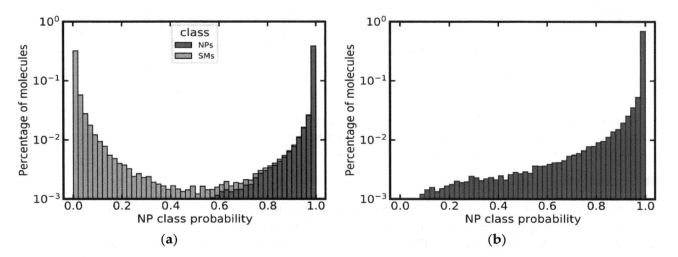

(a)   (b)

Figure 3. Predicted NP class probabilities distributions for (a) the independent test set (stacked histogram), (b) the DNP (after the removal of any compounds present in the training set). Note that the y-axis is in logarithmic scale.

The model's ability to identify NPs was also tested using the DNP as an external validation set. By definition, the DNP should consist exclusively of NPs. After the removal of any molecules present in the training data (based on canonicalized SMILES), the preprocessed DNP consisted of 60,502 compounds. Approximately 95% of these compounds were predicted as NPs by the model, demonstrating the model's capacity to identify NPs with high sensitivity (Figure 3b).

3.5. Comparison of Model Performance with the NP-Likeness Calculator

We compared the performance of the model derived from MACCS keys to the NP-likeness calculator (based on the Natural-Product-Likeness Scoring System; see Introduction), which we trained and tested on the identical data sets used for the development of our models. On the independent test set, the NP-likeness calculator performed equally well as our model, with an AUC of 0.997 and an MCC of 0.959 (Table 2). Approximately 95% of all compounds of the DNP were classified as NPs (i.e., having assigned an NP-likeness score greater than 0; see Figure S1), which is comparable to the classification obtained with our model based on MACCS keys.

3.6. Analysis of Class Probability Distributions for Different Data Sets

In addition to the above experiments, we used the model based on MACCS keys for profiling the ChEMBL database and a subset thereof. The ChEMBL database [44] primarily contains SMs, and 87% of all compounds stored in ChEMBL were predicted as such (Figure 4a). Interestingly, 42,949 molecules (~3%) were assigned an NP class probability of 1.0, and therefore likely are NPs. This finding is in agreement with our previous study, which identified approximately 40,000 NPs in the ChEMBL database, by overlapping the database with a comprehensive set of known NPs [19].

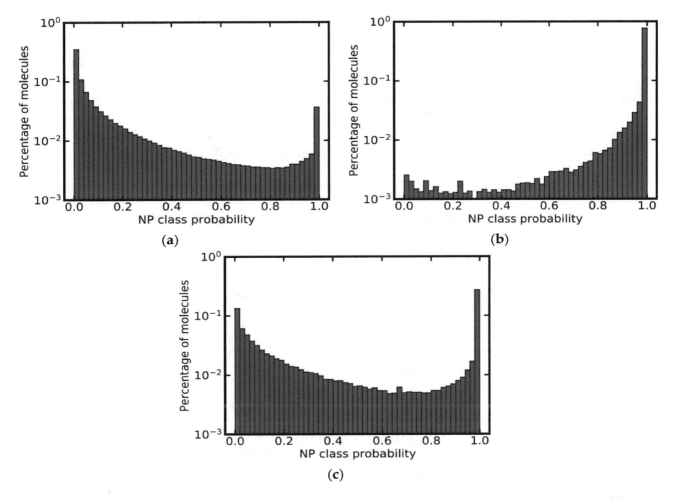

Figure 4. Predicted NP class probability distributions for (**a**) the ChEMBL database, (**b**) a subset of the ChEMBL database composed of molecules originating from the Journal of Natural Products, and (**c**) the natural products subset of ZINC. Note that the y-axis is in logarithmic scale.

A subset of the ChEMBL database containing molecules originating from the Journal of Natural Products [45] has been used as a source of genuine NPs to train models for the prediction of NP-likeness [31]. Our model based on MACCS keys predicts a small percentage of the molecules (less than 4%) in this data set as not NP-like (Figure 4b). Closer inspection of the compounds predicted as not NP-like reveals that these are, for example, SMs used as positive controls in biochemical assays. They include the drugs celecoxib, glibenclamide and linezolid, all of which are predicted with an NP class probability of 0.0. This experiment demonstrates that the classifiers can be used as powerful tools for the identification of NPs or SMs in mixed data sets with high accuracy.

A second example of a data set that by its name is assumed to consist exclusively of NPs is the natural products subset of ZINC [46]. The class probability distribution calculated for this subset however is similar to that obtained for the complete ChEMBL, indicating the presence of a substantial number of SMs (including NP derivatives and NP analogs) in this subset (Figure 4c): Only approximately 43% of all compounds in the NPs subset of ZINC were classified as NPs; around 23% were assigned an NP class probability of 1.0.

3.7. Analysis of Discriminative Features of Natural Products and Synthetic Molecules

The most discriminative features were determined, based on the feature_importances_ attributes computed with scikit-learn (see Methods for details). For the classifier based on MOE two-dimensional molecular descriptors, the three most important features were the number of nitrogen atoms (a large fraction of NPs has no nitrogen atom; see Figure 2e), the entropy of the element distribution in molecules (NPs have on average lower element distribution entropy than SMs; see Figure 2c), and the number of unconstrained chiral centers (NPs have on average more chiral centers than SMs; see Figure 2d). An overview of the ten most important features is provided in Table 3.

Table 3. Feature importance for the random forest classifier based on MOE two-dimensional descriptors.

Identifier Used by MOE	Feature Importance [1]	Description
a_nN	0.103	Number of nitrogen atoms.
a_ICM	0.051	Entropy of the element distribution in the molecule.
chiral_u	0.045	Number of unconstrained chiral centers.
GCUT_SLOGP_0	0.045	Descriptor derived from graph distance adjacency matrices utilizing atomic contribution to log P.
SlogP_VSA0	0.044	Surface area descriptor taking into account the contributions of individual atoms to log P.
chiral	0.042	Number of chiral centers.
GCUT_SLOGP_3	0.036	Descriptor derived from graph distance adjacency matrices utilizing atomic contribution to log P.
a_nO	0.025	The number of oxygen atoms.
GCUT_PEOE_0	0.025	Descriptor derived from graph distance adjacency matrices utilizing partial equalization of orbital electronegativities charges.
SlogP_VSA1	0.024	Surface area descriptor taking into account the contributions of individual atoms to log P.

[1] From the feature_importances_ attribute of the classifier based on MOE two-dimensional descriptors. The higher, the more important the feature is.

For the classifier based on MACCS keys, the 15 most important features are reported in Figure 5. In agreement with the differences observed in the physiochemical property distributions of NPs versus SMs (see Analysis of the Physicochemical Properties of Natural Products and Synthetic Molecules), the most important MACCS keys describe the presence or absence of nitrogen atoms, such as key 161, matching molecules containing at least one nitrogen atom, key 142, matching molecules with at least two nitrogen atoms, and keys 117, 158, 122, 156, 75, 110, 133, 92 and 80, matching molecules containing specific nitrogen-containing substructures. Also several oxy gen-containing substructures are among the most important features, such as keys 139, 117, 110, 92.

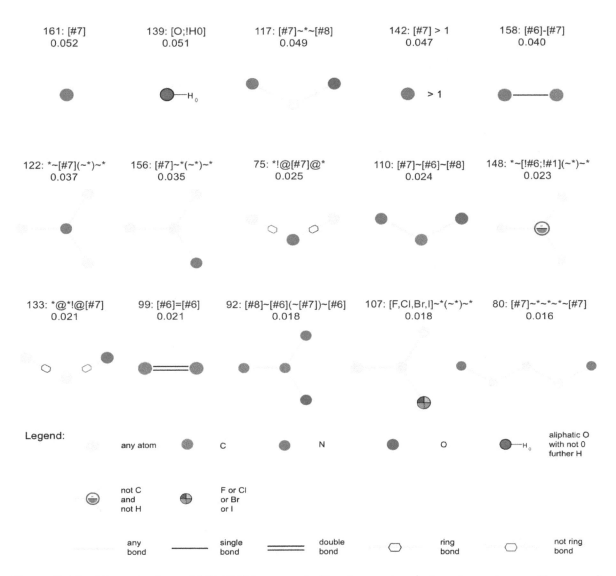

Figure 5. The 15 most relevant MACCS keys, sorted by decreasing feature importance. Above each diagram, the first line reports the index of the respective MACCS key and its SMARTS pattern. The second line reports the feature importance (feature_importances_ attribute). The figure was produced with SMARTSviewer [100,101].

3.8. Similarity Maps

Similarity maps [36] allow the visualization of the atomic contribution of molecular fingerprints and can be extended to visualize the "atomic weights" of the predicted probability of the machine learning model. During several test runs with different Morgan fingerprint, radii, and bit vector lengths, we identified a radius of 2 and a bit vector length of 1024 bits as the most suitable setup for generating fine-grained similarity maps. The examples of similarity maps, generated with this descriptor, and the random forest approach, are reported in Table 4 for representative molecules, none of which have been part of model training. In this similarity maps, green highlights mark atoms contributing to the classification of a molecule as NP, whereas orange highlights mark atoms contributing to the classification of a molecule as SM. As expected, the similarity maps for the NP arglabin are mostly green, whereas for the synthetic drugs, bilastine and perampanel, are mostly orange. For NP derivatives and mimetics, the similarity maps are more heterogeneous and show green, as well as orange areas. The thrombin receptor antagonist vorapaxar is a derivative of the piperidine alkaloid himbacine. Vorapaxar shares a decahydronaphtho[2,3-c]furan-1(3H)-one scaffold with himbacine, but has the piperidine ring replaced by a pyridine, besides other modifications. The similarity map generated for vorapaxar shows that the model correctly identifies the decahydronaphtho[2,3-c]furan-1(3H)-one as NP-like, whereas it associates the modified areas with synthetic molecules. In the case of empagliflozin, which mimics the flavonoid phlorozin, the model correctly recognizes the C-glycosyl moiety as NP-like, whereas other atoms in the molecule are associated with synthetic molecules.

Table 4. Examples of similarity maps generated by the NP classifier based on Morgan2 fingerprints.

Similarity Map [1]	Name	Source [2]	NP Class Probability	Disease Indication	Year Introduced
	arglabin	N	1.0	anticancer	1999
	cefonicid sodium	ND	0.34	antibacterial	1984
	dutaseride	ND	0.18	benign prostatic hypertrophy	2001
	vorapaxar	ND	0.30	coronary artery disease	2014
	empagliflozin	S*/NM	0.67	antidiabetic (diabetes 2)	2014
	belinostat	S*/NM	0.09	anticancer	2014
	febuxostat	S/NM	0.19	hyperuricemia	2009
	zalcitabine	S*	0.46	antiviral	1992

Table 4. *Cont.*

Similarity Map [1]	Name	Source [2]	NP Class Probability	Disease Indication	Year Introduced
	bilastine	S	0.17	antihistamine	2011
	perampanel	S	0.16	antiepileptic	2012

[1] Green highlights mark atoms contributing to the classification of a molecule as NP, whereas orange highlights mark atoms contributing to the classification of a molecule as SM. [2] N: Unaltered NP; ND: NP derivative; S*: Synthetic drug (NP pharmacophore); S: Synthetic drug; NM: Mimic of NP. Definitions according to ref [5].

3.9. NP-Scout Web Service

A web service named "NP-Scout" is accessible free of charge via http://npscout.zbh.uni-hamburg.de/npscout. It features the random forest model, based on MACCS keys for the computation of NP class probabilities and the random forest model, based on Morgan2 fingerprints (with 1024 bits) for the generation of similarity maps.

Users can submit molecular structures for calculation, by entering SMILES, uploading a file with SMILES or a list of SMILES, or drawing the molecule with the JavaScript Molecule Editor (JSME) [102]. The results page (Figure 6) presents the calculated NP class probabilities and similarity maps of submitted molecules in a tabular format. The results can be downloaded in CSV file format. Calculations of the NP class probabilities and the similarity maps take few seconds per compound and approximately 15 min for 1000 compounds. Users may utilize a unique link provided upon job submission to return to the website after all calculations have been completed.

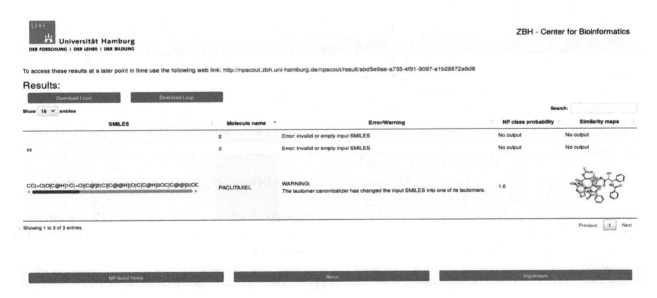

Figure 6. Screenshot of the result page of NP-Scout.

4. Conclusions

In this work, we introduced a pragmatic machine learning approach for the discrimination of NPs and SMs and for the quantification of NP-likeness. As shown by validation experiments using independent and external testing data, the models reach a very high level of accuracy. An interesting and relevant new aspect of this work is the utilization of similarity maps to visualize atoms in molecules making decisive contributions to the assignment of compounds to either class. A free web service for the classification of small molecules and the visualization of similarity maps is available at http://npscout.zbh.uni-hamburg.de/npscout.

Author Contributions: Conceptualization, Y.C. and J.K.; methodology, Y.C. and J.K.; software, Y.C., C.S., and S.H.; validation, Y.C.; formal analysis, Y.C; investigation, Y.C., C.S., and S.H.; resources, J.K.; data curation, Y.C.; writing—original draft preparation, Y.C., C.S., S.H., and J.K.; visualization, Y.C. and S.H.; supervision, J.K.; project administration, J.K.; funding acquisition, Y.C. and J.K.

Acknowledgments: Gerd Embruch from the Center of Bioinformatics (ZBH) of the Universität Hamburg is thanked for his technical support with the web service.

References

1. Cragg, G.M.; Newman, D.J. Biodiversity: A continuing source of novel drug leads. *J. Macromol. Sci. Part A Pure Appl. Chem.* **2005**, *77*, 7–24. [CrossRef]
2. Rodrigues, T.; Reker, D.; Schneider, P.; Schneider, G. Counting on natural products for drug design. *Nat. Chem.* **2016**, *8*, 531–541. [CrossRef] [PubMed]
3. Harvey, A.L.; Edrada-Ebel, R.; Quinn, R.J. The re-emergence of natural products for drug discovery in the genomics era. *Nat. Rev. Drug Discov.* **2015**, *14*, 111–129. [CrossRef]
4. Shen, B. A new golden age of natural products drug discovery. *Cell* **2015**, *163*, 1297–1300. [CrossRef] [PubMed]
5. Newman, D.J.; Cragg, G.M. Natural products as sources of new drugs from 1981 to 2014. *J. Nat. Prod.* **2016**, *79*, 629–661. [CrossRef] [PubMed]
6. Grabowski, K.; Baringhaus, K.-H.; Schneider, G. Scaffold diversity of natural products: Inspiration for combinatorial library design. *Nat. Prod. Rep.* **2008**, *25*, 892–904. [CrossRef]
7. Ertl, P.; Schuffenhauer, A. Cheminformatics analysis of natural products: Lessons from nature inspiring the design of new drugs. *Prog. Drug Res.* **2008**, *66*, 219–235.
8. Chen, Y.; de Lomana, M.G.; Friedrich, N.-O.; Kirchmair, J. Characterization of the chemical space of known and Readily Obtainable Natural Products. *J. Chem. Inf. Model.* **2018**, *58*, 1518–1532. [CrossRef]
9. Chen, H.; Engkvist, O.; Blomberg, N.; Li, J. A comparative analysis of the molecular topologies for drugs, clinical candidates, natural products, human metabolites and general bioactive compounds. *Med. Chem. Commun.* **2012**, *3*, 312–321. [CrossRef]
10. Camp, D.; Garavelas, A.; Campitelli, M. Analysis of physicochemical properties for drugs of natural origin. *J. Nat. Prod.* **2015**, *78*, 1370–1382. [CrossRef]
11. Koch, M.A.; Schuffenhauer, A.; Scheck, M.; Wetzel, S.; Casaulta, M.; Odermatt, A.; Ertl, P.; Waldmann, H. Charting biologically relevant chemical space: A structural classification of natural products (SCONP). *Proc. Natl. Acad. Sci. USA* **2005**, *102*, 17272–17277. [CrossRef] [PubMed]
12. Stratton, C.F.; Newman, D.J.; Tan, D.S. Cheminformatic comparison of approved drugs from natural product versus synthetic origins. *Bioorg. Med. Chem. Lett.* **2015**, *25*, 4802–4807. [CrossRef] [PubMed]

13. Wetzel, S.; Schuffenhauer, A.; Roggo, S.; Ertl, P.; Waldmann, H. Cheminformatic analysis of natural products and their chemical space. *CHIMIA Int. J. Chem.* **2007**, *61*, 355–360. [CrossRef]
14. López-Vallejo, F.; Giulianotti, M.A.; Houghten, R.A.; Medina-Franco, J.L. Expanding the medicinally relevant chemical space with compound libraries. *Drug Discov. Today* **2012**, *17*, 718–726. [CrossRef]
15. Feher, M.; Schmidt, J.M. Property distributions: Differences between drugs, natural products, and molecules from combinatorial chemistry. *J. Chem. Inf. Comput. Sci.* **2003**, *43*, 218–227. [CrossRef] [PubMed]
16. Clemons, P.A.; Bodycombe, N.E.; Carrinski, H.A.; Wilson, J.A.; Shamji, A.F.; Wagner, B.K.; Koehler, A.N.; Schreiber, S.L. Small molecules of different origins have distinct distributions of structural complexity that correlate with protein-binding profiles. *Proc. Natl. Acad. Sci. USA* **2010**, *107*, 18787–18792. [CrossRef] [PubMed]
17. Henkel, T.; Brunne, R.M.; Müller, H.; Reichel, F. Statistical investigation into the structural complementarity of natural products and synthetic compounds. *Angew. Chem. Int. Ed. Engl.* **1999**, *38*, 643–647. [CrossRef]
18. Lee, M.L.; Schneider, G. Scaffold architecture and pharmacophoric properties of natural products and trade drugs: Application in the design of natural product-based combinatorial libraries. *J. Comb. Chem.* **2001**, *3*, 284–289. [CrossRef]
19. Chen, Y.; de Bruyn Kops, C.; Kirchmair, J. Data resources for the computer-guided discovery of bioactive natural products. *J. Chem. Inf. Model.* **2017**, *57*, 2099–2111. [CrossRef]
20. Rupp, M.; Schroeter, T.; Steri, R.; Zettl, H.; Proschak, E.; Hansen, K.; Rau, O.; Schwarz, O.; Müller-Kuhrt, L.; Schubert-Zsilavecz, M.; et al. From machine learning to natural product derivatives that selectively activate transcription factor PPARγ. *ChemMedChem* **2010**, *5*, 191–194. [CrossRef]
21. Maindola, P.; Jamal, S.; Grover, A. Cheminformatics based machine learning models for AMA1-RON2 abrogators for inhibiting Plasmodium falciparum erythrocyte invasion. *Mol. Inform.* **2015**, *34*, 655–664. [CrossRef] [PubMed]
22. Chagas-Paula, D.A.; Oliveira, T.B.; Zhang, T.; Edrada-Ebel, R.; Da Costa, F.B. Prediction of anti-inflammatory plants and discovery of their biomarkers by machine learning algorithms and metabolomic studies. *Planta Med.* **2015**, *81*, 450–458. [CrossRef] [PubMed]
23. Reker, D.; Perna, A.M.; Rodrigues, T.; Schneider, P.; Reutlinger, M.; Mönch, B.; Koeberle, A.; Lamers, C.; Gabler, M.; Steinmetz, H.; et al. Revealing the macromolecular targets of complex natural products. *Nat. Chem.* **2014**, *6*, 1072–1078. [CrossRef] [PubMed]
24. Rodrigues, T.; Sieglitz, F.; Somovilla, V.J.; Cal, P.M.S.D.; Galione, A.; Corzana, F.; Bernardes, G.J.L. Unveiling (−)-englerin A as a modulator of L-type calcium channels. *Angew. Chem. Int. Ed. Engl.* **2016**, *55*, 11077–11081. [CrossRef] [PubMed]
25. Merk, D.; Grisoni, F.; Friedrich, L.; Gelzinyte, E.; Schneider, G. Computer-assisted discovery of retinoid X receptor modulating natural products and isofunctional mimetics. *J. Med. Chem.* **2018**, *61*, 5442–5447. [CrossRef] [PubMed]
26. Schneider, P.; Schneider, G. De-orphaning the marine natural product (±)-marinopyrrole A by computational target prediction and biochemical validation. *Chem. Commun.* **2017**, *53*, 2272–2274.
27. Merk, D.; Grisoni, F.; Friedrich, L.; Schneider, G. Tuning artificial intelligence on the de novo design of natural-product-inspired retinoid X receptor modulators. *Commun. Chem.* **2018**, *1*, 68.
28. Friedrich, L.; Rodrigues, T.; Neuhaus, C.S.; Schneider, P.; Schneider, G. From complex natural products to simple synthetic mimetics by computational de novo design. *Angew. Chem. Int. Ed. Engl.* **2016**, *55*, 6789–6792. [CrossRef]
29. Grisoni, F.; Merk, D.; Consonni, V.; Hiss, J.A.; Tagliabue, S.G.; Todeschini, R.; Schneider, G. Scaffold hopping from natural products to synthetic mimetics by holistic molecular similarity. *Commun. Chem.* **2018**, *1*, 44.
30. Ertl, P.; Roggo, S.; Schuffenhauer, A. Natural product-likeness score and its application for prioritization of compound libraries. *J. Chem. Inf. Model.* **2008**, *48*, 68–74. [CrossRef]
31. Jayaseelan, K.V.; Moreno, P.; Truszkowski, A.; Ertl, P.; Steinbeck, C. Natural product-likeness score revisited: An open-source, open-data implementation. *BMC Bioinform.* **2012**, *13*, 106. [CrossRef] [PubMed]
32. Jayaseelan, K.V.; Steinbeck, C. Building blocks for automated elucidation of metabolites: Natural product-likeness for candidate ranking. *BMC Bioinform.* **2014**, *15*, 234. [CrossRef] [PubMed]
33. RDKit NP_Score. Available online: https://github.com/rdkit/rdkit/tree/master/Contrib/NP_Score (accessed on 27 November 2018).

34. Yu, M.J. Natural product-like virtual libraries: Recursive atom-based enumeration. *J. Chem. Inf. Model.* **2011**, *51*, 541–557. [CrossRef] [PubMed]

35. Zaid, H.; Raiyn, J.; Nasser, A.; Saad, B.; Rayan, A. Physicochemical properties of natural based products versus synthetic chemicals. *Open Nutraceuticals J.* **2010**, *3*, 194–202. [CrossRef]

36. Riniker, S.; Landrum, G.A. Similarity maps—A visualization strategy for molecular fingerprints and machine-learning methods. *J. Cheminform.* **2013**, *5*, 43. [CrossRef] [PubMed]

37. RDKit Version 2017.09.3: Open-source cheminformatics software. Available online: http://www.rdkit.org (accessed on 22 May 2018).

38. Stork, C.; Wagner, J.; Friedrich, N.-O.; de Bruyn Kops, C.; Šícho, M.; Kirchmair, J. Hit Dexter: A machine-learning model for the prediction of frequent hitters. *ChemMedChem* **2018**, *13*, 564–571. [CrossRef]

39. MolVs Version 0.1.1. Available online: https://github.com/mcs07/MolVS (accessed on 12 July 2018).

40. Sterling, T.; Irwin, J.J. ZINC 15-Ligand discovery for everyone. *J. Chem. Inf. Model.* **2015**, *55*, 2324–2337. [CrossRef]

41. ZINC "in-stock" subset. ZINC15. Available online: http://zinc15.docking.org/ (accessed on 21 August 2018).

42. *Dictionary of Natural Products*, version 19.1; Chapman & Hall/CRC: London, UK, 2010.

43. Bento, A.P.; Gaulton, A.; Hersey, A.; Bellis, L.J.; Chambers, J.; Davies, M.; Krüger, F.A.; Light, Y.; Mak, L.; McGlinchey, S.; et al. The ChEMBL bioactivity database: An update. *Nucleic Acids Res.* **2014**, *42*, D1083–D1090. [CrossRef]

44. ChEMBL Version 24_1. Available online: https://www.ebi.ac.uk/chembl/ (accessed on 30 July 2018).

45. ChEMBL Version 23. Available online: https://www.ebi.ac.uk/chembl (accessed on 6 June 2017).

46. Natural products subset of ZINC. ZINC15. Available online: http://zinc15.docking.org/substances/subsets/ (accessed on 7 November 2018).

47. *Molecular Operating Environment (MOE)*, version 2016.08; Chemical Computing Group: Montreal, QC, Canada, 2016.

48. Morgan, H.L. The generation of a unique machine description for chemical structures-A technique developed at Chemical Abstracts Service. *J. Chem. Doc.* **1965**, *5*, 107–113. [CrossRef]

49. Rogers, D.; Hahn, M. Extended-connectivity fingerprints. *J. Chem. Inf. Model.* **2010**, *50*, 742–754. [CrossRef]

50. Pedregosa, F.; Varoquaux, G.; Gramfort, A.; Michel, V.; Thirion, B.; Grisel, O.; Blondel, M.; Prettenhofer, P.; Weiss, R.; Dubourg, V.; et al. Scikit-learn: Machine learning in Python. *J. Mach. Learn. Res.* **2011**, *12*, 2825–2830.

51. Scikit-Learn: Machine Learning in Python. version 0.19.1.

52. Natural Product Likeness Calculator Version 2.1. Available online: https://sourceforge.net/projects/np-likeness/ (accessed on 5 October 2018).

53. Natural Products Atlas. Available online: https://www.npatlas.org/ (accessed on 20 August 2018).

54. Gu, J.; Gui, Y.; Chen, L.; Yuan, G.; Lu, H.-Z.; Xu, X. Use of natural products as chemical library for drug discovery and network pharmacology. *PLoS ONE* **2013**, *8*, e62839. [CrossRef]

55. Universal Natural Products Database (UNPD). Available online: http://pkuxxj.pku.edu.cn/UNPD (accessed on 17 October 2016).

56. Chen, C.Y.-C. TCM Database@Taiwan: The world's largest traditional Chinese medicine database for drug screening in silico. *PLoS ONE* **2011**, *6*, e15939. [CrossRef] [PubMed]

57. TCM Database@Taiwan. Available online: http://tcm.cmu.edu.tw (accessed on 17 October 2016).

58. Xue, R.; Fang, Z.; Zhang, M.; Yi, Z.; Wen, C.; Shi, T. TCMID: Traditional Chinese medicine integrative database for herb molecular mechanism analysis. *Nucleic Acids Res.* **2013**, *41*, D1089–D1095. [CrossRef] [PubMed]

59. Traditional Chinese Medicine Integrated Database (TCMID). Available online: www.megabionet.org/tcmid (accessed on 19 October 2016).

60. Lin, Y.-C.; Wang, C.-C.; Chen, I.-S.; Jheng, J.-L.; Li, J.-H.; Tung, C.-W. TIPdb: A database of anticancer, antiplatelet, and antituberculosis phytochemicals from indigenous plants in Taiwan. *Sci. World J.* **2013**, *2013*, 736386. [CrossRef]

61. Tung, C.-W.; Lin, Y.-C.; Chang, H.-S.; Wang, C.-C.; Chen, I.-S.; Jheng, J.-L.; Li, J.-H. TIPdb-3D: The three-dimensional structure database of phytochemicals from Taiwan indigenous plants. *Database* **2014**, *2014*, bau055. [CrossRef] [PubMed]

62. Taiwan Indigenous Plant Database (TIPdb). Available online: http://cwtung.kmu.edu.tw/tipdb (accessed on 19 October 2016).

63. Ambinter. Available online: www.ambinter.com (accessed on 2 June 2017).

64. GreenPharma. Available online: www.greenpharma.com (accessed on 2 June 2017).

65. AnalytiCon Discovery. Available online: www.ac-discovery.com (accessed on 14 November 2017).

66. Ntie-Kang, F.; Telukunta, K.K.; Döring, K.; Simoben, C.V.; A Moumbock, A.F.; Malange, Y.I.; Njume, L.E.; Yong, J.N.; Sippl, W.; Günther, S. NANPDB: A resource for natural products from Northern African sources. *J. Nat. Prod.* **2017**, *80*, 2067–2076. [CrossRef]

67. Northern African Natural Products Database (NANPDB). Available online: www.african-compounds.org/nanpdb (accessed on 5 April 2017).

68. Klementz, D.; Döring, K.; Lucas, X.; Telukunta, K.K.; Erxleben, A.; Deubel, D.; Erber, A.; Santillana, I.; Thomas, O.S.; Bechthold, A.; et al. StreptomeDB 2.0—An extended resource of natural products produced by streptomycetes. *Nucleic Acids Res.* **2015**, *44*, D509–D514. [CrossRef]

69. StreptomeDB. Available online: http://132.230.56.4/streptomedb2/ (accessed on 13 April 2017).

70. Ming, H.; Tiejun, C.; Yanli, W.; Stephen, B.H. Web search and data mining of natural products and their bioactivities in PubChem. *Sci. China Chem.* **2013**, *56*, 1424–1435.

71. Natural products subset. PubChem Substance Database. Available online: http://ncbi.nlm.nih.gov/pcsubstance (accessed on 7 April 2017).

72. Pilon, A.C.; Valli, M.; Dametto, A.C.; Pinto, M.E.F.; Freire, R.T.; Castro-Gamboa, I.; Andricopulo, A.D.; Bolzani, V.S. NuBBE: An updated database to uncover chemical and biological information from Brazilian biodiversity. *Sci. Rep.* **2017**, *7*, 7215. [CrossRef]

73. Núcleo de Bioensaios, Biossíntese e Ecofisiologia de Produtos Naturais (NuBBE). Available online: http://nubbe.iq.unesp.br/portal/nubbedb.html (accessed on 19 April 2017).

74. PI Chemicals. Available online: www.pipharm.com (accessed on 5 May 2017).

75. Choi, H.; Cho, S.Y.; Pak, H.J.; Kim, Y.; Choi, J.-Y.; Lee, Y.J.; Gong, B.H.; Kang, Y.S.; Han, T.; Choi, G.; et al. NPCARE: Database of natural products and fractional extracts for cancer regulation. *J. Cheminform.* **2017**, *9*, 2. [CrossRef] [PubMed]

76. Database of Natural Products for Cancer Gene Regulation (NPCARE). Available online: http://silver.sejong.ac.kr/npcare (accessed on 20 February 2017).

77. Mangal, M.; Sagar, P.; Singh, H.; Raghava, G.P.S.; Agarwal, S.M. NPACT: Naturally Occurring Plant-based Anti-cancer Compound-Activity-Target database. *Nucleic Acids Res.* **2013**, *41*, D1124–D1129. [CrossRef] [PubMed]

78. Naturally Occurring Plant-based Anti-cancer Compound-Activity-Target database (NPACT). Available online: http://crdd.osdd.net/raghava/npact (accessed on 13 April 2017).

79. InterBioScreen. Available online: www.ibscreen.com (accessed on 14 November 2017).

80. Ntie-Kang, F.; Zofou, D.; Babiaka, S.B.; Meudom, R.; Scharfe, M.; Lifongo, L.L.; Mbah, J.A.; Mbaze, L.M.; Sippl, W.; Efange, S.M.N. AfroDb: A select highly potent and diverse natural product library from African medicinal plants. *PLoS ONE* **2013**, *8*, e78085. [CrossRef] [PubMed]

81. AfroDb. Available online: http://african-compounds.org/about/afrodb (accessed on 18 October 2016).

82. TargetMol. Available online: www.targetmol.com (accessed on 17 May 2017).

83. Kang, H.; Tang, K.; Liu, Q.; Sun, Y.; Huang, Q.; Zhu, R.; Gao, J.; Zhang, D.; Huang, C.; Cao, Z. HIM-herbal ingredients in-vivo metabolism database. *J. Cheminform.* **2013**, *5*, 28. [CrossRef] [PubMed]

84. Herbal Ingredients In-Vivo Metabolism database (HIM). Available online: http://binfo.shmtu.edu.cn:8080/him (accessed on 13 April 2017).

85. Hatherley, R.; Brown, D.K.; Musyoka, T.M.; Penkler, D.L.; Faya, N.; Lobb, K.A.; Tastan Bishop, Ö. SANCDB: A South African natural compound database. *J. Cheminform.* **2015**, *7*, 29. [CrossRef] [PubMed]

86. South African Natural Compound Database (SANCDB). Available online: http://sancdb.rubi.ru.ac.za (accessed on 8 February 2017).

87. UEFS Natural Products Catalog. ZINC15. Available online: http://zinc15.docking.org (accessed on 26 May 2017).

88. Ntie-Kang, F.; Amoa Onguéné, P.; Fotso, G.W.; Andrae-Marobela, K.; Bezabih, M.; Ndom, J.C.; Ngadjui, B.T.; Ogundaini, A.O.; Abegaz, B.M.; Meva'a, L.M. Virtualizing the p-ANAPL library: A step towards drug discovery from African medicinal plants. *PLoS ONE* **2014**, *9*, e90655. [CrossRef]

89. Natural Products Set IV of the Developmental Therapeutic Program of the National Cancer Institute/National Institutes of Health. Available online: http://dtp.cancer.gov/organization/dscb/obtaining/available_plates.htm (accessed on 20 October 2016).

90. Ye, H.; Ye, L.; Kang, H.; Zhang, D.; Tao, L.; Tang, K.; Liu, X.; Zhu, R.; Liu, Q.; Chen, Y.Z.; et al. HIT: Linking herbal active ingredients to targets. *Nucleic Acids Res.* **2011**, *39*, D1055–D1059. [CrossRef]

91. Herbal Ingredients' Targets database (HIT). Available online: http://lifecenter.sgst.cn/hit (accessed on 13 April 2017).

92. Ntie-Kang, F.; Nwodo, J.N.; Ibezim, A.; Simoben, C.V.; Karaman, B.; Ngwa, V.F.; Sippl, W.; Adikwu, M.U.; Mbaze, L.M. Molecular modeling of potential anticancer agents from African medicinal plants. *J. Chem. Inf. Model.* **2014**, *54*, 2433–2450. [CrossRef]

93. AfroCancer. Available online: http://african-compounds.org/about/afrocancer (accessed on 10 February 2017).

94. Onguéné, P.A.; Ntie-Kang, F.; Mbah, J.A.; Lifongo, L.L.; Ndom, J.C.; Sippl, W.; Mbaze, L.M. The potential of anti-malarial compounds derived from African medicinal plants, part III: An *in silico* evaluation of drug metabolism and pharmacokinetics profiling. *Org. Med. Chem. Lett.* **2014**, *4*, 6. [CrossRef]

95. AfroMalariaDB. Available online: http://african-compounds.org/about/afromalariadb (accessed on 10 February 2017).

96. Natural products subset of AK Scientific. AK Scientific. Available online: www.aksci.com (accessed on 19 April 2017).

97. Natural products of Selleck Chemicals. Selleck Chemicals. Available online: www.selleckchem.com (accessed on 14 November 2017).

98. Breiman, L. Random forests. *Machine Learning* **2001**, *45*, 5–32. [CrossRef]

99. Matthews, B.W. Comparison of the predicted and observed secondary structure of T4 phage lysozyme. *Biochim. Biophys. Acta* **1975**, *405*, 442–451. [CrossRef]

100. Schomburg, K.; Ehrlich, H.-C.; Stierand, K.; Rarey, M. From structure diagrams to visual chemical patterns. *J. Chem. Inf. Model.* **2010**, *50*, 1529–1535. [CrossRef] [PubMed]

101. SMARTSview. Available online: http://smartsview.zbh.uni-hamburg.de/ (accessed on 30 November 2018).

102. Bienfait, B.; Ertl, P. JSME: A free molecule editor in JavaScript. *J. Cheminform.* **2013**, *5*, 24. [CrossRef] [PubMed]

13

Terpene Derivatives as a Potential Agent against Antimicrobial Resistance (AMR) Pathogens

Nik Amirah Mahizan [1], Shun-Kai Yang [1], Chew-Li Moo [1], Adelene Ai-Lian Song [2],
Chou-Min Chong [3], Chun-Wie Chong [4], Aisha Abushelaibi [5], Swee-Hua Erin Lim [5]
and Kok-Song Lai [1,5,*]

[1] Department of Cell and Molecular Biology, Faculty of Biotechnology and Biomolecular Sciences, Universiti Putra Malaysia, 43400 Serdang, Selangor, Malaysia
[2] Department of Microbiology, Faculty of Biotechnology and Biomolecular Sciences, Universiti Putra Malaysia, 43400 Serdang, Selangor, Malaysia
[3] Department of Aquaculture, Faculty of Agriculture, Universiti Putra Malaysia, 43400 Serdang, Selangor, Malaysia
[4] School of Pharmacy, Monash University Malaysia, Jalan Lagoon Selatan, Bandar Sunway 47500, Selangor, Malaysia
[5] Health Sciences Division, Abu Dhabi Women's College, Higher Colleges of Technology, 41012 Abu Dhabi, UAE
* Correspondence: laikoksong@upm.edu.my;

Academic Editor: Pinarosa Avato

Abstract: The evolution of antimicrobial resistance (AMR) in pathogens has prompted extensive research to find alternative therapeutics. Plants rich with natural secondary metabolites are one of the go-to reservoirs for discovery of potential resources to alleviate this problem. Terpenes and their derivatives comprising of hydrocarbons, are usually found in essential oils (EOs). They have been reported to have potent antimicrobial activity, exhibiting bacteriostatic and bactericidal effects against tested pathogens. This brief review discusses the activity of terpenes and derivatives against pathogenic bacteria, describing the potential of the activity against AMR followed by the possible mechanism exerted by each terpene class. Finally, ongoing research and possible improvisation to the usage of terpenes and terpenoids in therapeutic practice against AMR are discussed.

Keywords: terpenes; terpenoids; antimicrobial resistance; synergy

1. Introduction

The increase of antimicrobial resistance (AMR) in microbiological pathogens has spurred a global mandate to identify potentially effective alternatives [1]. AMR is defined as inefficacious infection-associated treatment with an antimicrobial agent that used to be effective [2]. The rise of AMR is contributed by both intrinsic and extrinsic factors. For instance, evolution of intrinsic factors in microbes include development of structural attributes [3] such as microbial biofilm production [4], and insertion of transposons [5]. On the other hand, extrinsic contributing factors include excessive antibiotic usage resulting from non-judicious prescribing practices, fueled by increased competition in the production and marketing of antimicrobials within the pharmaceutical industry [6]. As a whole there is also inadequate public education, in tandem with a lack of consistent regulatory systems in place. Both of these, coupled with improper infection control in healthcare, poor sanitation, and water hygiene in low-middle income countries (LMIC), are expanding the AMR challenge [1,7].

Laxminarayan et al. [7] reported that the antibiotic usage in growth and disease prevention on veterinary, agriculture, aquaculture, and horticulture are the main contributors in the non-clinical setting. In the clinical settings however, lack of antibiotic stewardship and uncertain diagnoses by physicians add to emerging pathogen resistance. In fact, as far back as in 1959, the potentially adverse consequences related to antibiotic misuse resulting in selection pressure to the development of resistance were observed. Recent genetic mutations in pathogens which were aided by chromosomal genes and inter species gene transmission has resulted in the rise of resistant microbes such as methicillin resistant *Staphylococcus aureus* (MRSA), *Escherichia coli* ST131 and *Klebsiella* ST258; this further contributes to the dissemination of resistant genes such as *Klebsiella pneumoniae* carbapenemase (KPC), NDM-1, and Enterobacteriaceae-producing extended-spectrum β-lactamases (ESBL) [7].

The continuous dissemination of AMR not only contributes to new resistance mechanisms; it will also have a detrimental impact whereby the efficacy of current antibiotics are drastically reduced, leading to therapeutic failure [8]. It is worrisome to note that in 2010, there were almost 1000 resistant cases worldwide associated with β-lactamases, a 10-fold increase since 1990 [9]. Correlation between antibiotic misuse and AMR is clearly evidenced when quinolone misuse caused the revival of MRSA 30 years after it was first introduced in 1962, while carbapenem misconduct via overuse causing resistance in Enterobacteriaceae has significantly increased over the past decade [7]. In addition, loss of function of ampicillin and gentamicin under the World Health Organisation (WHO) recommended dosage in neonatal infection-related pathogens such as *Klebsiella* spp. and *E. coli* was common in the hospitals of developing countries [10]. This was attributed to the high mortality rates of sepsis cases caused by carbapenem-resistant *Enterobacteriaceae* and *Acinetobacter* spp. in neonatal nurseries. It was also noted by Saleem [11] that in Pakistan, common oral antibiotics such as cefixime and ciprofloxacin have become inefficient in Gram-negative pathogens such as *E. coli*, bacteria commonly associated with urinary infection. Barbieri [2] stated in his review that dissemination of AMR inadvertently affected health systems in the community in LMICs due to the escalating cost of accessing necessary therapies and the prolonged duration of illness caused by AMR which increases treatment time.

Bacterial resistance is commonly mediated by transfer of resistance genes [12]. Overall, there are four main ways in which resistance is acquired, firstly, via inactivation of the drug (Figure 1) as reported by Shen [13]. The modification of the antibiotics which occurred based on their target location (bacterial cell wall, cytoplasm, and genome) rendered ineffective to that antibiotic [14]. The second method is the specific modification (Figure 1) at the target such as penicillin-binding protein (PBPs) in MRSA [15]. Similar modifications may arise from mutational or post-translational modifications [3]. Furthermore, porin mutation causes reduction in the number of porins, preventing antibiotic entry and thus increased resistance to antibiotics [16]. Mutations can either be acquired from existing genes (vertical transfer) or new genes can be acquired from other cells (horizontal gene transfer) [17]. Third is the ability of the bacteria to obtain genes for metabolic pathways, these genes then prevent antimicrobial agents from binding to their target. For instance, mobile genes in resistant *Enterococcus* spp. can be disseminated to susceptible strains via horizontal transfer mediated by conjugative plasmids [18]. Finally, the fourth method of bacterial resistance is the reduction of antimicrobial agent intracellularly due to the presence of a bacterial efflux pump. In fact, some resistant bacteria increase impermeability in the cell membrane or increase active efflux, both of which result in reduced drug concentration (Figure 1) in the bacterial cell [19]. The up-regulation in expression of efflux pump has been found to be a major resistance mechanism in many bacteria [20].

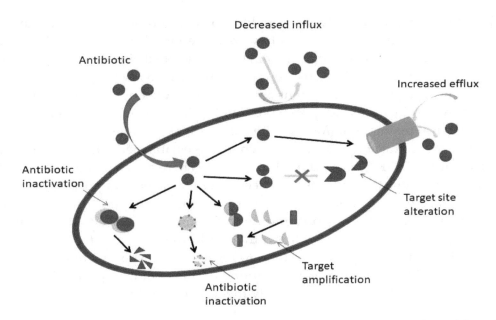

Figure 1. Overall mechanisms of antibiotic resistance in bacteria. Picture adapted from [17].

Strategies to curb the ongoing emergence of AMR require the involvement from various parties. They include policy makers to develop antibiotic regulations, pharmacists and physicians to practice proper antibiotic stewardship, the pharmaceutical industry to invest in new antibiotic discovery, as well as academics to provide adequate public education [7]. Some strategies for control and containment of AMR included extensive surveillance of antimicrobials, especially for antibiotic prescriptions amongst health care providers, avoiding unnecessary use of antimicrobials in the agricultural sectors, limiting drugs advertising, improvising on sanitation, in tandem with continuous research of novel drugs and invention of nanotechnology; these were some of the measures to be implemented [7]. A shift in focus towards alternative therapies targeting AMR mechanisms would also be an important aspect and these include incorporation of antimicrobial peptides (AMPs), phage therapy, metalloantibiotics, lipopolysaccharides, efflux pump inhibitors, and phytochemicals [1].

Antimicrobial agents may comprise of naturally-occurring compounds such as phytochemicals and essential oils (EOs) [21]. They can also be either semi-synthetic or synthetic [22] in nature. Natural secondary metabolites which have a molecular weight ≤500 g/mol may have the ability to act as adjuvants for antimicrobials and exhibit synergy effects [2,23]. Exploration of new antimicrobial agents via biotransformation such as through microbial modification may present an important alternative [24]. Combination therapy of an antimicrobial agent with a low molecular weight natural product, such as terpene derivatives have shown promising effects, with the ability to eliminate fungal and bacterial biofilm production [4]. Terpenes and their derivatives are secondary metabolites which are commonly found in EOs and have been shown to have antimicrobial activities against susceptible and resistant pathogens [25]. Combination therapy between natural compounds and drugs may be able to recover the loss of function for existing antimicrobial agents [26], potentiating the action of drugs. Wagner and Merzenich [27] reported that the potentiation of antimicrobial agents was accomplished via several mechanisms in combinatorial therapy; these provide a multi-targeted pharmacokinetic effect, allowing simultaneous destruction of existing resistance mechanisms in a specific pathogen.

EOs are naturally produced from aromatic plants such as herbs as their secondary metabolites. Usually EOs exist in liquid form, are volatile and exhibit good solubility in lipids and inorganic compounds that are less dense compared to water. They can be extracted from various parts of the plant organ such as flowers, buds, leave, bark, twigs, stem, wood, seed, or root [28] by various methods which include solvent extraction (solvent, supercritical CO_2, subcritical water), distillation (steam, hydrodistillation, hydrodiffusion), solvent-free (microwave) and combination method (solvent + steam) [29]. Generally, plants store their EOs in specific cellular compartments such as in the secretory cells, cavities, or glandular trichomes. EOs primarily function as protection against plant pests and infections [30]. In particular, EOs have been reported to be a prominent antimicrobial, antioxidant, and insecticidal agent, significantly inhibiting microbial biofilm production and the growth of bacteria, yeasts, and molds [31]. Previously our group has also focused on the bacterial membranous disruption effect when subjected to treatment with EOs [32]. A list of reports summarized in Table 1 indicate various antimicrobial activities possessed by EOs. In 2018, our research group demonstrated synergistic activity when peppermint (*Mentha x piperita* L. Carl) essential oil was added to meropenem against resistant *E. coli* [33]. Recently, our research group established a mode of action of EO from cinnamon bark against KPC-KP via oxidative stress [34]. There are challenges involved in working with EOs. They are laborious to handle as they need to be extracted and purified before being tested and manipulated. Furthermore, despite EOs being used for testing, it is difficult to ascertain as to which bioactive component in EOs is contributing to the antimicrobial activity. Acquisition of EOs will also require higher cost as compared to synthetic additives because they need to be processed prior to screening for their activity. One method to resolve the cost issue involves downscaling the volume via extraction of the antimicrobial compounds. This review in particular will focus on one such compound commonly found in EOs, namely the terpenes and their antimicrobial potential and their possible mechanisms of action.

Table 1. Essential oils extracted from plant against tested pathogens.

Plants spp.	Common Name	Pathogens Tested	MIC/Sensitivity/Inhibition Zone	Citation
Eugenia caryophyllata	Clove	*Burkholderia cepacia* complex	ES	[35]
Origanum vulgare	Oregano	*B. cepacia* complex	ES	[35]
Thymus vulgaris	Thyme	*B. cepacia* complex	ES	[35]
Eucalyptus camadulensis	Eucalyptus	*Streptococcus pyogenes*	1 mg mL^{-1}	[36]
		Fusarium oxysporum f. sp. *lycopersici*	15.93% to 72.5%	[37]
Mentha spicata	Spearmint	*S. pyogenes*	2 mg mL^{-1}	[36]
		E. coli	21 mm at 150 µL	[38]
		Salmonella thyphi	13 mm at 150 µL	
		S. aureus	12 mm at 150 µL	
Cymbopogon citratus	Lemongrass	*Acinetobacter baumannii*	0.65% (v/v)	[39]
		F. oxysporum f. sp. *lycopersici*	250 ppm	[37]
Syzygium aromaticum	Clove	*Candida albicans*	360 µg mL^{-1}	[40]
		F. oxysporum f. sp. *lycopersici*	125 ppm	[37]
Pelargonium graveolens	Geranium	*B. cepacia* complex	0.4% (v/v)	[41]
		Prototheca zopfii	3.5 to 4.0 µL mL^{-1}	[42]
Laurus nobilis	Bay laurel	*S. typhimurium*	3 % (v/v)	[43]
		E. coli	1 % (v/v)	[44]
		Candida spp.	250 to 500 µg mL^{-1}	
Melaleuca alternifolia	Tea tree	*Campylobacter* spp.	0.00%	[45]
Leptospermum petersonii	Manuka	*Campylobacter* spp.	0.01%	[45]
Backhousia citriodora	Lemon myrtle	*Campylobacter* spp.	0.01%	[45]
Lavandula angustifolia	Lavender	*S. aureus*	2 mg mL^{-1}	[46]
		Pseudomonas aeruginosa	2 mg mL^{-1}	
		C. albicans	3 mg mL^{-1}	
Mentha x piperita	Peppermint	*Clostridium perfringens Fusarium oxysporum* f. sp. *lycopersici*	10 mg mL^{-1}	[47]
			500 ppm	[37]
Chamaemelum nobile	Roman chamomile	*Porphyromonas gingivalis*	20.5 ± 0.5 mm	[48]
Origanum majorana	Marjoram	*Micrococcus luteus*	0.097 mg mL^{-1}	[49]
		Vibrio alginolyticus	0.39 mg mL^{-1}	
Foeniculum vulgare	Fennel	*Candida* spp.	1.56 to 12.48 mg mL^{-1}	[50]
Pinus sylvestris	Pine	*Pseudomonas* spp.	4.33 ± 0.58 mm	[51]
Cedrus atlantica	Cedarwoood	*E. coli*	0.4 µL mL^{-1}	
		Bacillus subtilis	0.2 µL mL^{-1}	[52]
		Bacillus cereus	0.4 µL mL^{-1}	
Aniba rosaeodora	Rosewood	*Trichophyton mentagrophytes*	0.002 M	[53]

ES: extremely sensitive.

2. Terpenes and Their Derivatives

Terpenes are large hydrocarbon groups that consist of 5-carbon isoprene (C5H8) units as their basic building block. They are synthesized via two pathways which are the non-mevalonate pathway; the Methylerythritol Phosphate (MEP) and the mevalonate pathway from Acetyl CoA precursor. Their backbones can be reorganized into cyclic structure by cyclases. The commonly found terpenes which differ in numbers of isoprene units are the monoterpenes and sesquiterpenes; however longer chains such as diterpenes and triterpenes also exist [47,54]. P-Cymene, limonene, sabinene, terpinene, carene, and pinene are examples belonging to the terpene groups. Most terpenes possess reduced antimicrobial activities [54]. Terpenoids are derivatives of terpenes which takes place when modification of terpenes occur, such as with the addition/removal of functional groups [2]. Therefore, the antimicrobial activity of terpenoids are determined from their functional group [55]. For instance, the shifting or removal of a methyl group and addition of oxygen by a specific enzyme result in derivation of terpenes. The hydroxyl group of the phenolic terpenoids and delocalized electrons are amongst the antimicrobial determining factors. Linalool, menthol, carvacrol, thymol, linalyl acetrate, piperitone, geraniol, and citronella are amongst the best studied terpenoids.

2.1. Bioactive Terpenes and Terpenoids

Terpenoids represent a large group of phytochemicals with promising antimicrobial activity [2]. The chemical diversity of terpenoids have led to discovery of over 40,000 structural varieties, with a few classes serving as pharmaceutical agents, some of which include terpenoid derived indole alkaloids [56]. There are a total of eight different classes of terpenoids (hemiterpenoids, monoterpenoids, sesquiterpenoids, diterpenoids, sesterpenoids, triterpenoids, tetrapenoids, and polyterpenoids) which differ in the number of isoprene (C5H8) units. Recently in 2017, it was reported that 67% of potentiators belong to monoterpenes and sesquiterpenes [4]. Meanwhile, specifically among the discovered potentiators of antibacterial drugs, 75% were terpenes; these include classes of mono-, di-, and tri-terpenes [4].

Although the antibacterial mode of action of terpenes remains largely unknown, Griffin et al. [55] reported in his study that most terpenoids are able to inhibit two crucial processes which are essential to microbial survival, this includes oxygen uptake and oxidative phosphorylation. Aerobic microbes require oxygen in order to yield energy for their growth. Previously, it was proven that low oxygen concentrations caused limitation in bacterial respiration rates [57]. Meanwhile, oxidative phosphorylation is a crucial biochemical process responsible for cellular respiration that takes place in the cytoplasmic membrane. Thus, terpene interaction leads to alteration in cellular respiration which later causes uncoupling of oxidative phosphorylation in the microbe [58]. Additionally, carbonylation of terpenoids was believed to increase bacteriostatic activity but not necessarily the bactericidal activity. A bacteriostatic agent is an agent that stops or inhibits microbial growth, while a bactericidal is responsible for killing the microbe. Terpenoids have also been found to exhibit antiseptic potential according to their solubility in water. Lipophilicity and/or hydrophobicity and presence of hydroxyl groups in the terpenes are amongst the determining elements of their antibacterial action [58]. In skin barrier-associated treatment, terpenes have also been reported to affect the lipid membrane activity by interacting with lipophilic tails of intermembrane lipid and polar head groups which, at the end, affects the lipodial intermembrane and polar transmembrane pathways [59].

2.1.1. Monoterpenes and Monoterpenoids

Monoterpenes comprise of two isoprene units and exist in many plants. It has been reported by Griffin et al. [55] that monotepenes possess antimicrobial activity. For instance, carvacrol, thymol, menthol, and geraniol were able to work against Gram-positive and Gram-negative bacteria. Geraniol was also later claimed to efficiently increase the susceptibility of the Gram-negative multi-drug resistant (MDR) *Enterobacter aerogenes* by becoming a potent efflux pump inhibitor [60]. Trombetta et al. [61]

claimed in his study that three monoterpenes linalyl acetate, (+) menthol and thymol showed positive responses against *S. aureus* and *E. coli*. Other compounds such as carvacrol, trans-cinnamaldehyde and (+)-carvone were reported to possess potent inhibitory activity against *E. coli* and *S. typhimurium* [30]. In addition, other types of monoterpenes such as halogenated monoterpenes recorded good cytotoxic, antimalarial, and antialgal effects while monocyclic monoterpenes had been reported to exhibit potent insecticidal, as well as antifungal effects [62].

In fact, in as early as 1979, Kurita et al. [63] had listed a total of 13 monoterpenes ((+)-terpinen-4-ol, γ-terpinene, α-terpinene, terpinolene, α-pinene 1,8-cineole, ρ-cymene, (+)-limonene, β-myrcene, (+)-β-pinene, (±)-linalool, α-phellandrene, α-terpinoel) which exhibited antifungal properties against 14 fungal strains. The phenolic monoterpenes such as carvacrol, eugenol and thymol were found to be highly active against bacteria [64]. There were twenty one monoterpenes (borneol, d-3-carene, carvacrol, carvacrol methyl ester, *cis/trans* citral, eugenol, geraniol, Geranyl acetate, *cis*-hex-3-en-1-ol, R(+)limonene, (2)-linalool, menthone, nerol, α-pinene, β-pinene, (+)sabinene, α-terpinene, terpinen-4-ol, α-terpineole, (−)-thujone, thymol) which were previously reported regarding their antimicrobial activity against 25 bacterial strains [65]. Phenol monoterpenes, such as carvacrol were also reported to inhibit biofilm development of *S.aureus* and *S. typhimurium* [66]. Recently, our research group found one monoterpene compound, linalool, extracted from lavender essential oil which exhibited strong antimicrobial activity against resistant *K. pneumoniae* [34]. The proposed mechanism of action for the compound was membrane disruption [34].

Monoterpene ketones were also found to exhibit antimicrobial properties [67]. In comparison, alcoholic monoterpenes are more bactericidal agents rather than bacteriostatic agents. In line with this, Bhatti et al. [67] reported that monoterpenes alcohol of terpinen-4-ol, α-terpineol, 1, 8-cineole and linalool exhibited good antifungal activity and suggested alcohol moieties as determinants of antifungal activity. In addition, myrcene, one of the acyclic monoterpene alcohols showed a negative response against fungal specimens; this infers that the cyclic structure of monoterpenes may also be the structure responsible for this activity [68]. Monoterpenes consisting of aldehydes, however, possessed a potent antimicrobial activity which can be explained through its carbon double bond arrangements; this creates high electronegativity. The observations of nine monoterpenes (α-terpinene, γ-terpinene, α-pinene, ρ-cymene, terpinen-4-ol, α-terpineol, thymol, citral and 1, 8-cineole) against *Herpes simplex virus* type 1 (HSV-1) were made by Thompson in 1989. Later in 2010, Dunkic et al. [69] listed a few more monoterpenes having considerable activity against HSV-1 which are borneol, bornyl acetate, and isoborneol, 1, 8-cineole, thujone, and camphor. Thymol and carvacrol were also noted to be powerful agents against the *Tobacco mosaic virus* (TMV) and *Cucumber mosaic virus* (CMV) [70].

2.1.2. Sesquiterpenes and Sesquiterpenoids

It has been long recognized that sesquiterpenes possess antimicrobial activites [55]. Back in 2011, Torres-Romero et al. [71] identified one of dihydro-β agarofuran sesquiterpenes, namely 1α-acetoxy-6β, 9β-dibenzoyloxy-dihydro-β-agarofuran inhibits the growth of *Bacillus* spp. [71]. Farnesol, which is an isoprenoid natural acyclic sesquiterpene alcohol showed moderate effects against *Streptococcus mutans* and *Streptococcus sobrinus* biofilm formation [72]. Farnesol also showed antibacterial activity against *S. aureus* and *S. epidermidis* whereby it inhibited the biofilm development [73]. Two studies conducted by Masako [74] evidenced that combinations of farnesol with xylitol have positive effects against atopic dermatitis caused by *S. aureus* without altering the microbial flora and successfully inhibited the biofilm production of *S. aureus*. Sesquiterpenes were also incorporated in the combination therapy using existing drugs.

A recent study conducted by Castelo-Branco et al. [75] showed potentiation effects of a combination therapy of farnesol with amoxicillin, doxycycline, ceftazidime, and sulfamethoxazole-trimethoprim against *B. pseudomallei*. A phenol sesquiterpene, xanthorrhizol was found to reduce 60% of *Staphylococcus mutans* cell adherence ability [76], and inhibited the growth of *Mycobacterium smegmatis* [77]. Recently, it was discovered that sesquiterpenes have potent antibiotic enhancement against MRSA and also

Gram-negative bacteria [4]. In 2011, Gonçalves et al. [78] reported a significantly larger inhibition zone when sesquiterpenes were incorporated into antibiotic discs. The experiment was conducted against MDR strains of *S. aureus* with a combination of sets of available antibiotics such as tetracycline, erythromycin, penicillin, and vancomycin.

2.1.3. Diterpenes and Diterpenoids

Diterpene is a class of terpene with broad biological activities [79]. Previously, 60 terpenoids have been tested for their minimum inhibitory concentration (MIC) against *P. aeruginosa, E. coli, S. aureus*, and *C. albicans* [55]. They were then classified into five groups to determine their activity patterns. Hydrogen bond was found to be the factor that determines the positive antimicrobial activity. On the other hand, low water solubility was discovered to be the factor of antimicrobial inactivity. Griffin [55] suggested that inhibition of microbial oxygen uptake and oxidative phosphorylation are likely mechanisms of action responsible for the antimicrobial properties of the diterpene class. Separately, diterpene derivatives such as ent-kaurane and ent-pimarane are able to inhibit growth of the dental caries pathogens. The MIC value of 2–10 mg/mL confirmed the antibacterial potential of the compounds [80]. Additionally, the diterpenoid salvipisone prevented cell adherence and biofilm developments of *S. aureus* and *S. epidermidis* [81].

Besides sesquiterpenes, diterpenes also function as a good antibiotic enhancer against MRSA. Moreover, diterpenes have been widely used in combination therapy with antibiotics [82]. For instance, clerodane diterpenoid 16αhydroxycleroda-3, 13 (14)-Z-dien-15, 16-olide (CD) extracted from leaves of *Polyathia longifolia* enhanced the efficacy of oxacillin, tetracycline, daptomycin, and linezolid against clinical isolates of MRSA. All MICs of the antibiotic dropped significantly between 10–80, 4–16, 2–8 and 2–4-folds respectively when combined with CD. Gupta et al. [82] then proposed the in vivo mechanism of CD in reversing the resistance of clinical isolates of MRSA. The same clinical MRSA isolates were tested with CD combined with norfloxacin, ciprofloxacin, and ofloxacin. qRT-PCR analysis showed that the expression of genes coding for efflux pumps were significantly modulated in cells treated with CD alone and in combination with antimicrobial drugs. In fact, the results of time-kill assay showed the MIC in combination of CD with norfloxacin was half of the MIC of CD and norfloxacin alone, undoubtedly decreasing the viability of bacterial cells. Unfortunately, despite the promising effects offered by CD, sourcing to obtain CD became the bottleneck for further testing [4].

Salvipisone and aethiopinone are diterpenoids isolated from roots of *Salvia sclarea* [81]. They were shown to express antibacterial and antibiofilm activities against *S. aureus, Enterococcus faecalis* and *S. epidermidis*. Both salvipisone and aethiopinone were also tested for their synergistic activity when combined with antimicrobial drugs alongside oxacillin, vancomycin, and linezolid against MRSA and Methicillin resistant *Staphylococcus epidermidis* (MRSE). It was discovered that they were either bactericidal or bacteriostatic against planktonic cultures of tested MRSA and MRSE [83]. Remarkably, the MIC was achieved with 50% reduction in the dose of antibiotic when diterpenoids were used in combination.

2.1.4. Triterpenes and Triterpenoids

Triterpenes comprises of six isoprene units. It was reported that *Pandanaceae* containing triterpenes in the form of 24, 24-dimethyl-5β-tirucall-9 [11], 25-dien-3-one showed promising activities against tubercular strains. Another triterpene, Oleanic acid (OA) is potent against pathogens such as *Mycobacterium tuberculosis*. OA also had promising synergy against MDR when combined with rifampicin, isoniazide, and ethambutol with significant MIC reduction of 128–16 fold, 32–4 fold, and from 128 to 16 fold, respectively [2].

Besides OA, bonianic acid A and B are two triterpenoids that were extracted from *Radermachera boniana*. Both compounds were found to be active against *M. tuberculosis*. There are at least six known molecules which include OA, ergosterol peroxide, and ursolic acid (UA). In fact, the combination of both ergosterol peroxide and UA showed synergistic activity against *M. tuberculosis* [84]. The reports conducted by Cunha et al. [85] depicted that OA and UA that were isolated from *Miconia ligustroides*, resulted in significant antibacterial activity when tested on selected bacteria (*B. cereus, Vibrio cholerae, S. choleraesuis, K. pneumoniae and S. pneumoniae*). When UA was used against *B. cereus*, the MIC value was 20 µg/mL and OA showed MIC value of 80 µg/mL against *B. cereus* and *S. pneumoniae*. In 2013, a study conducted by Zhou et al. [86] showed that UA and OA were active against planktonic cariogenic microorganism and their biofilm. Later in 2015, Liu et al. [31] expanded the research and reported the combinatory effects of UA and xylitol against biofilm produced by *S. mutans and S. sobrinus*. Moreover, OA and UA were reported to enhance antimicrobial activity against *Listeria monocytogenes* without affecting toxin secretion; this influenced the virulence factors of *L. monocytogenes* and inhibited the capacity of biofilm production from these bacteria [45].

OA also exhibited strong interactions alongside aminoglycoside (gentamicin and kanamycin) against *A. baumanii*, but not with other classes of which ampicillin, norfloxacin, chloramphenicol, tetracycline, and rifampicin are examples [4]. Based on time-kill assay, the bactericidal effects of gentamicin were significantly greater when combined with OA compared to gentamicin alone [4]. Three triterpenoids, amyrin, betulinic acid, and betulinaldehyde were extracted from the bark of *Callicarpa farinose* Roxb (Verbenaceae) and were shown to exhibit potent antimicrobial activity against clinical methicillin-resistant (MRSA) and methicillin-susceptible (MSSA) with MICs ranging from 2 to 512 µg/mL [87].

While there is no firm report specifically on modes of action by terpenoids, the mechanisms of action of phytochemicals found in nature have been proposed. Typically, phytochemicals aim either for disruption of the bacterial cell membranes, modulation of bacterial efflux pump, suppression of bacterial biofilm development or inhibition of some virulence factors which include enzymes and toxins [2]. For instance, carvacrol was found to be responsible for sub-lethal injury to bacterial cells due to alteration of fatty acid compositions, while other reports state that carvacrol and thymol caused disintegration of the outer membrane and disruption of the cytoplasmic membrane of Gram-negative bacteria [30]. Antimicrobial activity effects of some terpenoids are summarized in Table 2 while the postulated mode of action of terpenes on antibiotic resistance pathogens and as combination therapies are depicted in Figure 2.

Table 2. Summary of antimicrobial activity effects of some terpenoid class.

Terpenoids Class	Chemical Compounds	Tested Microorganism	Antimicrobial Effect	Reference
Monoterpenes and monoterpenoids	Carvacrol Thymol Geraniol	Resistant *Enterobacter aerogenes*	Efflux pump inhibition	[60]
	Linalyl acetate (+)- Menthol Thymol	*S. aureus* *E. coli*	Growth inhibition	[61]
	Carvacrol Trans-cinnamaldehyde (+)-Carvone	*E. coli* *S. typhimurium*	Growth inhibition	[30]
	(+)-Terpinen-4-ol γ-Terpinene α-Terpinene Terpinolene α-Pinene 1,8-Cineole ρ-Cymene (+)-Limonene β-Myrcene (+)-β-Pinene (±)-Linalool α-Phellandrene α-Terpinoel	*T. mentagrophytes* *Trichophyton violaceum* *Microsporium gypseum* *Histoplasma capsulatum* *Blastomyces dermatitidis* ... etc.	Growth inhibition	[63]

Table 2. *Cont.*

Terpenoids Class	Chemical Compounds	Tested Microorganism	Antimicrobial Effect	Reference
	Carvacrol Eugenol Thymol	*Acinetobacter calcoacetica Aeromonas hydrophila B. subtilis*	Growth inhibition	[64]
	Borneol d-3-Carene Carvacrol Carvacrol methyl ester *cis/trans* Citral Eugenol Geraniol Geranyl acetate *cis*-hex-3-en-1-ol R(+)Limonene (2)-Linalool Menthone Nerol α-Pinene β-Pinene (+)sabinene α-Terpinene Terpinen-4-ol α-terpineole (−)-Thujone Thymol	*S. aureus E. coli Salmonella typhia S. typhimurium Salmonella enteritidis A. hydrophila Yersinia* sp. *Vibrio anguillarum Shigella* sp. *Vibrio parahaemolyticus C. albicans Penicillium expansum Aspergillus niger . . .* etc.	Growth inhibition	[65]
	Carvacrol	*S.aureus S. typhimurium*	Biofilm inhibition	[66]
	Linalool	Resistant *K. pneumoniae carbapenemase* (KPC)	Cell membrane disruption	[34]
	Terpinen-4-ol α-Terpineol 1, 8-Cineole Linalool	*A. niger Botrytis cinerea*	Growth inhibition	[67]
	α-Terpinene γ-Terpinene α-Pinene ρ-Cymene Terpinen-4-ol α-Terpineol Thymol Citral 1, 8-Cineole Borneol Bornyl acetate Isoborneol 1, 8-Cineole Thujone Camphor	*Herpes simplex virus* type 1 (HSV-1)	Growth inhibition	[69]

Table 2. *Cont.*

Terpenoids Class	Chemical Compounds	Tested Microorganism	Antimicrobial Effect	Reference
	Thymol Carvacrol	*Tobacco mosaic virus* (TMV) *Cucumber mosaic virus* (CMV)	Growth inhibition	[70]
Sesquiterpenes and Sesquiterpenoids	1α-Acetoxy-6β, 9β-dibenzoyloxy-dihydro-β-agarofuran	*Bacillus* spp.	Growth inhibition	[71]
	Farnesol	*Streptococcus mutans* *Streptococcus sobrinus*	Biofilm formation inhibition	[72]
		S. aureus *S. epidermidis*		[73] [74]
		B. pseudomallei	Potentiation effect—combination therapy	[75]
	Xanthorrhizol	*Staphylococcus mutans*	Reduction of cell adherence ability	[76]
		Mycobacterium smegmatis	Growth inhibition	[77]
Diterpenes and diterpenoids	(-)-Carvone Thymol Dihydrocarveol (-)-Perilla alcohol Carvacrol (-)-Carveol ... etc.	*P. aeruginosa* *E. coli* *S. aureus* *C. albicans*	Growth inhibition	[55]
	Ent-kaurane Ent-pimarane	Dental carries pathogens	Growth inhibition	[80]
	Salvipisone	*S. aureus* *S. epidermidis*	Bacterial cell adherence prevention Biofilm development inhibition	[81]
	16αHydroxycleroda-3, 13 (14)-Z-dien-15, 16-olide (CD)	MRSA	Antibiotic potentiation Efflux pump modulation	[82]
	Salvipisone Aethiopinone	*S. aureus* *Enterococcus faecalis* *S. epidermidis*	Biofilm production inhibition	[81]
		MRSA MRSE	Synergistic activity alongside antibiotic	[83]

Table 2. *Cont.*

Terpenoids Class	Chemical Compounds	Tested Microorganism	Antimicrobial Effect	Reference
Triterpenes and triterpenoids	24, 24-Dimethyl-5β-tirucall-9	Tubercular strains	Growth inhibition	[11]
	25-Dien-3-one Oleanic acid (OA) Bonianic acid A Bonianic acid B	*Mycobacterium tuberculosis*	Synergistic activity alongside antibiotic	[2]
	OA Ergosterol peroxide Ursolic acid (UA)		Synergistic activity—combination therapy	
	OA UA	*B. cereus* Vibrio cholerae S. choleraesuis K. pneumoniae S. pneumoniae	Growth inhibition	[85]
		Planktonic cariogenic microorganism S. mutans S. sobrinus	Biofilm inhibition	[86] [31]
		Listeria monocytogenes		[45]
	OA	*A. baumanii*	Antibiotic potentiation	[4]
	Amyrin Betulinic acid Betulinaldehyde	MRSA MMSA	Growth inhibition	[87]

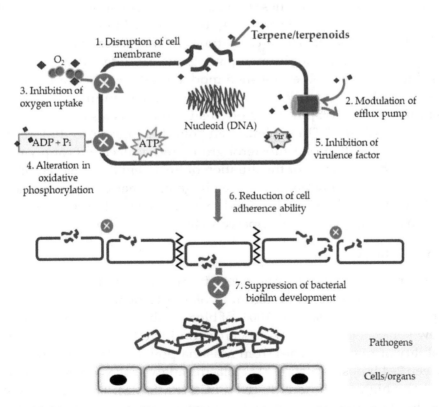

Figure 2. Postulated mode of action of terpene/terpenoids on antibiotic resistance pathogens and as combination therapies.

2.2. Therapeutic Implementation

2.2.1. Drugs and Antibiotics

Combination therapy with terpenes have been widely seen in current therapeutic practice especially in antifungal drugs [26]. It was shown that fluconazole which had once lost its efficacy, had been potentiated by monoterpenes, thymol, and carvacrol when subjected against 38 fluconazole-sensitive *C. albicans*, *C. tropicalis*, and *C. glabrata* and 11 fluconazole-resistant *C. albicans*, *C. krusei*, *C. glabrata*, *C. tropicalis*, and *C. parapsilopsis*. The combination analysis showed that of the strains tested, 32 out of 38 strains and eight out of 10 strains have obtained a Fractional Inhibitory Concentration (FIC) index of less than 0.5 [88]. FIC is a term used to express the degree of synergy interaction between antibacterial drugs whereby FIC < 0.5 shows positive synergism while FIC > 0.5 shows negative synergism [89]. The sequiterpene, farnesol, also showed potentiation activity with fluconazole against candidiasis [88]. Previously, it was reported that three diterpene compounds, ent-clerodanes (bacchotricuneatin, bacrispine and hawtriwaic acid) which were isolated from *Baccharis* extract synergistically reduced the dose of the anti-fungal drug Terbinafine against *Trichophyton rubrum* [90]. Another triterpene, retigeric acid, found in the lichenized fungi family, Lobariaceae exhibited strong potentiation when combined with either fluconazole, itraconazole or ketoconazole against azole-resistant *C. albicans* strains [91]. It was proposed that facilitation of azole uptake or membranous repair associated with azoles were the modes of action of retigeric acid.

Prior to the development of novel drugs, in vitro and in vivo testing are usually performed to ascertain the safety and efficacy of the compound to better understand the physiological effects. Despite a number of published in vitro reports pertaining to terpenes antimicrobial testing, incorporation of various terpenes in clinical trials focusing on antimicrobial activity is still lacking due to insufficient data on the in vivo system. Most in vivo testing for terpenes and its derivatives has been conducted for human health associated with anti-inflammatory, anti-tumorigenic, anti-cancer, transdermal delivery medium and neuroprotective [92] aspects. However, incorporation of terpenes into household products and cosmetics due to antibacterial properties showed increasing assurance in vivo, inhibiting multiple species of bacteria [93]. In 2006, Mondello et al. [94] demonstrated in vivo activity of the monoterpene terpinen-4-ol which is the main bioactive constituent of *Malaleuca alternifolia* Cheel (tea tree) oil against azole-susceptible and resistant human pathogenic candida species. In this demonstration, terpinen-4-ol was able to clear a well-established model of rat vaginal candidiasis. Terpenes which were found in *Cassia occidentalis* and *Phyllanthus niruri* showed antimalarial activity in vivo using mice against *Plasmodium berghei* [95]. In addition, β-sitosterol was tested in the treatment of culture proven pulmonary tuberculosis (PTB) patients using blinded randomized placebo-controlled trials. Two groups of patients consisting of a sitosterol group and a placebo group were set up upon the treatment. Patients were hospitalized for the duration of treatment and checked monthly with regards to sputum culture positivity, chest radiography, weight gain, hematology, liver function, and Mantoux test response. At the end of trials, it was reported that the sitosterol group marked a greater weight gain, lymphocyte and eosinophils count compared to the other group [96].

2.2.2. Terpenes Bioavailability

In order to ensure greater therapeutic effect from drugs, terpene bioavailability should be determined. It was reported that while natural volatile terpenes from 1,8-cineole of uncrushed capsule from the plasma yielded relatively 100% of bioavailability, limomene and α-pinene were only detectable for a few subjects [97]. In 2017, research conducted by Papada et al. [98] demonstrated positive bioavailability of major terpenes from Mastiha powder after 30 min of ingestion with the highest peak between 2–4 h post ingestion. The plasma analysis was done using ultra-high-pressure liquid chromatography high-resolution MS (UHPLC-HRMS/MS). The bioavailability bottleneck of medicinal herbs including terpenes, however, had been improved ever since phytosome technology arrival. It was reported that the bioavailability of *Ginkgo biloba* extract (GBE) which constitutes of the terpene, lactone, was improved significantly with 2–4 times greater plasma concentration compared to a non-phytosome delivery method [99].

2.2.3. Evaluation of Compounds Interaction in Combination Therapies

Combination therapies using natural products such as the terpenoids may synergistically, additively, or antagonistically affect the treatments. Zacchino et al. [4] reported in a review that the nature of interaction between phytochemical and antimicrobial drugs can be determined using the median-effect method of Chou [89] which permits the calculation of combination index (CI). As for combination therapy, both agents at a fixed ratio will result in IC_{50} respectively; these are mixed with two-fold dilutions of both agents with a fixed ratio. The CI will resolve synergistic (CI < 1), additive (CI = 1) and antagonistic effects (CI > 1). In addition, another method that contributed significantly in synergistic activity was to calculate the Dose Reduction Index (DRI), also known as the reversal enhancement ratio, that measures how many folds the dose of antimicrobial drugs may be cut down when used in combination rather than alone. One of the measures that can be used to evaluate synergism is through checkerboard assay.

In our previous study, through this method, peppermint essential oil was proven to synergistically react with meropenem. MIC of individual peppermint oil and meropenem were 8% and 4 µg/mL respectively. Meanwhile when used in combination, the MIC of peppermint oil and meropenem were reduced to 1% and 0.5 µg/mL respectively. The CI value of 0.26 obtained in checkerboard assay had portrayed a high synergism. Last year, our group carried out extensive analysis to investigate the additive interaction of cinnamon bark oil and meropenem. The shift of attention towards synergism between compounds and antibiotics have caused researchers to overlook the additive effects, thus we conducted the study to understand additive interaction which focused on the effect on the bacterial membrane [100].

2.2.4. Methods for Antimicrobial Evaluation

Both in vitro and in vivo experimental systems can be used to evaluate the antimicrobial activity of either synthetic compounds or naturally-acquired compounds. Nevertheless, in vitro approaches have been more commonly used due to their feasibility. In vivo studies, however, are seldom applied due to limitations in detecting the actual mechanism of action. Susceptibility testing which determines the MIC of a compound against bacteria is routinely done using variations in the methods of MIC assay such as rapid p-Iodonitrotetrazolium chloride (INT) colorimetric assay, micro- or macro-dilution and disc diffusion methods. However, Griffin et al. [55] stated in his study that the disc diffusion method is prone to problems as the method was highly dependent on water solubility and suitability of the test agent to be diffused through the agar. In combination therapy, however, the effects are assessed through the checkerboard assay which investigated the interaction between agents. The checkerboard antibiofilm microsomal triglyceride transfer protein (MTP) assay through which the checkerboard microdilution was seeded with biofilm have also been used in an experiment associated with biofilm producing bacteria [88]. By performing the checkerboard assay, an important index called the FIC will reveal the potential of an individual compound [4]. The Dose Reduction Index (DRI) [89] can also be conducted in a compound combination analysis in order to find out the dosage reductions ruled out by individual compounds that affected the MIC of the second compound. A greater DRI disclosed better adjuvant capabilities for a given effect level [89]. More extensively, further analysis usually includes isobolograms and time-kill studies.

3. Perspectives

3.1. Ongoing Research

Effective management and treatment of microbial resistance are among the main priorities in healthcare. Terpene derivatives are an important and promising source of novel antibiotics. Indeed, ent-kaurenoids (ent-kaur-15-en-18, 20-diol and ent-kaur-15-en-18-ol) extracted from *Senegalia nigrescens* are among the novel terpene derivatives discovered recently. Both in vitro and in silico anti-quorum sensing evaluation have demonstrated potential anti-quorum sensing against *Chromobacterium violaceum* [101]. In addition, it was reported that antiquorum sensing does not contribute towards evolution of MDR pathogens as there is no enforcement of selection pressure [32]. Additionally, terpenoids found in microbial volatile compounds (MVCs) have exhibited the ability to combat and modulate antibiotic resistance in human and animal pathogens [102].

With the success of terpenoids in the treatment of microbial resistance, the hunt for new terpenoids has been an important quest amongst the scientific community as a potential application. For instance, screening for terpenoids was conducted on semi-arid plants such as *Caesalpinia pulcherrima*, *Lawsonia inermis*, *Pithecellobium dulce*, *Euphorbia tithymaloides*, *Punica granatum*, *Plumeria obtusa*, *Carica papaya*, *Cassia fistula*, *Cordia dichotoma*, *Euphorbia prostrate*, *Nerium oleander*, and *Cyanthillium cinereum* [103]. A separate study conducted in 2018 identified three terpenoid derivatives (α-pinene—45.44%, 3-carene—38.34%, and terpinolene—5.36%) of *Cupressus torulosa* essential oil. The compounds are effective against pathogens including *B.subtilis*, *Pseudomonas alcaligenes*, *M. luteus*, and *B. cereus* [104]. This can mitigate AMR problems by manipulating combinatory therapeutics of existing antimicrobial agents with terpenoid derivatives. *Ganoderma lucidum* (Reishi) which is a medicinal mushroom, contains several triterpenoid substances such as ganoderic acid and lucidenic acid. The compounds were then evaluated for their therapeutic effects whereby they exhibited anti-human immunodeficiency virus (HIV) activity by inhibiting the effects of HIV progression [105].

3.2. Application of Terpenoids in Clinical Settings: Challenges

As mentioned previously, terpenes and terpenoids had been known to exert antimicrobial activity against a wide variety of bacteria, both Gram-positive and Gram-negative. Clinical trials regarding highlighting the application of terpenes had been performed in several studies. In addition, β-sitosterol had also demonstrated immune enhancing ability in tuberculosis patients, demonstrating significant weight gain and higher white blood cell counts which resulted in faster recovery [106]. However, the application of terpenes as antimicrobials in the clinical phase is yet to be explored. This can be attributed to several factors, as the mode of actions of terpenes is not fully understood and the amount of time and resources required for clinical trials are limited and not always rewarding [107]. Terpenes consist of a diverse group of lipophilic organic compounds, resulting in different structures which affect their mode of action. β-caryophyllene showed poor antimicrobial activity against a panel of bacteria [108]. In the event whereby terpenes with efficient antimicrobial activities have been discovered, the safety of the terpenes would often be the next obstacle prior to clinical trials. Certain terpenes are reported to be toxic at low dosage and thus not preferred [109]. For instance, even at 1% dose of eugenol, it was reported to effectively inhibit growth of *Dermanyssus gallinae* at 20% of the pathogen population. Eugenol, geraniol, and citral found in plant essential oils were able to administer 100% mortality when used undiluted. This shows that some undiluted terpenes are highly toxic upon direct usage [110]. Generally, the unfavorable toxicity of terpenes towards whole cells takes place due to disturbance; primarily disrupting cell membrane integrity which eventually leads to cell lysis [111]. Due to the lipophilic nature of terpenes, upon ingestion, they are easily absorbed by epidermal cells before reaching the site of infection. Thus, delicate drug delivery systems are required for their application into clinical trials.

3.3. Future Prospects

The evidenced antimicrobial activity of terpenes and their derivatives need to be further expounded with the aid of automation and advancement in technology. Experimental analyses will need to be more streamlined to become more precise, resulting in less ambiguity so that the results obtained can be ensured and are consistent. This will reduce the time taken for experimental work and more time can be spent for extended analyses. Researchers may then study the modification effects of natural products with a special focus on terpenoids. Structural modifications of natural compounds produced either synthetically or via biotransformation may offer a new facet in finding novel AMR solutions as it explores new antimicrobial agents. In addition, delivery methods involving existing treatments against AMR should be improved and new inventions can be investigated. Combination therapeutics may be enhanced by exploring more antimicrobial adjuvants which will synergistically affect treatment outcomes with greater efficiency and less side effects. Natural terpenes and terpenoids which are available at very low prices such as carvacrol, thymol, and geraniol [4], should be optimally used for development of good antibacterial combination drugs. However, application at the pharmaceutical level remains challenging as the in vivo after effect is, currently, still very much unexplored. Extended analysis involving well-designed clinical trials should be improved in order to manipulate potent compounds of terpenoids to the best of their functional potential.

4. Conclusions

From this review, it has been evidenced that some terpenes and their derivatives were proven to be potent antimicrobial agents against drug resistant pathogens which mainly include bacteria and fungi. Specific mechanisms of each class of terpenes have also been highlighted and as a whole, terpenes provide a possible mitigation route for AMR and navigating the dead end of the diminishing antibiotic pipeline, hence, an appropriate match between terpenoids and existing antimicrobial agents may provide ultimate therapeutic options for AMR-associated infections.

Author Contributions: Authors would also like to thank all the members of Floral Biotechnology Laboratory, UPM. K.-S.L. designed the manuscript. N.A.M. drafted the manuscript. S.-H.E.L. significantly refined the manuscript whereas K.-S.L., S.-K.Y., C.-L.M., A.A.-L.S., C.-M.C. and C.-W.C. edited the draft. All authors read and approved the final manuscript.

Acknowledgments: Special thanks are given to the HCT Research Grant for financial support of the research.

References

1. Mandal, S.M.; Roy, A.; Ghosh, A.K.; Hazra, T.K.; Basak, A.; Franco, O.L. Challenges and future prospects of antibiotic therapy: From peptides to phages utilization. *Front. Pharmacol.* **2014**, *5*, 105. [CrossRef] [PubMed]
2. Barbieri, R.; Coppo, E.; Marchese, A.; Daglia, M.; Sobarzo-Sánchez, E.; Nabavi, S.F. Phytochemicals for human disease: An update on plant-derived compounds antibacterial activity. *Microbiol. Res.* **2017**, *196*, 44–68. [CrossRef] [PubMed]
3. Blair, J.M.; Webber, M.A.; Baylay, A.J.; Ogbolu, D.O.; Piddock, L.J. Molecular mechanisms of antibiotic resistance. *Nat. Rev. Microbiol.* **2015**, *1*, 42. [CrossRef] [PubMed]
4. Zacchino, S.A.; Butassi, E.; Cordisco, E.; Svetaz, L.A. Hybrid combinations containing natural products and antimicrobial drugs that interfere with bacterial and fungal biofilms. *Phytomedicine* **2017**, *37*, 14–26. [CrossRef] [PubMed]
5. Rajagopal, M.; Martin, M.J.; Santiago, M.; Lee, W.; Kos, V.N.; Meredith, T.; Gilmore, M.S.; Walker, S. Multidrug intrinsic resistance factors in *Staphylococcus aureus* identified by profiling fitness within high-diversity transposon libraries. *MBio* **2016**, *7*, 4. [CrossRef]
6. Lewis, K. Persister cells, dormancy and infectious disease. *Nat. Rev. Microbiol.* **2007**, *5*, 48–56. [CrossRef]
7. Laxminarayan, R.; Duse, A.; Wattal, C.; Zaidi, A.K.M.; Wertheim, H.F.L.; Sumpradit, N.; Vlieghe, E.; Hara, G.L.; Gould, I.M.; Goossens, H.; et al. Antibiotic resistance-the need for global solutions. *Lancet Infect. Dis.* **2013**, *13*, 1057–1098. [CrossRef]
8. Touani, F.K.; Seukep, A.J.; Djeussi, D.E.; Fankam, A.G.; Noumedem, J.A.K.; Kuete, V. Antibiotic-potentiation activities of four Cameroonian dietary plants against multidrug-resistant Gram-negative bacteria expressing efflux pumps. *BMC Complement. Altern. Med.* **2014**, *1*, 258. [CrossRef]

9.   Davies, J.; Davies, D. Origins and Evolution of Antibiotic Resistance. *Microbiol. Mol. Biol. Rev.* **2010**, *3*, 417–433. [CrossRef]

10. Zaidi, A.K.M.; Huskins, W.C.; Thaver, D.; Bhutta, Z.A.; Abbas, Z.; Goldmann, D.A. Hospital-acquired neonatal infections in developing countries. *Lancet* **2005**, *365*, 1175–1188. [CrossRef]

11. Saleem, A.F.; Ahmed, I.; Mir, F.; Ali, S.R.; Zaidi, A.K.M. Pan-resistant Acinetobacter infection in neonates in Karachi, Pakistan. *J. Infect. Dev. Ctries.* **2010**, *4*, 30–37. [CrossRef]

12. Bush, K.; Courvalin, P.; Dantas, G.; Davies, J.; Eisenstein, B.; Huovinen, P.; Jacoby, G.A.; Kishony, R.; Kreiswirth, B.N.; Kutter, E.; et al. Tackling antibiotic resistance. *Nat. Rev. Microbiol.* **2011**, *9*, 894–896. [CrossRef]

13. Shen, J.; Davis, L.E.; Wallace, J.M.; Cai, Y.; Lawson, L.D. Enhanced diallyl trisulfide has in vitro synergy with amphotericin B against *Cryptococcus neoformans*. *Planta Med.* **1996**, *62*, 415–418. [CrossRef]

14. Yang, S.K.; Low, L.Y.; Yap, P.S.X.; Yusoff, K.; Mai, C.W.; Lai, K.S.; Lim, S.H. Plant-derived antimicrobials: Insights into mitigation of antimicrobial resistance. *Rec. Nat. Prod.* **2018**, *12*, 295–316. [CrossRef]

15. Spratt, B.G. Resistance to antibiotics mediated by target alterations. *Science* **1994**, *264*, 388–393. [CrossRef]

16. Baroud, M.; Dandache, I.; Araj, G.F.; Wakim, R.; Kanj, S.; Kanafani, Z.; Khairallah, M.; Sabra, A.; Shehab, M.; Dbaibo, G.; et al. Underlying mechanisms of carbapenem resistance in extended-spectrum β-lactamase-producing *Klebsiella pneumoniae* and *Escherichia coli* isolates at a tertiary care centre in Lebanon: Role of OXA-48 and NDM-1 carbapenemases. *Int. J. Antimicrob. Agents* **2013**, *41*, 75–79. [CrossRef]

17. Schmieder, R.; Edwards, R. Insights into antibiotic resistance through metagenomic approaches. *Future Microbiol.* **2012**, *7*, 73–89. [CrossRef]

18. Palmer, K.L.; Kos, V.N.; Gilmore, M.S. Horizontal gene transfer and the genomics of enterococcal antibiotic resistance. *Curr. Opin. Microbiol.* **2010**, *13*, 632–639. [CrossRef]

19. Nikaido, H. Prevention of drug access to bacterial targets: Permeability barriers and active efflux. *Science* **1994**, *264*, 382–388. [CrossRef]

20. Hancock, R.E.W. Mechanisms of action of newer antibiotics for Gram-positive pathogens. *Lancet Infect. Dis.* **2005**, *5*, 209–218. [CrossRef]

21. Moo, C.L.; Yang, S.K.; Yusoff, K.; Ajat, M.; Thomas, W.; Abushelaibi, A.; Lim, S.H.; Lai, K.S. Mechanisms of antimicrobial resistance (AMR) and alternative approaches to overcome AMR. *Curr. Drug Discov. Technol.* **2019**, *16*. [CrossRef]

22. Rudramurthy, G.R.; Swamy, M.K.; Sinniah, U.R.; Ghasemzadeh, A. Nanoparticles: Alternatives against drug-resistant pathogenic microbes. *Molecules* **2016**, *21*, 836. [CrossRef]

23. Langeveld, W.T.; Veldhuizen, E.J.A.; Burt, S.A. Synergy between essential oil components and antibiotics: A review. *Crit. Rev. Microbiol.* **2014**, *40*, 76–94. [CrossRef]

24. Yu, H.; Zhang, L.; Li, L.; Zheng, C.; Guo, L.; Li, W.; Sun, P.; Qin, L. Recent developments and future prospects of antimicrobial metabolites produced by endophytes. *Microbiol. Res.* **2010**, *165*, 437–449. [CrossRef]

25. Thapa, D.; Louis, P.; Losa, R.; Zweifel, B.; Wallace, R.J. Essential oils have different effects on human pathogenic and commensal bacteria in mixed faecal fermentations compared with pure cultures. *Microbiology* **2015**, *161*, 441–449. [CrossRef]

26. Lewis, R.E.; Kontoyiannis, D.P. Rationale for combination antifungal therapy. *Pharmacotherapy* **2001**, *21*, 149S–164S. [CrossRef]

27. Wagner, H.; Ulrich-Merzenich, G. Synergy research: Approaching a new generation of phytopharmaceuticals. *Phytomedicine* **2009**, *16*, 97–110. [CrossRef]

28. Oussalah, M.; Caillet, S.; Saucier, L.; Lacroix, M. Inhibitory effects of selected plant essential oils on the growth of four pathogenic bacteria: *E. coli* O157:H7, *Salmonella Typhimurium*, *Staphylococcus aureus* and *Listeria monocytogenes*. *Food Control* **2007**, *18*, 414–420. [CrossRef]

29. Tongnuanchan, P.; Benjakul, S. Essential oils: Extraction, bioactivities, and their uses for food preservation. *J. Food Sci.* **2014**, *7*. [CrossRef]

30. Helander, I.M.; Alakomi, H.L.; Latva-Kala, K.; Mattila-Sandholm, T.; Pol, I.; Smid, E.J.; Gorris, L.G.; Wright, A. Characterization of the action of selected essential oil components on Gram-negative bacteria. *Agric. Food Chem.* **1998**, *46*, 590–595. [CrossRef]

31. Liu, Q.; Niu, H.; Zhang, W.; Mu, H.; Sun, C.; Duan, J. Synergy among thymol, eugenol, berberine, cinnamaldehyde and streptomycin against planktonic and biofilm-associated food-borne pathogens. *Lett. Appl. Microbiol.* **2015**, *60*, 21–30. [CrossRef]

32. Yap, P.S.X.; Yang, S.K.; Lai, K.S.; Lim, S.H. Essential oils: The ultimate solution to antimicrobial resistance in *Escherichia coli*? In *Escherichia coli-Recent Advances on Physiology, Pathogenesis and Biotechnological Applications*; Samie, A., Ed.; Intech Open: Rijeka, Croatia, 2017; pp. 299–313.

33. Yang, S.K.; Yap, P.S.X.; Krishnan, T.; Yusoff, K.; Chan, K.G.; Yap, W.S.; Lai, K.S.; . Lim, S.H. Mode of action: Synergistic interaction of peppermint (*Mentha x piperita* L. Carl) essential oil and meropenem against plasmid-mediated resistant *E. coli*. *Rec. Nat. Prod.* **2018**, *12*, 582–594. [CrossRef]

34. Yang, S.K.; Yusoff, K.; Ajat, M.; Thomas, W.; Abushelaibi, A.; Akseer, R.; Lim, S.E.; Lai, K.S. Disruption of KPC-producing *Klebsiella pneumoniae* membrane via induction of oxidative stress by cinnamon bark (*Cinnamomum verum* J. Presl) essential oil. *PLoS ONE* **2019**, 1–20. [CrossRef]

35. Maida, I.; Lo Nostro, A.; Pesavento, G.; Barnabei, M.; Calonico, C.; Perrin, E.; Chiellini, C.; Fondi, M.; Mengoni, A.; Maggini, V.; et al. Exploring the anti- *Burkholderia cepacia* complex activity of essential oils: A preliminary analysis. *Evidence-Based Complement. Altern. Med.* **2014**, *2014*. [CrossRef]

36. Rasooli, I.; Shayegh, S.; Astaneh, S.D.A. The effect of *Mentha spicata* and *Eucalyptus camaldulensis* essential oils on dental biofilm. *Int. J. Dent. Hyg.* **2009**, *7*, 196–203. [CrossRef]

37. Sharma, A.; Rajendran, S.; Srivastava, A.; Sharma, S.; Kundu, B. Antifungal activities of selected essential oils against *Fusarium oxysporum* f. sp. lycopersici 1322, with emphasis on *Syzygium aromaticum* essential oil. *J. Biosci. Bioeng.* **2017**, *123*, 308–313. [CrossRef]

38. Shrigod, N.M.; Swami Hulle, N.R.; Prasad, R.V. Supercritical fluid extraction of essential oil from mint leaves (*Mentha spicata*): Process optimization and its quality evaluation. *J. Food Process Eng.* **2017**, *40*, 12488. [CrossRef]

39. Adukwu, E.C.; Bowles, M.; Edwards-Jones, V.; Bone, H. Antimicrobial activity, cytotoxicity and chemical analysis of lemongrass essential oil (*Cymbopogon flexuosus*) and pure citral. *Appl. Microbiol. Biotechnol.* **2016**, *100*, 9619–9627. [CrossRef]

40. De Andrade, F.B.; Midena, R.Z.; Koga-Ito, C.Y.; Duarte, M.A. Conventional and natural products against oral infections. Microbial pathogens and strategies for combating them: Science, technology and education. In *Pathogens and Strategies for Combating Them: Science, Technology and Education*; Méndez-Vilas, A., Ed.; FORMATEX Research Center: Badajoz, Spain, 2013; pp. 1574–1583.

41. Vasireddy, L.; Bingle, L.E.H.; Davies, M.S. Antimicrobial activity of essential oils against multidrug-resistant clinical isolates of the *Burkholderia cepacia* complex. *PLoS ONE* **2018**, *13*. [CrossRef]

42. Grzesiak, B.; Głowacka, A.; Krukowski, H.; Lisowski, A.; Lassa, H.; Sienkiewicz, M. The in vitro efficacy of essential oils and antifungal drugs against *Prototheca zopfii*. *Mycopathologia* **2016**, *181*, 609–615. [CrossRef]

43. Rafiq, R.; Hayek, S.; Anyanwu, U.; Hardy, B.; Giddings, V.; Ibrahim, S.; Tahergorabi, R.; Kang, H. Antibacterial and antioxidant activities of essential oils from *Artemisia herba-alba* Asso., *Pelargonium capitatum* radens and *Laurus nobilis* L. *Foods* **2016**, *5*, 28. [CrossRef]

44. Peixoto, L.R.; Rosalen, P.L.; Ferreira, G.L.S.; Freires, I.A.; de Carvalho, F.G.; Castellano, L.R.; Castro, R.D. Antifungal activity, mode of action and anti-biofilm effects of *Laurus nobilis Linnaeus* essential oil against *Candida* spp. *Arch. Oral Biol.* **2017**, *73*, 179–185. [CrossRef]

45. Kurekci, C.; Padmanabha, J.; Bishop-Hurley, S.L.; Hassan, E.; Al Jassim, R.A.M.; McSweeney, C.S. Antimicrobial activity of essential oils and five terpenoid compounds against *Campylobacter jejuni* in pure and mixed culture experiments. *Int. J. Food Microbiol.* **2013**, *166*, 450–457. [CrossRef]

46. De Rapper, S.; Viljoen, A.; Van Vuuren, S. The in vitro antimicrobial effects of *Lavandula angustifolia* essential oil in combination with conventional antimicrobial agents. *Evidence-Based Complement. Altern. Med.* **2016**. [CrossRef]

47. Swamy, M.K.; Akhtar, M.S.; Sinniah, U.R. Antimicrobial properties of plant essential oils against human pathogens and their mode of action: An updated review. *Evid.-Based Complement. Altern. Med.* **2016**. [CrossRef]

48. Al-Snafi, A.E. Medical importance of *Anthemis nobilis*—A review. *As. J. Pharm. Sci. Technol.* **2016**, *6*, 89–95.

49. Hajlaoui, H.; Mighri, H.; Aouni, M.; Gharsallah, N.; Kadri, A. Chemical composition and in vitro evaluation of antioxidant, antimicrobial, cytotoxicity and anti-acetylcholinesterase properties of Tunisian *Origanum majorana* L. essential oil. *Microb. Pathog.* **2016**, *95*, 86–94. [CrossRef]

50. Garzoli, S.; Božović, M.; Baldisserotto, A.; Sabatino, M.; Cesa, S.; Pepi, F.; Vicentini, C.B.; Manfredini, S.; Ragno, R. Essential oil extraction, chemical analysis and anti-Candida activity of *Foeniculum vulgare* Miller—new approaches. *Nat. Prod. Res.* **2018**, *32*, 1254–1259. [CrossRef]

51. Kačániová, M.; Terentjeva, M.; Vukovic, N.; Puchalski, C.; Roychoudhury, S.; Kunová, S.; Klūga, A.; Tokár, M.; Kluz, M.; Ivanišová, E. The antioxidant and antimicrobial activity of essential oils against Pseudomonas spp. isolated from fish. *Saudi Pharm. J.* **2017**, *25*, 1108–1116. [CrossRef]

52. Zrira, S.; Ghanmi, M. Chemical composition and antibacterial activity of the essential of *Cedrus atlantica* (Cedarwood oil). *J. Essent. Oil-Bearing Plants.* **2016**, *19*, 1267–1272. [CrossRef]

53. El Omari, K.; Hamze, M.; Alwan, S.; Jama, C.; Chihib, N.E. Antifungal activity of the essential oil of *Micromeria barbata* an endemic lebanese micromeria species collected at North Lebanon. *J. Mater. Environ. Sci.* **2016**, *7*, 4158–4167.

54. Nazzaro, F.; Fratianni, F.; De Martino, L.; Coppola, R.; De Feo, V. Effect of essential oils on pathogenic bacteria. *Pharmaceuticals* **2013**, *6*, 1451–1474. [CrossRef]

55. Griffin, S.G.; Wyllie, S.G.; Markham, J.L.; Leach, D.N. The role of structure and molecular properties of terpenoids in determining their antimicrobial activity. *Flavour Fragr. J.* **1999**, *14*, 322–332. [CrossRef]

56. Roberts, S.C. Production and engineering of terpenoids in plant cell culture. *Nat. Chem. Biol.* **2007**, *3*, 387–395. [CrossRef]

57. Shaw, M.K.; Ingraham, J.L. Synthesis of macromolecules by *Escherichia coli* near the minimal temperature for growth. *J. Bacteriol.* **1967**, *1*, 157–164.

58. Zengin, H.; Baysal, A. Antibacterial and antioxidant activity of essential oil terpenes against pathogenic and spoilage-forming bacteria and cell structure-activity relationships evaluated by SEM microscopy. *Molecules* **2014**, *11*, 17773–17798. [CrossRef]

59. Chen, J.; Jiang, Q.D.; Chai, Y.P.; Zhang, H.; Peng, P.; Yang, X.X. Natural terpenes as penetration enhancers for transdermal drug delivery. *Molecules* **2016**, *12*, 1709. [CrossRef]

60. Lorenzi, V.; Muselli, A.; Bernardini, A.F.; Berti, L.; Pagès, J.M.; Amaral, L.; Bolla, J.L. Geraniol restores antibiotic activities against multidrug-resistant isolates from Gram-negative species. *Antimicrob. Agents Chemother.* **2009**, *53*, 2209–2211. [CrossRef]

61. Trombetta, D.; Castelli, F.; Sarpietro, M.G.; Venuti, V.; Cristani, M.; Daniele, C.; Saija, A.; Mazzanti, G.; Bisignano, G. Mechanisms of antibacterial action of three monoterpenes. *Antimicrob. Agents Chemother.* **2005**, *49*, 2474–2478. [CrossRef]

62. De Inés, C.; Argandoña, V.H.; Rovirosa, J.; San-Martín, A.; Díaz-Marrero, A.R.; Cueto, M.; González-Coloma, A. Cytotoxic activity of halogenated monoterpenes from *Plocamium cartilagineum*. *Zeitschrift fur Naturforsch-Sect. C J. Biosci.* **2004**, *59*, 339–344. [CrossRef]

63. Kurita, N.; Miyaji, M.; Kuraney, R.; Takahara, Y.; Ichimura, K. Antifungal activity and molecular orbital energies of aldehyde compounds from oils of higher plants. *Agric. Biol. Chem.* **1979**, *43*, 2365–2371.

64. Dorman, H.J.D.; Deans, S.G. Antimicrobial agents from plants: Antibacterial activity of plant volatile oils. *J. Appl. Microbiol.* **2000**, *88*, 308–316. [CrossRef]

65. Liu, X.; Dong, M.; Chen, X.; Jiang, M.; Lv, X.; Zhou, J. Antimicrobial activity of an endophytic Xylaria sp. YX-28 and identification of its antimicrobial compound 7-amino-4-methylcoumarin. *Appl. Microbiol. Biotechnol.* **2008**, *78*, 241–247. [CrossRef]

66. Knowles, J.R.; Roller, S.; Murray, D.B.; Naidu, A.S. Antimicrobial action of carvacrol at different stages of dual-species biofilm development by *Staphylococcus aureus* and *Salmonella enterica* serovar typhimurium. *Appl. Environ. Microbiol.* **2005**, *71*, 797–803. [CrossRef]

67. Bhatti, H.N.; Khan, S.S.; Khan, A.; Rani, M.; Ahmad, V.U.; Choudhary, M.I. Biotransformation of monoterpenoids and their antimicrobial activities. *Phytomedicine.* **2014**, *21*, 1597–1626. [CrossRef]

68. Smid, E.J.; de Witte, Y.; Gorris, L.G.M. Secondary plant metabolites as control agents of postharvest Penicillium rot on tulip bulbs. *Postharvest Biol. Technol.* **1995**, *6*, 303–312. [CrossRef]

69. Dunkic, V.; Bezic, N.; Vuko, E.; Cukrov, D. Antiphytoviral activity of *Satureja montana* L. ssp. variegata (host) P. W. Ball essential oil and phenol compounds on CMV and TMV. *Molecules* **2010**, *15*, 6713–6721. [CrossRef]

70. Astani, A.; Reichling, J.; Schnitzler, P. Comparative study on the antiviral activity of selected monoterpenes derived from essential oils. *Phytother. Res.* **2010**, *24*, 673–679. [CrossRef]

71. Torres-Romero, D.; Jiménez, I.A.; Rojas, R.; Gilman, R.H.; López, M.; Bazzocchi, I.L. Dihydro-β-agarofuran sesquiterpenes isolated from *Celastrus vulcanicola* as potential anti-*Mycobacterium tuberculosis* multidrug-resistant agents. *Bioorganic Med. Chem.* **2011**, *19*, 2182–2189. [CrossRef]

72. Koo, H.; Pearson, S.K.; Scott-Anne, K.; Abranches, J.; Cury, J.A.; Rosalen, P.L.; Park, Y.; Marquis, R.E.; Bowen, W.H. Effects of apigenin and tt-farnesol on glucosyltransferase activity, biofilm viability and caries development in rats. *Oral Microbiol. Immunol.* **2002**, *17*, 337–343. [CrossRef]

73. Gomes, F.I.A.; Teixeira, P.; Azeredo, J.; Oliveira, R. Effect of farnesol on planktonic and biofilm cells of *Staphylococcus epidermidis*. *Curr. Microbiol.* **2009**, *59*, 118–122. [CrossRef]

74. Masako, K.; Yusuke, K.; Hideyuki, I.; Atsuko, M.; Yoshiki, M.; Kayoko, M.; Makoto, K. Corrigendum to "A novel method to control the balance of skin microflora. Part 2. A study to assess the effect of a cream containing farnesol and xylitol on atopic dry skin". *J. Dermatol. Sci.* **2005**, *39*, 197. [CrossRef]

75. Castelo-Branco, D.S.C.M.; Riello, G.B.; Vasconcelos, D.C.; Guedes, G.M.M.; Serpa, R.; Bandeira, T.J.P.G.; Monteiro, A.J.; Cordeiro, R.A.; Rocha, M.F.; Sidrim, J.J.; et al. Farnesol increases the susceptibility of *Burkholderia pseudomallei* biofilm to antimicrobials used to treat melioidosis. *J. Appl. Microbiol.* **2016**, *120*, 600–606. [CrossRef]

76. Rukayadi, Y.; Hwang, J.K. Effect of coating the wells of a polystyrene microtiter plate with xanthorrhizol on the biofilm formation of *Streptococcus mutans*. *J. Basic Microbiol.* **2006**, *46*, 410–415. [CrossRef]

77. Jin, J.; Guo, N.; Zhang, J.; Ding, Y.; Tang, X.; Liang, J.; Li, L.; Deng, X.; Yu, L. The synergy of honokiol and fluconazole against clinical isolates of azole-resistant *Candida albicans*. *Lett. Appl. Microbiol.* **2010**, *51*, 351–357. [CrossRef]

78. Gonçalves, O.; Pereira, R.; Gonçalves, F.; Mendo, S.; Coimbra, M.A.; Rocha, S.M. Evaluation of the mutagenicity of sesquiterpenic compounds and their influence on the susceptibility towards antibiotics of two clinically relevant bacterial strains. *Mutat. Res. -Genet. Toxicol. Environ. Mutagen.* **2011**, *723*, 18–25. [CrossRef]

79. Ambrosio, S.R.; Tirapelli, C.R.; da Costa, F.B.; de Oliveira, A.M. Kaurane and pimarane-type diterpenes from the Viguiera species inhibit vascular smooth muscle contractility. *Life Sci.* **2006**, *79*, 925–933. [CrossRef]

80. Souza, A.B.; Martins, C.H.G.; Souza, M.G.M.; Furtado, N.A.J.C.; Heleno, V.C.G.; De Sousa, J.P.B.; Rocha, E.M.; Bastos, J.K.; Cunha, W.R.; Veneziani, R.C.; et al. Antimicrobial activity of terpenoids from *Copaifera langsdorffii* Desf. against cariogenic bacteria. *Phythother. Res.* **2011**, *25*, 215–220. [CrossRef]

81. Różalski, M.; Walencka, E.; Różalska, B.; Wysokińska, H. Antimicrobial activity of diterpenoids from hairy roots of *Salvia sclarea* L.: Salvipisone as a potential anti-biofilm agent active against antibiotic resistant Staphylococci. *Phytomedicine.* **2007**, *14*, 31–35.

82. Gupta, V.K.; Tiwari, N.; Gupta, P.; Verma, S.; Pal, A.; Srivastava, S.K.; Darokar, M.P. A clerodane diterpene from *Polyalthia longifolia* as a modifying agent of the resistance of methicillin resistant *Staphylococcus aureus*. *Phytomedicine.* **2016**, *23*, 654–661. [CrossRef]

83. Walencka, E.; Rozalska, S.; Wysokinska, H.; Rozalski, M.; Kuzma, L.; Rozalska, B. Salvipisone and aethiopinone from *Salvia sclarea* hairy roots modulate staphylococcal antibiotic resistance and express anti-biofilm activity. *Planta Med.* **2007**, *73*, 545–551. [CrossRef]

84. Jiménez-Arellanes, A.; Luna-Herrera, J.; Cornejo-Garrido, J.; López-García, S.; Castro-Mussot, M.E.; Meckes-Fischer, M.; Mata-Espinosa, D.; Marquina, B.; Torres, J.; Hernández-Pando, R. Ursolic and oleanolic acids as antimicrobial and immunomodulatory compounds for tuberculosis treatment. *BMC Complement. Altern. Med.* **2013**, *13*, 258. [CrossRef]

85. Cunha, W.R.; De Matos, G.X.; Souza, M.G.M.; Tozatti, M.G.; Andrade, E.; Silva, M.L.; Martins, C.H.G.; Silva, R.D.; Da Silva Filho, A.A. Evaluation of the antibacterial activity of the methylene chloride extract of *Miconia ligustroides*, isolated triterpene acids, and ursolic acid derivatives. *Pharm. Biol.* **2010**, *48*, 166–169. [CrossRef]

86. Zhou, L.; Ding, Y.; Chen, W.; Zhang, P.; Chen, Y.; Lv, X. The in vitro study of ursolic acid and oleanolic acid inhibiting cariogenic microorganisms as well as biofilm. *Oral Dis.* **2013**, *19*, 494–500. [CrossRef]

87. Chung, P.Y.; Chung, L.Y.; Navaratnam, P. Potential targets by pentacyclic triterpenoids from *Callicarpa farinosa* against methicillin-resistant and sensitive *Staphylococcus aureus*. *Fitoterapia.* **2014**, *94*, 48–54. [CrossRef]

88. Lewis, R.E.; Diekema, D.J.; Messer, S.A.; Pfaller, M.A.; Klepser, M.E. Comparison of Etest, chequerboard dilution and time – kill studies for the detection of synergy or antagonism between antifungal agents tested against Candida species. *J. Antimicrob. Chemother.* **2002**, *49*, 345–351. [CrossRef]

89. Chou, T.C. Theoretical basis, experimental design, and computerized simulation of synergism and antagonism in drug combination studies. *Pharmacol. Rev.* **2006**, *58*, 621–681. [CrossRef]

90. Rodriguez, M.V.; Sortino, M.A.; Ivancovich, J.J.; Pellegrino, J.M.; Favier, L.S.; Raimondi, M.P.; Gattuso, M.A.; Zacchino, S.A. Detection of synergistic combinations of Baccharis extracts with Terbinafine against *Trichophyton rubrum* with high throughput screening synergy assay (HTSS) followed by 3D graphs. Behavior of some of their components. *Phytomedicine* **2013**, *13*, 1230–1239. [CrossRef]

91. Zacchino, S.A.; Butassi, E.; Di Liberto, M.; Raimondi, M.; Postigo, A.; Sortino, M. Plant phenolics and terpenoids as adjuvants of antibacterial and antifungal drugs. *Phytomedicine* **2017**, *37*, 27–48. [CrossRef]

92. Cho, K.S.; Lim, Y.R.; Lee, K.; Lee, J.; Lee, J.H.; Lee, I.S. Terpenes from forests and human health. *Toxicol. Res.* **2017**, *2*, 97. [CrossRef]

93. Schwab, W.; Fuchs, C.; Huang, F.C. Transformation of terpenes into fine chemicals. *Eur. J. Lipid Sci. Tech.* **2013**, *1*, 3–8. [CrossRef]

94. Mondello, F.; De Bernardis, F.; Girolamo, A.; Cassone, A.; Salvatore, G. In vivo activity of terpinen-4-ol, the main bioactive component of *Melaleuca alternifolia* Cheel (tea tree) oil against azole-susceptible and-resistant human pathogenic Candida species. *BMC infectious diseases* **2006**, *1*, 158. [CrossRef]

95. Tona, L.; Mesia, K.; Ngimbi, N.P.; Chrimwami, B.; Okond'Ahoka; Cimanga, K.; Bruyne, T.D.; Apers, S.; Hermans, N.; Totte, J.; et al. In-vivo antimalarial activity of *Cassia Occidentalism, Morinda morindoides* and *Phyllanthus niruri*. *Ann. Trop. Med. Parasitol.* **2001**, *1*, 47–57. [CrossRef]

96. Donald, P.R.; Lamprecht, J.H.; Freestone, M.; Albrecht, C.F.; Bouic, P.J.; Kotze, D.; Van Jaarsveld, P.P. A randomised placebo-controlled trial of the efficacy of beta-sitosterol and its glucoside as adjuvants in the treatment of pulmonary tuberculosis. *Int. J. Tuberc. Lung Dis.* **1997**, *6*, 518–522.

97. Kohlert, C.; Van Rensen, I.; März, R.; Schindler, G.; Graefe, E.U.; Veit, M. Bioavailability and pharmacokinetics of natural volatile terpenes in animals and humans. *Planta Med.* **2000**, *6*, 495–505. [CrossRef]

98. Papada, E.; Gioxari, A.; Brieudes, V.; Amerikanou, C.; Halabalaki, M.; Skaltsounis, A.L.; Smyrnioudis, I.; Kaliora, A.C. Bioavailability of terpenes and postprandial effect on human antioxidant potential. An open-label study in healthy subjects. *Mol. Nutr. Food Res.* **2018**, *3*, 1700751. [CrossRef]

99. Amin, T.; Bhat, S.V. A review on phytosome technology as a novel approach to improve the bioavailability of nutraceuticals. *Int. J. Adv. Res. Technol.* **2012**, *3*, 1–5.

100. Yang, S.K.; Yusoff, K.; Mai, C.W.; Lim, W.M.; Yap, W.S.; Lim, S.H.E.; Lai, K.S. Additivity vs. synergism: Investigation of the additive interaction of cinnamon bark oil and meropenem in combinatory therapy. *Molecules* **2017**, *22*, 1733. [CrossRef]

101. Bodede, O.; Shaik, S.; Chenia, H.; Singh, P.; Moodley, R. Quorum sensing inhibitory potential and in silico molecular docking of flavonoids and novel terpenoids from *Senegalia nigrescens*. *J. Ethnopharmacol.* **2018**, *216*, 134–146. [CrossRef]

102. Avalos, M.; van Wezel, G.P.; Raaijmakers, J.M.; Garbeva, P. Healthy scents: Microbial volatiles as new frontier in antibiotic research? *Curr. Opin. Microbiol.* **2018**, *45*, 84–91. [CrossRef]

103. Chudasama, R.G.; Dhanani, N.J.; Amrutiya, R.M.; Chandni, R.; Jayanthi, G.; Karthikeyan, K. Screening of selected plants from semi-arid region for its phytochemical constituents and antimicrobial activity. *J. Pharmacog. Phytochem.* **2018**, *7*, 2983–2988.

104. Gupta, S.; Bhagat, M.; Sudan, R.; Rajput, S.; Rajput, K. Analysis of chemical composition of *Cupressus torulosa* (D.Don) essential oil and bioautography guided evaluation of its antimicrobial fraction. *Indian J. Exp. Biol.* **2018**, *56*, 252–257.

105. Cör, D.; Knez, Ž.; Hrnčič, M.K. Antitumour, antimicrobial, antioxidant and antiacetylcholinesterase effect of *Ganoderma Lucidum* terpenoids and polysaccharides: A review. *Molecules* **2018**, *23*, 649. [CrossRef]

106. Bin Sayeed, M.; Karim, S.; Sharmin, T.; Morshed, M. Critical analysis on characterization, systemic effect, and therapeutic potential of beta-sitosterol: A plant-derived orphan phytosterol. *Medicines* **2016**, *3*, 29. [CrossRef]

107. Silver, L.L. Challenges of antibacterial discovery. *Clin. Microbiol. Rev.* **2011**, *24*, 71–109. [CrossRef]

108. Fidyt, K.; Fiedorowicz, A.; Strządała, L.; Szumny, A. β-caryophyllene and β-caryophyllene oxide—Natural compounds of anticancer and analgesic properties. *Cancer Medicine* **2016**, *5*, 3007–3017. [CrossRef]

109. De Moraes, M.M.; da Camara, C.A.G.; Da Silva, M.M.C. Comparative toxicity of essential oil and blends of selected terpenes of Ocotea species from Pernambuco, Brazil, against *Tetranychus urticae* Koch. *An. Acad. Bras. Cienc.* **2017**, *89*, 1417–1429. [CrossRef]

110. Sparagano, O.; Khallaayoune, K.; Duvallet, G.; Nayak, S.; George, D. Comparing terpenes from plant essential oils as pesticides for the poultry red mite (*Dermanyssus gallinae*). *Transbound. Emerg. Dis.* **2013**, *60*, 150–153. [CrossRef]

111. Van der Werf, M.J.; de Bont, J.A.; Leak, D.J. Opportunities in microbial biotransformation of monoterpenes. In *Biotechnology of Aroma Compounds*; Springer: Berlin/Heidelberg, Germany, 1997; pp. 147–177.

14

Carotenoids: How Effective are they to Prevent Age-Related Diseases?

Bee Ling Tan [1] **and Mohd Esa Norhaizan** [1,2,3,*]

[1] Department of Nutrition and Dietetics, Faculty of Medicine and Health Sciences, Universiti Putra Malaysia, Serdang 43400, Selangor, Malaysia; tbeeling87@gmail.com
[2] Laboratory of Molecular Biomedicine, Institute of Bioscience, Universiti Putra Malaysia, Serdang 43400, Selangor, Malaysia
[3] Research Centre of Excellent, Nutrition and Non-Communicable Diseases (NNCD), Faculty of Medicine and Health Sciences, Universiti Putra Malaysia, Serdang 43400, Selangor, Malaysia
* Correspondence: nhaizan@upm.edu.my;

Abstract: Despite an increase in life expectancy that indicates positive human development, a new challenge is arising. Aging is positively associated with biological and cognitive degeneration, for instance cognitive decline, psychological impairment, and physical frailty. The elderly population is prone to oxidative stress due to the inefficiency of their endogenous antioxidant systems. As many studies showed an inverse relationship between carotenoids and age-related diseases (ARD) by reducing oxidative stress through interrupting the propagation of free radicals, carotenoid has been foreseen as a potential intervention for age-associated pathologies. Therefore, the role of carotenoids that counteract oxidative stress and promote healthy aging is worthy of further discussion. In this review, we discussed the underlying mechanisms of carotenoids involved in the prevention of ARD. Collectively, understanding the role of carotenoids in ARD would provide insights into a potential intervention that may affect the aging process, and subsequently promote healthy longevity.

Keywords: aging; cancer; cardiovascular disease; dementia; diabetes; inflammation; oxidative stress

1. Introduction

The average life expectancy has been rising rapidly in recent decades, with an average of 72.0 years in 2016 globally [1]. However, the healthy life expectancy was 63.3 years in 2016 worldwide [1]. In view of the demographics of the global population from 2000 to 2050, the population aged 60 years or more is estimated to increase from 605 million to 2 billion people [2]. In many countries, the average life expectancy aged 60 years could expect to live another 20.5 years in 2016 [1]. This longevity accounts for a growing share of age-related diseases (ARD) and their consequent economic and social burden [3]. In fact, aging is positively associated with biological and cognitive degeneration including cognitive decline, psychological impairment, and physical frailty [4].

Reactive oxygen species (ROS) are continuously generated in normal aerobic metabolism as a by-product; however, when the amount is elevated under stress, it may cause potential biological damage [5]. Oxidative stress emerges from an imbalance of either pro- and/or antioxidant molecules, being characterized by the decreased capacity of endogenous systems to combat an oxidative attack and subsequently leading to molecular and cellular damage [6]. Oxidative stress has been recognized as the main contributor to the pathophysiology and pathogenesis of ARD [7] such as metabolic syndromes, atherosclerosis, osteoporosis, obesity, dementia, diabetes, cancer, and arthritis [8,9].

ARD have become the most common health threats in recent decades. ARD have been linked to structural changes in mitochondria, accompanied by an alteration of biophysical properties of the membrane such as reduced fluidity and altered electron transport chain complex activity, which in turn contribute to mitochondrial failure and energy imbalance. This perturbation impairs mitochondrial function and cellular homeostasis, and increases susceptibility to oxidative stress [10,11]. The elderly population is susceptible to oxidative stress due to the inefficiency of their endogenous antioxidant systems [12]. An irreversible progression of oxidative decay due to ROS also causes a negative impact on the biology of aging such as reducing lifespan, increasing disease incidence, and the impairment of physiological functions [13]. Several organs, for example the heart and brain, with a high consumption of oxygen and limited replication rate are vulnerable to these phenomena, suggesting the high prevalence of neurological disorders and cardiovascular disease (CVD) in elderly populations [14,15]. Increased ROS has been linked to the progression and onset of aging. Although ROS generation may not be an essential factor for aging [16], they are more likely to aggravate ARD development through interaction with mitochondria and cause oxidative damage [17]. Due to their reactivity, high levels of ROS can generate oxidative stress by interrupting the balance of prooxidant and antioxidant levels [18]. Substantial evidence highlights that carotenoids can decrease oxidative stress and the progression of ARD [19]. Lycopene, a carotenoid that is abundantly found in tomatoes, is a crucial antioxidant source. A meta-analysis study has demonstrated an inverse relationship between lycopene intake and cardiovascular disease (CVD) risk [20]. This favorable effect could be attributed to the decreased inflammatory response and cholesterol level, as well as the reduced oxidation of biomolecules [21]. Besides CVD, several studies have also found that consumption of carotenoid-rich fruits and vegetables can prevent cancers such as prostate and cervical [22–24]. As many studies show that carotenoid intake is negatively associated with ARD by disrupting the formation of free radicals and subsequently reduces oxidative stress, carotenoid has been foreseen as a promising nutritional approach for ARD. Therefore, the role of carotenoids that combat oxidative stress and promote healthy longevity is worth to discuss further. Of particular interest in this review, we discussed the underlying mechanisms of carotenoids involved in the prevention of ARD. Understanding the role of carotenoids in ARD would provide insight for potential interventions that may affect the aging process, and subsequently promoting healthy longevity.

2. Carotenoids

Carotenoids are a family of naturally occurring organic pigmented compounds that are produced by the fungi, several bacteria, and plastids of algae and plants [25]. Notably, red pea aphid (*Acyrthosiphon pisum*) and spider mite (*Tetranychus urticae*) are the only animals that produce carotenoids from fungi through gene transfer [26]. In plants, carotenoids contribute to the photosynthetic machinery and protect them from photo-damage [27]. They occur in all organisms capable of photosynthesis, a process to convert into chemical energy in the presence of sunlight. Generally, carotenoids absorb wavelengths between 400 and 550 nanometers, and hence the compounds are present in red, orange, or yellow color [28].

Nearly 600 carotenoids have been identified in nature to modulate a broad spectrum of functions [29]. However, only about 50 carotenoids are found in a typical human diet [30], while about 20 carotenoids are present in human tissues and blood [31]. Carotenoids are classified into two groups, namely xanthophylls and carotenes, according to their chemical constituents [32]. Oxygenated derivatives are known as xanthophylls; while hydrocarbon only carotenoids (lycopene, β-carotene, and α-carotene) are called carotenes. Additionally, aldehyde groups (β-citraurin), epoxide groups (neoxanthin, antheraxanthin, and violaxanthin), oxo/keto groups (canthaxanthin and echinenone), and oxygen substituents (zeaxanthin and lutein) are categorized as complex xanthophylls [33].

3. Chemical Structures

In particular, most of the carotenoids are tetraterpenoids, containing 40 carbon atoms and derived from eight isoprene molecules [34]. All carotenoids have a polyisoprenoid structure, accompanied by a long-conjugated chain adjacent with multiple double bonds and symmetry on the central double bonds. The molecular structures of carotenes and xanthophylls are shown in Figures 1 and 2, respectively.

Alteration of the basic acyclic structure acquired oxygen-rich functional groups [35]. One of the features of carotenoid is a strong coloration, which is a consequence of light absorption in the presence of a conjugated chain [36]. Due to the presence of the electron-rich conjugated system of the polyene structure, carotenoids scavenge the free radicals by trapping peroxyl radicals and quenching the singlet oxygen [37]. Indeed, the conjugated double bond is critical for the proper functioning of carotenoids, for example in light absorption for photosynthetic organisms [36].

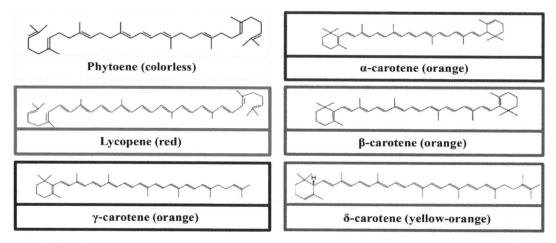

Figure 1. Molecular structures of carotenes (Phytoene, lycopene, γ-carotene, α-carotene, β-carotene, and δ-carotene).

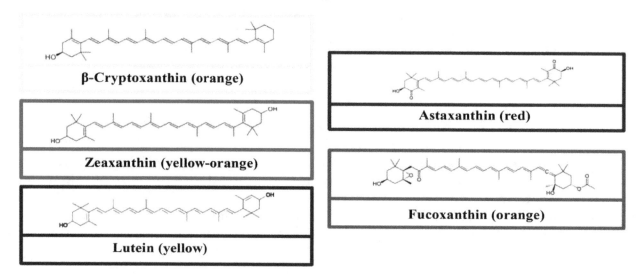

Figure 2. Molecular structures of some common xanthophylls (β-cryptoxanthin, zeaxanthin, lutein, astaxanthin, and fucoxanthin).

4. Dietary Sources

Carotenoids are abundantly found in deeply pigmented fruits and vegetables (Table 1), in which the orange-yellow vegetables and fruits are rich in β-carotene and α-carotene. While, α-cryptoxanthin, lycopene, and lutein are found in orange fruits, tomatoes and tomato products, and dark green vegetables, respectively [38]. Egg yolk is a highly bioavailable source of zeaxanthin and lutein [39]. The unsaturated nature of the carotenoids makes them prone to oxidation [40]. Other factors like pH, light, and temperature can also affect the color and nutritional value of foods [41]. Some common household cooking methods, for example boiling, steaming, and microwave cooking, do not markedly change the extent of the carotenoid content in food [42]. However, extreme heat can cause oxidative damage to carotenoids [42].

Table 1. Carotenoids content in some common foods.

Food Source	Carotenoids (μg/100 g)							References
	Lutein	Zeaxanthin	Lutein and Zeaxanthin	Lycopene	α-Carotene	β-Carotene	β-Cryptoxanthin	
Apples (with skin)	100–840				30			[40,43,44]
Apricot, raw	0–141				0–37	140–6939	28–231	[45]
Asparagus, raw	610–750				12	493		[40,44,46]
Avocados			270		28	53	36	[40,47]
Basil, raw			7050					[48]
Blackberry	270				9	100		[49]
Blueberry	230					49		[49]
Broccoli, raw	830–4300				1	414–2760		[45]
Brussels sprouts, boiled			1541					[45,47]
Carrot, raw	110–2097				530–35,833	1161–64,350		[50]
Corn, cooked	202	202						[51]
Cress, raw	7540							[47]
Frozen corn, boiled from frozen			684					[40,44,46]
Cucumbers (with skin)	160					138		[47,50]
Egg whole, cooked	237	216	353					[50]
Egg yolk, cooked	645	587						[47,50]
Egg whole, raw	288	279	504					[47,50]
Egg yolk, raw	787	762	1094					[47]
Frozen green beans, cooked			564					[52]
Jackfruit				37–111		40–772		[47]
Kale, cooked			18,246					[48]
Leek, raw			3680					[48]
Lettuce, raw	1000–4780							[40,45]
Mango	100				27	300–4200	0–1640	[40]
Melon, cantaloupe					8	1595	0	[40,53]
Orange juice	67					13	34	[40,45,47]
Orange	64–350		129		0–400	0–500	14–1395	[50]
Orange pepper, raw		1665						[40,45]
Papaya	20–820			2080–4750	0–60	71–1210	60–1483	[47,50]
Parsley, raw	4326		5562					[47]
Peas, green, boiled			2593					[54]
Pepper, bell, green, raw	340–660				22	198	1	[40]
Pineapple			1404					[47]
Pistachio nuts, raw			1014					[47]
Pumpkin, cooked						171–476		[47]
Spinach, raw	2047–20,300		12,197			840–24,070		[40,47]
Sweet potatoes, white flesh (cooked)						25–157		[55]

Table 1. *Cont.*

Food Source	Lutein	Zeaxanthin	Lutein and Zeaxanthin	Lycopene	α-Carotene	β-Carotene	β-Cryptoxanthin	References
			Carotenoids (µg/100 g)					
Squash, boiled			2249					[47]
Strawberry	6–21					5		[40],43]
Tomato, raw	40–1300			21–62,273		36–2232		[45]
Watermelon	0–40			2300–7200	0–1	44–324	62–457	[45]

5. Metabolism and Bioavailability

There are several factors that affect the carotenoid absorption, bioavailability, breakdown, transport, and storage. For example, the dietary intake of fat (in the form of salad dressing, cooking oil for instance extra virgin olive oil or whole egg) at the same meal with carotenoid consumption (cooked vegetables or raw vegetable salad) has been found to effectively increase the absorption of some carotenoids [56–59]. The bioavailability of carotenoids may reduce when consumed within the same meal due to the competition between carotenoids during absorption [60]. In addition, dietary fiber from plant sources, for example guar gum and pectin, were found to decrease carotenoid absorption [61], and the localization of carotenoids with the chromoplasts and chloroplasts of plants may reduce the bioavailability [62]. A study reported by Hornero-Mendez and Mínguez-Mosquera [63] evaluated the impact of cooking on carotenoids in the plant. The data showed that although heat reduces the carotenoid content, the bioavailability of the carotenoids was enhanced compared to the control (uncooked) [63]. Furthermore, Baskaran et al. [64] evaluated the micellar phospholipid in relation to the intestinal uptake of carotenoids in in vivo study. The data showed that phosphatidylcholine suppressed the accumulation of lutein and β-carotene in plasma and liver, suggesting the phospholipids derived from food and bile could influence the cellular uptake of carotenoids solubilized in mixed micelles formed in the intestinal tract. In addition, the rate of bioaccessibility of carotenoids is highly affected by the food matrix. The previous study revealed that in vitro transfer rate of β-cryptoxanthin, zeaxanthin, and lutein is nearly 100% from fruits such as sweet potato, grapefruit, kiwi, and orange compared to the vegetables such as spinach and broccoli, which is between 19 to 38% [65]. This observation indicates that the release of carotenoids from a food matrix followed by absorption is a determining factor for delivering potential health benefits.

The release of carotenoids from the food matrix is highly dependent on their state, as well as their associations with other food components such as protein [66]. As an example, the microcrystalline form of carotenoids, for instance lycopene in tomato and β-carotene in carrot, reduces their bioavailability compared to those that are immersed entirely in lipid droplets [36]. The bioavailability of carotenoids is markedly varied in food. The previous data stated that nearly 5% of carotenoids (whole, raw vegetables) are absorbed by the intestine whereas up to 50% of the carotenoid is absorbed from the micellar solutions [67]. This finding implies that the physical form of carotenoids present in intestinal mucosal cells is vitally important. Many studies have revealed that thermal treatment increases the bioaccessibility of carotenoids and improves their absorption due to the bond loosening and disruption of cell walls [68]. They are absorbed into gastrointestinal mucosal cells and remain unchanged in the tissues and circulations [69,70]. In the intestine, carotenoids are absorbed via passive diffusion after being incorporated into the micelles formed by the bile acid and dietary fat. Subsequently, these micellular carotenoids are incorporated into the chylomicrons and released into the lymphatic system. Ultimately, they bind with the lipoprotein at the liver and are released into the bloodstream [71]. Carotenoids are predominantly accumulated in adipose tissue and the liver; whereas in brain stem tissue, the carotenoid concentration is below the detection limit [72,73]. Other factors such as gender, aging, nutritional status, genetic factor, and infection may also influence the bioavailability of carotenoids [74,75]. It has been demonstrated that any disease with an abnormal absorption of fat from the digestive tract markedly alters the incorporation of carotenoids. Additionally, interaction with drugs such as aspirin and sulphonamides has been found to reduce the bioavailability of β-carotene [74].

6. Physiological Changes in Aging

Aging is characterized by a progressive loss and decline of tissues and organ systems. The degeneration rate is varied between individuals and is highly dependent on genetics and environmental factors, for instance exercise, ionizing radiation, pollutant exposure, and diet. In general, the physiological changes of aging are divided into three groups that include (1) changes in cellular homeostatic mechanisms, such as extracellular fluid volume, blood, and body temperature; (2) a decrease in organ mass; and (3) the loss and decline of the functional reserve of the body system [76]. The loss of functional reserve may impair the ability of an individual to cope with external challenges, for instance trauma and surgery.

Cardiovascular aging attenuates contractile and mechanical efficiency. The specific changes include an increase in smooth muscle tone, promotion of collagenolytic and elastolytic activity, and arterial wall thickening [77]. Subsequently, vessels stiffen progressively with age and contribute to the elevation of systolic arterial pressure and increase cardiac afterload and systemic vascular resistance. This phenomenon is usually demonstrated in isolated systolic hypertension, in which the left ventricle has to work harder to eject blood into the stiffer aorta, and hence increase the workload and contribute to the left ventricular hypertrophy. Hypertrophy of myocytes in response to increased afterload may promote contraction time as well as the cardiac cycle. Ventricular relaxation is delayed at the time of mitral valve opening and leads to diastolic dysfunction. Further, the early diastolic filling rate is also decreased with age and partly compensated by an elevated rate of late diastolic filling. Aging is also linked to the reduction of cardiac output in the face of falls in blood pressure [77].

In the context of the central nervous system, aging reduces the neural density, accounting for nearly a 30% loss of brain mass by the age of 80 years, largely grey matter. Growing older is linked to a reduction of central neurotransmitters such as acetylcholine, serotonin, and catecholamine. In addition, aging may also reduce dopamine uptake transporters and decrease γ-aminobutyric acid, β-adrenergic, α_2-adrenergic, and cortical serotonergic binding sites. All these changes may reduce the speed of memory and processing [77].

The greatest change in gastrointestinal physiology affecting nutrient bioavailability is atrophic gastritis, which presents in nearly 20% of the elderly population [78]. It has been shown that a slight decline in the secretion of pepsin and hydrochloric acid occurs with advancing age. Nutrient absorption is affected by low acid conditions in the stomach. Research evidence revealed that growing older is associated with the age-associated decline in the absorption of certain substances absorbed by active mechanisms such as vitamin B_{12}, β-carotene, iron, and calcium [79]. For example, dietary vitamin B_{12} is linked to the food protein, in which the vitamin B_{12} molecules must be digested before bound to the endogenous R binders. This digestion takes place in the presence of pepsin and acid. If stomach acid is low, the digestion of vitamin B_{12} cannot take place effectively [78].

In addition to the effects mentioned above, aging may reduce the number of fibroblasts and keratinocytes, decrease epidermal cell turnover, and impair the barrier function [80]. Moreover, aging can also decrease the vascular network such as round hair glands and bulbs (skin atrophy and fibrosis). Notably, elderly people are susceptible to the changes in cutaneous function due to the reduction in vitamin D synthesis. These changes increase their susceptibility to skin injuries such as skin tear and pressure ulcer [77].

7. The Role of Carotenoids in the Prevention of ARD

Antioxidant plays a predominant role in the termination of oxidative chain reactions by disrupting the free radical intermediates [81]. Antioxidants control autoxidation by disrupting the formation of free radicals or suppressing the propagation of free radicals through several mechanisms. This compound facilitates in quenching $\bullet O_2^-$, breaking the autoxidative chain reaction, inhibiting the formation of peroxides, and scavenging the species that promote the peroxidation [82].

Carotenoids are known as a highly effective physical and chemical singlet oxygen quencher and a potent scavenger of ROS [83]. The previous study stated that the antioxidant activity of lycopene is superior to α-tocopherol and β-carotene [84]. This favorable effect is attributed to the singlet oxygen quenching ability [85], suggesting that a tetraterpene hydrocarbon polyene accompanied with two unconjugated and eleven conjugated double bonds readily interact with electrophilic reagents, and subsequently affect the reactivity of oxygen and oxygenated free radical species [85]. The previous finding has revealed that a high consumption of carotenoids is inversely associated with ARD [86]. It has been suggested that the alleviation of chronic diseases is mainly due to the antioxidant properties of carotenoids [87]. Figure 3 shows the effect of oxidative stress and the interaction of carotenoids in relation to ARD.

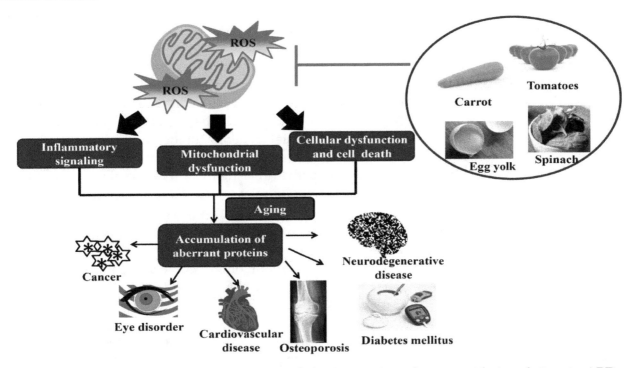

Figure 3. The effect of oxidative stress and the interaction of carotenoids in relation to ARD. Accumulation of reactive oxygen species (ROS) leads to inflammation, cellular dysfunction and cell death, and mitochondrial dysfunction. Mitochondria function decline, oxidative stress response in aging, and accumulation of aberrant proteins may contribute to ARD. The consumption of carotenoids may block ROS production.

7.1. Eye Disorders

Visual impairment has become the second most common cause of lived with disability [88]. Diabetic retinopathy, glaucoma, cataract, and age-related macular degeneration (AMD) are the most common types of vision loss among the elderly [89]. The development of AMD is not only due to the age factor, other factors, for example diet, oxidative stress, and smoking, may also increase the risk [90]. Tosini et al. [91] revealed that prolonged exposure to blue light emitted by energy-efficient lightbulbs and electronics enhanced retinal cell damage. This study further demonstrated that long-term exposure to energy-efficient lightbulbs and electronics can reduce visual function and promote AMD [91].

AMD is the predominant contributor of blindness among the elderly aged 75 years and above in developed countries [92,93]. AMD contributes approximately 8.7% of all blindness globally [94]. Notably, some research has emerged to predict that the percentage of AMD patients will double between 2010 and 2050 [95]. Non-proliferative postmitotic cells including retinal pigment epithelium cell and photoreceptors are particularly sensitive to oxidative damage due to the absence of DNA damage detection systems compared to other cells [96]. In the context of cataracts, zeaxanthin and lutein therapy has provided significant beneficial outcomes [97]. Zeaxanthin/lutein (2 mg/10 mg) significantly reduced the risk of cataract surgery [98]. Moreover, AMD is inversely correlated with the dietary intake of a carotenoid-rich diet (5–10 mg/day) compared to those individuals who rarely or never consume carotenoids [98].

Carotenoids have been demonstrated as an eye-sight protecting agent [99]. Such carotenoids are categorized as pro-vitamin A comprised of the unsubstituted β-ionone ring (γ-carotene, α-carotene, β-carotene, and β-cryptoxanthin) which can be converted into retinal [100]. Two dietary carotenoids, namely zeaxanthin and lutein, are macular pigments found in the human retina [101]. Macular pigments exert antioxidant properties, which can absorb short wavelengths and high energy blue light, and subsequently protect the retina from photochemical damage [86]. This pigment can protect against UV-induced peroxidation and neutralize ROS [101].

Deficiency of vitamin A affects immunity, which can damage the light-sensitive receptors [102]. Further, vitamin A deficiency may also lead to permanent blindness called xerophthalmia [103]. The previous study stated that supplementation with carotenoids such as zeaxanthin (2 mg/day/year) and lutein (10–20 mg/day/year) can increase macular pigment optical density levels [104,105]. Several studies reported by Hammond et al. [104] and Nolan et al. [106] also showed that zeaxanthin/lutein (2 mg/10 mg/day/year) can enhance visual performance such as photostress recovery, glare tolerance, and contrast sensitivity. Collectively, carotenoid intake could be a potential approach for the amelioration of oxidative stress and provide potential benefits for ocular health and function. The potential implication of carotenoids on AMD, as well as the dosage of the zeaxanthin and lutein when combined with other nutrients is worthy of further investigation in randomized clinical trials.

7.2. Neurodegenerative Diseases

Dementia is a chronic and progressive neurodegenerative disease in which there is deterioration in behavior, thinking, memory, and the ability to perform daily activities [107]. Dementia has become one of the major causes of disability and dependency among older people and contributes to nearly 60% of the total cases. It is projected that by 2050 there will be 152 million dementia cases in low- and middle-income countries [107]. Alzheimer's disease is the most common form of dementia and accounts for nearly 60–70% of cases [107].

The data from the previous study revealed that the concentration of carotenoids is passively associated with cognitive performance in both cognitively intact and cognitively impaired people [108,109]. A human study involving 91 healthy individuals suggested that twelve months supplementation with lutein (10 mg/day), zeaxanthin (2 mg/day), and meso-zeaxanthin (10 mg/day) improved the memory compared to the placebo control group [110]. A study reported by Rubin et al. [111] also demonstrated that carotenoids (16 mg/day for 26 days) are inversely associated with inflammatory markers, for instance interleukin (IL)-1β, tumor necrosis factor-α (TNF-α), IL-6, vascular cell adhesion molecule-1 (VCAM-1), and monocyte chemoattractant protein 1 (MCP-1) in both human and animal models. A study analyzed of 3031 participants aged 40–75 years revealed that total carotenoids (1.63 μmol/L) were negatively correlated with retinol binding protein 4 (RBP4) [112]. RBP4 also known as adipose-derived cytokine is a sole retinol transporter in the blood which is secreted from the adipocyte and liver [113]. RBP4 plays a crucial role as a proinflammatory marker by activating c-Jun N-terminal kinase (JNK) and nuclear factor-kappa B (NF-κB) pathways [114,115], as well as increasing the secretion of IL-1β, IL-6, and TNF-α expression. Thus, controlling systemic inflammation could be a targetable tool for the prevention of ARD.

Much information indicates that carotenoids may limit neuronal damage from free radicals, which is potentially served as a modifiable risk factor for cognitive decline. The data from 2011–2014 National Health and Nutrition Examination Survey involving 2796 participants aged ≥60 years demonstrated that lutein and zeaxanthin supplementation (2.02 mg/day) may prevent cognitive decline [116]. Carotenoids delay neurodegenerative diseases progression through several pathways, for example suppress proinflammatory cytokines [117], trigger Aβ peptide production [118], and reduce oxidative stress [119]. Due to its high binding energy with Alzheimer's disease-associated receptors (histone deacetylase and P53 kinase receptors) [120], β-carotene is potential to be an Alzheimer' disease antagonist. Fucoxanthin, a marine carotenoid, destabilizes Aβ fibril and inhibits Aβ formation [121]. Likewise, Ono and Yamada [122] reported that both β-carotene and vitamin A can block the oligomerization of Aβ42 and Aβ40 during Aβ peptide formation. Further, lycopene (1–4 mg/kg body weight/14 days) also decreases the Aβ42-induced inflammatory cytokine, for instance TNF-α, NF-κB, IL-1β, and transforming growth factor beta (TGF-β) in the brain [123]. High serum carotenoid levels such as lycopene, zeaxanthin, and lutein were found to reduce Alzheimer's disease mortality [124]. Collectively, carotenoids play a significant role as an antioxidant to delay the progression of neurodegenerative disease.

7.3. Cardiovascular Disease

According to the World Health Organization [125], nearly 17.9 million people die from CVD, represents 31% of all deaths worldwide. About 85% of all CVD deaths are due to strokes and heart attacks [125]. CVD is the disorder of blood vessels and the heart such as cerebrovascular disease, rheumatic heart disease, and coronary heart disease [125]. CVD is the major clinical concern in the elderly, with 68% of individuals aged 60–79 years having CVD and the prevalence is increased to 85% among people aged 80 years and above [126]. Oxidative stress is implicated in the development and progression of CVD [127]. High oxidative stress in the heart is one of the common characteristics of CVD [128]. Indeed, reduced antioxidant defense and enhanced ROS accumulation can cause systemic oxidative damage in CVD patients [129].

Carotenoids have been reported to prevent oxidative stress-induced diseases including CVD [130]. The implication of carotenoids against pathophysiology of CVD has been widely studied in both in vivo and in vitro models [131,132]. Lutein suppresses the NF-κB activation which plays a prominent role in the pathogenesis of several human diseases [133]. The anti-inflammatory and antioxidant properties of lutein (1–25 µM/24 h) reduced the risk of coronary artery disease [134] and CVD [135] in the elderly population. Lutein consumption (one soft boiled egg per day for 4 weeks) was shown to reduce the oxidized low-density lipoprotein (LDL), implies that lutein may prevent the development of atherosclerosis [136]. High plasma lutein levels were found to protect the myocardium from ischemia injury by decreasing oxidative stress and apoptosis [135]. A meta-analysis involving 387,569 participants suggested that a high lutein intake or high lutein concentration in the blood reduced the risk of stroke and coronary heart disease [137]. The previous study reported by Costa-Rodrigues et al. [138] further revealed that carotenoids (lycopene) are of benefit in the protection of vascular, endothelial, and cardiac. Moreover, research evidence also indicates that carotenoids reduce LDL-cholesterol plasma levels [139] and promote high-density lipoprotein (HDL) functionality (three eggs for 30 days) [140]. Compared to those who rarely or deficient in lycopene, individuals who supplemented with lycopene may trigger a significant reduction in coronary artery disease [141]. Although most of the studies have reported a positive effect of lycopene on cardiovascular health, not all data demonstrated such a link. Several human intervention studies failed to identify an inverse relationship between lycopene intake and CVD markers [140,142–145]. There are many reasons underlying these negative associations. Both the metabolism and bioavailability of lycopene are highly affected by genetic variability, as they are found in more than 28 single nucleotide polymorphisms in 16 genes [146,147]. In addition, the cardiovascular markers utilized in different studies also varied significantly, which makes detailed comparisons difficult. A difference in lycopene sources and doses may also reduce the lycopene effects, which in turn influence the observed effects. Further, most of the studies used less than 100 subjects, which reduce the statistical power of the results. Therefore, further studies should be performed in large populations, preferably from the same geographic location to avoid high genetic variability. The processing method and amount of tomatoes ingested also should be strictly controlled [138]. Taken together, carotenoid intake might be a promising strategy to enhance cardiovascular health.

7.4. Cancer

Cancer represents the second most common cause of death worldwide, with nearly 9.6 million deaths and 18.1 million new cases in 2018 [148,149]. Emerging research evidence has suggested that 30–50% of cancer deaths could be prevented by modifying the key risk factors, for instance exercise regularly, maintaining healthy body weight, reducing alcohol consumption, and avoiding tobacco [148].

Carotenoids have been reported to decrease the risk of certain cancers such as colon [150], prostate [151], and lung [152]. Several carotenoids, for instance lutein, zeaxanthin, and lycopene, have been reported to decrease the inflammatory mediator's production through the blockage of NF-κB pathway [153,154]. Lutein was found to negatively link to several types of cancer. A study obtained by Chang et al. [133] reported that lutein decreases the proliferation of breast cancer cells, ameliorates ROS, and improves the expression of cellular antioxidant enzymes via activation of nuclear factor E2-related factor 2 (Nrf2)/antioxidant responsive element (ARE) and inhibition of NF-κB pathways. In prostate cancer patients aged 64–75 years, high carrot, tomatoes, and lycopene intakes were shown to decrease the risk of prostate cancer compared to those with low carrot, tomatoes, and lycopene consumption [22]. The data from a human population-based study involving 638 independently living elderly aged 65–85 years revealed that increased serum carotenoid levels are inversely associated with cancer mortality [155]. The preventive role of carotenoids against cancer could be attributed to their antioxidant activity. In fact, the anticancer ability of carotenoids such as lycopene is modulated via several mechanisms such as apoptosis, cell cycle arrest, phase II detoxifying enzymes, and growth factor signaling [156]. However, a previous study revealed that smokers who supplemented with β-carotene (20 mg/day for 5–8 years) experienced increased lung cancer incidence, and these findings were not associated with the nicotine or tar level of cigarettes smoked, suggesting that all smokers should continue to avoid β-carotene supplementation [157]. The detrimental effect of β-carotene supplementation in smokers could be due to the instability of the β-carotene molecule in the lung after exposure to cigarette smoke. Oxidized β-carotene metabolites diminish retinoic acid levels and thus enhance lung carcinogenesis [158]. Taken together, regular consumption of carotenoids may become a useful approach to ameliorate oxidative stress. The beneficial effect of carotenoids in relation to cancer is worth attention.

7.5. Diabetes Mellitus

Diabetes mellitus is a chronic disease due to the deficiency or ineffective of the pancreas to produce insulin. The prevalence of diabetes has risen from 108 million in 1980 to 422 million in 2014 [159]. Nearly 1.6 million people worldwide died due to diabetes in 2016 [159]. Type 2 diabetes is the most common form of the disease, accounting nearly 90% of all diabetes mellitus cases worldwide [159]. Diabetes mellitus is a progressive disease, accompanied by complications including macro- and microvascular damage, neuropathy, retinopathy, and nephropathy [160].

Oxidative stress has been recognized as a key risk factor in the development of diabetes [161]. Several risk factors for instance aging, obesity, and unhealthy dietary intake, all contribute to an oxidative environment and subsequently alter the insulin sensitivity via impairment of glucose tolerance or promote the insulin resistance [162]. Hyperglycemia is commonly related to diabetes and leads to the progression and an overall oxidative environment [163]. The dysregulation of cellular and molecular process is common in type 2 diabetes, particularly in β-cells. Reactive nitrogen species (RNS) and ROS, for instance hydroxyl radical ($OH\cdot$), peroxynitrite ($ONOO-$), NO, superoxide anion ($O_2^{\bullet-}$), and H_2O_2, all contribute to key metabolic and physiologic processes [164,165].

Another common carotenoid, astaxanthin, is a potent antioxidant for the prevention and treatment of diabetes. An animal study has shown that astaxanthin (1.0 mg/mouse/day for 13 weeks) decreases blood glucose levels, improves insulin serum levels, and reduces glucose tolerance in type 2 diabetes mellitus rodent models [166]. A 10-year prospective study involving 37,846 men and women revealed that high dietary intake of β-carotene (10 ± 4 mg/day) can reduce the risk of type 2 diabetes mellitus [167]. A low serum β-carotene level has also been associated with impaired insulin sensitivity [168]. Another common carotenoid, fucoxanthin has been demonstrated to prevent diabetes mellitus. Maeda et al. [169] revealed that feeding obese mice Fucoxanthin-rich Wakame lipids (1.06–2.22%) may restore insulin and blood glucose levels via the upregulation of glucose transporter type 4 (GLUT4) mRNA expression in the skeletal muscle. A previous study reported by Manabe et al. [170] evaluated astaxanthin in relation to inflammatory markers and proinflammatory cytokine production. The data showed that astaxanthin ($10^{-7}–10^{-4}$ M) reduces high glucose-induced ROS production in the mitochondria and downregulates the expression of cyclooxygenase-2 (COX-2), TGF-β, NF-κB, and MCP-1. In a further study focused on inflammation outcomes, Kim et al. [171] found that astaxanthin inhibits the peroxynitrite ($ONOO^-$), nitric oxide (NO), and superoxide (O_2^-) induced by high glucose concentration. These data suggest that astaxanthin may exert the potential in the prevention of diabetic nephropathy. The Epidemiology of Vascular Aging Study involving 127 diabetes cases and 1389 volunteers aged 59–71 years revealed that individuals with high plasma carotenoid levels were significantly reduced the risk of dysglycemia [172]. Collectively, carotenoids may be a useful nutritional intervention for diabetes and its complications.

7.6. Osteoporosis

Osteoporosis is the most common metabolic bone disease, which is characterized by low bone mass and increase bone fragility [173]. Osteoporosis has become a global epidemic, affecting more than 8.9 million fractures annually worldwide [174]. Nearly 75% of the distal forearm, spine, and hip fractures occur in patients aged 65 years and above [175]. By 2050, the incidence of hip fracture is expected to increase by 240% and 310% in women and men, respectively [176].

Studies in both in vivo and in vitro models have suggested that carotenoids could prevent bone loss via the reduction of oxidative stress. Osteoclastogenesis and the apoptosis of osteocytes and osteoblasts are accelerated with the presence of oxidative stress, and subsequently lead to bone resorption [177,178]. A study found that a high intake of β-carotene, β-cryptoxanthin, and lutein/zeaxanthin reduces the risk of hip fracture in the middle-aged and elderly population [179]. Further, epidemiological studies have also found that a dietary intake of carotenoids may decrease the risk of osteoporosis [180] and improve bone mineral density [181]. The in vivo study further demonstrated that lutein (50 mg/kg for 4 weeks) protects the ovariectomized rats against oxidative stress and osteoporosis by downregulating the inflammation and osteoclast-specific marker (NFATc1) expression via Nrf2 activation [182]. Likewise, Tominari et al. [183] also showed that lutein (3, 10, and 30 μM) suppresses osteoclastic bone resorption and enhances bone formation. High serum lutein and zeaxanthin levels increase bone density in young healthy adults, suggesting that lutein and zeaxanthin play a pivotal role in optimal bone health [184].

8. Carotenoids and Aging

Numerous animal and clinical studies suggest that a diet rich in antioxidants can prevent aging [185]. In support of this, an animal study has revealed that lutein could prolong the lifespan and ameliorate the mortality rate induced by hydrogen peroxide and paraquat in Drosophila melanogaster [186]. The data showed that supplementation with 0.1 mg/mL lutein significantly increased the mean lifespan of Oregon-R-C (OR) wild type flies by 11.35% compared to the control group [186]. This study further revealed that the maximum lifespan is increased more than 11.23 days after supplementation with 0.1 mg/mL lutein compared to the control [186]. Similarly, the study obtained by Neena et al. [187] has also demonstrated that lutein (0.5, 1.5, 5, 15 μM) could reduce the age-associated decline in human skin cells. Despite none of the clinical study demonstrating that a diet high in lutein could promote human lifespan, several human clinical studies revealed that a dosage ranging from 2.4–30 mg/day is beneficial to human health without undesirable outcomes [188]. In another study, Yazaki et al. [189] showed that astaxanthin (0.1–1 mM) can prolong the lifespan in the wild-type and long-lived mutant age-1 of C. elegans. The data revealed that astaxanthin increased DAF-16 gene expression and reduced mitochondrial production of ROS, suggesting that carotenoid is partially involved in the modulation of insulin-like growth factor 1 (IGF-1) signaling [189]. Indeed, IGF-1 plays a predominant role in biological aging [190]. Fucoxanthin (0.3–1.0 μM) has also been reported to prolong lifespan and promote the viability of the organism such as Drosophila melanogaster and C. elegans [191]. An adequate intake of lutein-rich food is vitally important throughout the lifespan. The previous finding suggests that carotenoids such as lutein play an important role in neural health (cognitive and visual function) in adults [192], implying that carotenoids may provide an optimal or better health outcome.

9. Safety and Toxicity

In a well-balanced diet, the intake of carotenoids, such as lutein, is sufficient to maintain health. However, supplementation is needed in cases of chronic disease or the inadequate absorption of carotenoids. Several studies conducted in both in vitro [193] and animal models [193,194] have revealed that the use of lutein is safe without teratogenic and mutagenic outcomes. Despite the fact that no toxic effect was observed during lutein supplementation in both intervention and epidemiological studies [195], the Joint Expert Committee on Food Additives established an upper safety limit for daily lutein consumption of 2 mg/kg [196]. Whereas the European Food Safety Authority (EFSA) indicated an upper safety limit of 1 mg/kg [197]. EFSA further established an upper limit for lutein-enriched milk for infants of 250 µg/L [198]. Notably, the data showed that there is no interaction between lutein consumption and cytochrome P450 enzyme activity, suggesting that lutein may not modify the metabolism of endogenous or exogenous substances [199]. An animal study has shown that mice lacking β-carotene oxygenase 2 significantly increased the mitochondrial dysfunction and oxidative stress as well as developed pathologic carotenoid accumulation [200]. This finding implied that an excessive carotenoid intake may contribute to toxicity under certain circumstances. Olmedilla et al. [201] found that the supplementation of lutein at a dosage of 15 mg/day for 20 weeks increased the risk of skin yellowing (carotenodermia). Similarly, the data from the observational study revealed that lutein may increase the risk of lung cancer, particularly non-small cell lung cancer in smokers [202]. The population-based study has also reported that lutein supplementation increased the risk of crystalline maculopathy in old women. The adverse outcomes are reversed after lutein intake discontinuation [203]. Although research has demonstrated a positive association between lutein and the risk of several diseases, the survey conducted by EFSA concluded that the data obtained were insufficient to show an adverse outcome [197]. Consistent with the data reported by EFSA, the Age-Related Eye Disease Study 2 (AREDS2) intervention study did not identify any risk of lung cancer after lutein supplementation [204,205]. Based on the evidence, it is suggested that chronic lutein supplementation at the dosage of 10 mg/day is safe and non-toxic [204,205].

10. Conclusions

A high intake of fruits and leafy green vegetables is important to achieve adequate dietary levels of carotenoids among other nutrients. Based on the evidence, an adequate diet is recommended rather than supplementation in order to maintain physical health. The previous finding suggests that high dietary consumption of zeaxanthin and lutein are likely to protect against ARD such as AMD. Although the beneficial effects of carotenoids for reducing the risk of ARD have been demonstrated in both in vivo and in vitro studies, there are still some controversies surrounding certain effects of carotenoids in ARD that need to be elucidated by long-term clinical trials with large cohorts of the general population. Moreover, further studies are warranted to evaluate the precise mechanism of action under pathological and healthy conditions to enhance the implementation and acceptance of carotenoids for use in clinical practice. Therefore, researchers should further investigate the underlying mechanism of action to better elucidate the possible role of carotenoids on human health.

Author Contributions: B.L.T. conceived and designed the review and wrote the manuscript. M.E.N. edited the manuscript. All authors read and approved the final manuscript.

Acknowledgments: We would like to thank the Ministry of Science, Technology, and Innovation (MOSTI), Malaysia (project no. 02-01-04-SF2141) for financial support.

References

1.   World Health Organization. Global Health Observatory (GHO) data, Life Expectancy. 2019. Available online: https://www.who.int/gho/mortality_burden_disease/life_tables/en/ (accessed on 3 March 2019).

2. World Health Organization. World Health Statistics–Large Gains in Life Expectancy. 2014. Available online: http://www.who.int/mediacentre/news/releases/2014/world-health-statistics-2014/en/ (accessed on 3 March 2019).

3. Bruins, M.J.; Van Dael, P.; Eggersdorfer, M. The role of nutrients in reducing the risk for noncommunicable diseases during aging. *Nutrients* **2019**, *11*, 85. [CrossRef] [PubMed]

4. Jin, K.; Simpkins, J.W.; Ji, X.; Leis, M.; Stambler, I. The critical need to promote research of aging and aging-related diseases to improve health and longevity of the elderly population. *Aging Dis.* **2015**, *6*, 1. [CrossRef]

5. Rahal, A.; Kumar, A.; Singh, V.; Yadav, B.; Tiwari, R.; Chakraborty, S.; Dhama, K. Oxidative stress, prooxidants, and antioxidants: The interplay. *BioMed Res. Int.* **2014**, *2014*. [CrossRef]

6. Gudkov, S.V.; Guryev, E.L.; Gapeyev, A.B.; Sharapov, M.G.; Bunkin, N.F.; Shkirin, A.V.; Zabelina, T.S.; Glinushkin, A.P.; Sevost'yanov, M.A.; Belosludtsev, K.N.; et al. Unmodified hydrated C60 fullerene molecules exhibit antioxidant properties, prevent damage to DNA and proteins induced by reactive oxygen species and protect mice against injuries caused by radiation-induced oxidative stress. *Nanomedicine* **2019**, *15*, 37–46. [CrossRef] [PubMed]

7. Giudetti, A.M.; Salzet, M.; Cassano, T. Oxidative stress in aging brain: Nutritional and pharmacological interventions for neurodegenerative disorders. *Oxid. Med. Cell. Longev.* **2018**, *2018*. [CrossRef]

8. Tan, B.L.; Norhaizan, M.E.; Huynh, K.; Heshu, S.R.; Yeap, S.K.; Hazilawati, H.; Roselina, K. Water extract of brewers' rice induces apoptosis in human colorectal cancer cells via activation of caspase-3 and caspase-8 and downregulates the Wnt/β-catenin downstream signaling pathway in brewers' rice-treated rats with azoxymethane-induced colon carcinogenesis. *BMC Complement. Altern. Med.* **2015**, *15*, 205.

9. Liu, Z.; Zhou, T.; Ziegler, A.C.; Dimitrion, P.; Zuo, L. Oxidative stress in neurodegenerative diseases: From molecular mechanisms to clinical applications. *Oxid. Med. Cell. Longev.* **2017**, *2017*. [CrossRef]

10. Chistiakov, D.A.; Sobenin, I.A.; Revin, V.V.; Orekhov, A.N.; Bobryshev, Y.V. Mitochondrial aging and age-related dysfunction of mitochondria. *BioMed Res. Int.* **2014**, *2014*. [CrossRef]

11. Eckmann, J.; Eckert, S.H.; Leuner, K.; Muller, W.E.; Eckert, G.P. Mitochondria: Mitochondrial membranes in brain ageing and neurodegeneration. *Int. J. Biochem. Cell Biol.* **2013**, *45*, 76–80. [CrossRef] [PubMed]

12. Liguori, I.; Russo, G.; Curcio, F.; Bulli, G.; Aran, L.; Della-Morte, D.; Gargiulo, G.; Testa, G.; Cacciatore, F.; Bonaduce, D.; et al. Oxidative stress, aging, and diseases. *Clin. Interv. Aging.* **2018**, *13*, 757–772. [CrossRef] [PubMed]

13. Maulik, N.; McFadden, D.; Otani, H.; Thirunavukkarasu, M.; Parinandi, N.L. Antioxidants in longevity and medicine. *Oxid. Med. Cell. Longev.* **2013**, *2013*. [CrossRef] [PubMed]

14. Corbi, G.; Acanfora, D.; Iannuzzi, G.L.; Longobardi, G.; Cacciatore, F.; Furgi, G.; Filippelli, A.; Rengo, G.; Leosco, D.; Ferrara, N. Hypermagnesemia predicts mortality in elderly with congestive heart disease: Relationship with laxative and antacid use. *Rejuvenation Res.* **2008**, *11*, 129–138. [CrossRef]

15. Stadtman, E.R.; Berlett, B.S. Reactive oxygen–mediated protein oxidation in aging and disease. *Chem. Res. Toxicol.* **1997**, *10*, 485–494. [CrossRef] [PubMed]

16. López-Otín, C.; Blasco, M.A.; Partridge, L.; Serrano, M.; Kroemer, G. The hallmarks of aging. *Cell* **2013**, *153*, 1194–1217.

17. Dias, V.; Junn, E.; Mouradian, M.M. The role of oxidative stress in Parkinson's disease. *J. Parkinson's Dis.* **2013**, *3*, 461–491.

18. Zuo, L.; Zhou, T.; Pannell, B.K.; Ziegler, A.; Best, T.M. Biological and physiological role of reactive oxygen species–the good, the bad and the ugly. *Acta Physiol.* **2015**, *214*, 329–348. [CrossRef]

19. Tan, B.L.; Norhaizan, M.E.; Liew, W.-P.P.; Rahman, H.S. Antioxidant and oxidative stress: A mutual interplay in age-related diseases. *Front. Pharmacol.* **2018**, *9*, 1162. [CrossRef]

20. Cheng, H.M.; Koutsidis, G.; Lodge, J.K.; Ashor, A.W.; Siervo, M.; Lara, J. Lycopene and tomato and risk of cardiovascular diseases: A systematic review and meta-analysis of epidemiological evidence. *Crit. Rev. Food Sci. Nutr.* **2019**, *59*, 141–158. [CrossRef] [PubMed]

21. Palozza, P.; Catalano, A.; Simone, R.E.; Mele, M.C.; Cittadini, A. Effect of lycopene and tomato products on cholesterol metabolism. *Ann. Nutr. MeTable* **2012**, *61*, 126–134. [CrossRef] [PubMed]

22. Hoang, D.V.; Pham, N.M.; Lee, A.H.; Tran, D.N.; Binns, C.W. Dietary carotenoid intakes and prostate cancer risk: A case-control study from Vietnam. *Nutrients* **2018**, *10*, 70. [CrossRef]

23. Hou, L.L.; Gao, C.; Chen, I.; Hu, G.Q.; Xie, S.Q. Essential role of autophagy in fucoxanthin-induced cytotoxicity to human epithelial cervical cancer HeLa cells. *Acta Pharmacol. Sin.* **2013**, *34*, 1403–1410. [CrossRef]

24. Satomi, Y. Antitumor and cancer-preventative function of fucoxanthin: A marine carotenoid. *Anticancer Res.* **2017**, *37*, 1557–1562. [CrossRef]

25. Alós, E.; Rodrigo, M.J.; Zacarias, L. Manipulation of carotenoid content in plants to improve human health. In *Carotenoids in Nature*; Springer: Cham Switzerland, 2016; pp. 311–343.

26. Du, X.; Song, K.; Wang, J.; Cong, R.; Li, L.; Zhang, G. Draft genome and SNPs associated with carotenoid accumulation in adductor muscles of bay scallop (*Argopecten irradians*). *J. Genomics* **2017**, *5*, 83. [CrossRef]

27. Singh, G.; Sahota, H.K. Impact of benzimidazole and dithiocarbamate fungicides on the photosynthetic machinery, sugar content and various antioxidative enzymes in chickpea. *Plant Physiol. Biochem.* **2018**, *132*, 166–173. [CrossRef]

28. Gauger, T.; Konhauser, K.; Kappler, A. Protection of phototrophic iron (II)-oxidizing bacteria from UV irradiation by biogenic iron (III) minerals: Implications for early Archean banded iron formation. *Geology* **2015**, *43*, 1067–1070. [CrossRef]

29. Paliwal, C.; Ghosh, T.; George, B.; Pancha, I.; Maurya, R.; Chokshi, K.; Ghosh, A.; Mishra, S. Microalgal carotenoids: Potential nutraceutical compounds with chemotaxonomic importance. *Algal Res.* **2016**, *15*, 24–31. [CrossRef]

30. Khachik, F. Distribution and metabolism of dietary carotenoids in humans as a criterion for development of nutritional supplements. *Pure Appl. Chem.* **2006**, *78*, 1551–1557. [CrossRef]

31. Parker, R.S. Carotenoids in human blood and tissues. *J. Nutr.* **1989**, *119*, 101–104. [CrossRef]

32. Yaroshevich, I.; Krasilnikov, P.; Rubin, A. Functional interpretation of the role of cyclic carotenoids in photosynthetic antennas via quantum chemical calculations. *Comput. Theor. Chem.* **2015**, *1070*, 27–32. [CrossRef]

33. Berman, J.; Zorrilla-López, U.; Farré, G.; Zhu, C.; Sandmann, G.; Twyman, R.M.; Capell, T.; Christou, P. Nutritionally important carotenoids as consumer products. *Phytochem. Rev.* **2015**, *14*, 727–743. [CrossRef]

34. Harrison, E.H.; Curley, R.W. Carotenoids and retinoids: Nomenclature, chemistry, and analysis. In *The Biochemistry of Retinoid Signaling II*; Springer: Dordrecht, the Netherlands, 2016; pp. 1–19.

35. Gabriel, H.B.; Silva, M.F.; Kimura, E.A.; Wunderlich, G.; Katzin, A.M.; Azevedo, M.F. Squalestatin is an inhibitor of carotenoid biosynthesis in Plasmodium falciparum. *Antimicrob. Agents Chemother.* **2015**, *59*, 3180–3188. [CrossRef] [PubMed]

36. Fiedor, J.; Burda, K. Potential role of carotenoids as antioxidants in human health and disease. *Nutrients* **2014**, *6*, 466–488. [CrossRef]

37. Nishino, A.; Yasui, H.; Maoka, T. Reaction of paprika carotenoids, capsanthin and capsorubin, with reactive oxygen species. *J. Agric. Food Chem.* **2016**, *64*, 4786–4792. [CrossRef]

38. Langi, P.; Kiokias, S.; Varzakas, T.; Proestos, C. Carotenoids: From plants to food and feed industries. In *Microbial Carotenoids. Methods in Molecular Biology*; Barreiro, C., Barredo, J.L., Eds.; Humana Press: New York, NY, USA, 2018; Volume 1852, pp. 57–71.

39. Johnson, E.J. The role of carotenoids in human health. *Nutr. Clin. Care* **2002**, *5*, 56–65. [CrossRef]

40. Yahia, E.M.; Ornelas-Paz, J.d.J. Chemistry, stability, and biological actions of carotenoids. In *Fruit and Vegetable Phytochemicals Chemistry, Nutritional Value and Stability*; de la Rosa, L.A., Alvarez-Parrilla, E., González-Aguilar, G.A., Eds.; Wiley-Blackwell: Ames, IA, USA, 2010; pp. 177–222.

41. Lin, Q.; Liang, R.; Williams, P.A.; Zhong, F. Factors affecting the bioaccessibility of β-carotene in lipid-based microcapsules: Digestive conditions, the composition, structure and physical state of microcapsules. *Food Hydrocoll.* **2018**, *77*, 187–203. [CrossRef]

42. Thane, C.; Reddy, S. Processing of fruits and vegetables: Effect on carotenoids. *Nutr. Food Sci.* **1997**, *2*, 58–65. [CrossRef]

43. Hart, D.J.; Scott, K.J. Development and evaluation of an HPLC method for the analysis of carotenoids in foods, and the measurement of the carotenoid content of vegetables and fruits commonly consumed in the UK. *Food Chem.* **1995**, *54*, 101–111. [CrossRef]

44. Calva, M.M. Lutein: A valuable ingredient of fruit and vegetables. *Crit. Rev. Food Sci. Nutr.* **2005**, *45*, 671–696. [CrossRef] [PubMed]

45. Van den Berg, H.; Faulks, R.; Granado, H.F.; Hirschberg, J.; Olmedilla, B.; Sandmann, G.; Southon, S.; Stahl, W. The potential for the improvement of carotenoid levels in foods and the likely systemic effects. *J. Sci. Food Agric.* **2000**, *80*, 880–912. [CrossRef]

46. Granado, F.; Olmedilla, B.; Blanco, I.; Rojas-Hidalgo, E. Carotenoid composition in raw and cooked Spanish vegetables. *J. Agric. Food Chem.* **1992**, *40*, 2135–2140. [CrossRef]

47. US Department of Agriculture, Agricultural Research Service, Nutrient Data Laboratory. USDA National Nutrient Database for Standard Reference. 2016. Available online: http://www.ars.usda.gov/ba/bhnrc/ndl (accessed on 15 March 2016).

48. Maiani, G.; Periago Caston, M.J.; Catasta, G.; Toti, E.; Cambrodon, I.G.; Bysted, A.; Granado-Lorencio, F.; Olmedilla-Alonso, B.; Knuthsen, P.; Valoti, M.; et al. Carotenoids: Actual knowledge on food sources, intakes, stability and bioavailability and their protective role in humans. *Mol. Nutr. Food Res.* **2009**, *53*, S194–S218. [CrossRef]

49. Marinova, D.; Ribarova, F. HPLC determination of carotenoids in Bulgarian berries. *J. Food Comp. Anal.* **2007**, *20*, 370–374. [CrossRef]

50. Perry, A.; Rasmussen, H.; Johnson, E. Xanthophyll (lutein, zeaxanthin) content in fruits, vegetables and corn and egg products. *J. Food Comp. Anal.* **2009**, *22*, 9–15. [CrossRef]

51. Kimura, M.; Rodriguez-Amaya, D.B. Carotenoid composition of hydroponic leafy vegetables. *J. Agric. Food Chem.* **2003**, *51*, 2603–2607. [CrossRef]

52. Setiawan, B.; Sulaeman, A.; Giraud, D.W.; Driskell, J.A. Carotenoid content of selected Indonesian fruits. *J. Food Compost. Anal.* **2001**, *14*, 169–176. [CrossRef]

53. Lee, H.S.; Coates, G.A. Effect of thermal pasteurization on Valencia orange juice color and pigments. *LWT Food Sci. Technol.* **2003**, *36*, 153–156. [CrossRef]

54. Marín, A.; Ferreres, F.; Tomás-Barberán, F.A.; Gil, M.I. Characterization and quantitation of antioxidant constituents of sweet pepper (*Capsicum annuum* L.). *J. Agric. Food Chem.* **2004**, *52*, 3861–3869.

55. Ameny, M.A.; Wilson, P.W. Relationship between hunter color values and β-carotene contents in white-fleshed African sweet potatoes (*Ipomoea batatas* Lam). *J. Sci. Food Agric.* **1997**, *73*, 301–306. [CrossRef]

56. Brown, M.J.; Ferruzzi, M.G.; Nguyen, M.L.; Cooper, D.A.; Eldridge, A.L.; Schwartz, S.J.; White, W.S. Carotenoid bioavailability is higher from salads ingested with full-fat than with fat-reduced salad dressings as measured with electrochemical detection. *Am. J. Clin. Nutr.* **2004**, *80*, 396–403. [CrossRef] [PubMed]

57. Ghavami, A.; Coward, W.A.; Bluck, L.J. The effect of food preparation on the bioavailability of carotenoids from carrots using intrinsic labelling. *Br. J. Nutr.* **2012**, *107*, 1350–1366. [CrossRef] [PubMed]

58. Kim, J.E.; Gordon, S.; Ferruzzi, M.; Campbell, W. Effects of whole egg consumption on carotenoids absorption from co-consumed, carotenoids-rich mixed-vegetable salad. *FASEB J.* **2015**, *29*, 1.

59. Goltz, S.R.; Campbell, W.W.; Chitchumroonchokchai, C.; Failla, M.L.; Ferruzzi, M.G. Meal triacylglycerol profile modulates postprandial absorption of carotenoids in humans. *Mol. Nutr. Food Res.* **2012**, *56*, 866–877. [CrossRef]

60. Reboul, E.; Thap, S.; Tourniaire, F.; Andre, M.; Juhel, C.; Morange, S.; Amiot, M.J.; Lairon, D.; Borel, P. Differential effect of dietary antioxidant classes (carotenoids, polyphenols, vitamins C and E) on lutein absorption. *Br. J. Nutr.* **2007**, *97*, 440–446. [CrossRef]

61. Riedl, J.; Linseisen, J.; Hoffmann, J.; Wolfram, G. Some dietary fibers reduce the absorption of carotenoids in women. *J. Nutr.* **1999**, *129*, 2170–2176. [CrossRef]

62. Van Het Hof, K.H.; West, C.E.; Weststrate, J.A.; Hautvast, J.G. Dietary factors that affect the bioavailability of carotenoids. *J. Nutr.* **2000**, *130*, 503–506. [CrossRef]

63. Hornero-Mendez, D.; Mínguez-Mosquera, M.-M. Bioaccessibility of carotenes from carrots: Effect of cooking and addition of oil. *Innov. Food Sci. Emerg. Technol.* **2007**, *8*, 407–412. [CrossRef]

64. Baskaran, V.; Sugawara, T.; Nagao, A. Phospholipids affect the intestinal absorption of carotenoids in mice. *Lipids* **2003**, *38*, 705–711. [CrossRef]

65. O'Connell, O.F.; Ryan, L.; O'Brien, N.M. Xanthophyll carotenoids are more bioaccessible from fruits than dark green vegetables. *Nutr. Res.* **2007**, *27*, 258–264. [CrossRef]

66. Prince, M.R.; Frisoli, J.K. Beta-carotene accumulation in serum and skin. *Am. J. Clin. Nutr.* **1993**, *57*, 175–181. [CrossRef]

67. Olson, J.A. Absorption, transport, and metabolism of carotenoids in humans. *Pure Appl. Chem.* **1994**, *66*, 1011–1016. [CrossRef]

68. Fernandez-Garcia, E.; Carvajal-Lerida, I.; Jaren-Galan, M.; Garrido-Fernandez, J.; Perez-Galvez, A.; Hornero-Mendez, D. Carotenoids bioavailability from foods: From plant pigments to efficient biological activities. *Food Res. Int.* **2012**, *46*, 438–450. [CrossRef]

69. Parker, R.S. Absorption, metabolism and transport of carotenoids. *FASEB J.* **1996**, *10*, 542–551. [CrossRef]

70. Erdman, J.W., Jr.; Bierer, T.L.; Gugger, E.T. Absorption and transport of carotenoids. *Ann. N. Y. Acad. Sci.* **1993**, *691*, 76–85. [CrossRef]

71. Rao, A.V.; Rao, L.G. Carotenoids and human health. *Pharmacol. Res.* **2007**, *55*, 207–216. [CrossRef]

72. Stahl, W.; Schwarz, W.; Sundquist, A.R.; Sies, H. cis-trans Isomers of lycopene and β-carotene in human serum and tissues. *Arch. Biochem. Biophys.* **1992**, *294*, 173–177. [CrossRef]

73. Darvin, M.E.; Sterry, W.; Landemann, J.; Vergou, T. The role of carotenoids in human skin. *Molecules* **2011**, *16*, 10491–10506. [CrossRef]

74. Castenmiller, J.J.M.; West, C.E. Bioavailability of carotenoids. *Pure Appl. Chem.* **1997**, *69*, 2145–2150. [CrossRef]

75. Yeum, K.-J.; Russell, R.M. Carotenoid bioavailability and bioconversion. *Ann. Rev. Nutr.* **2002**, *22*, 483–504. [CrossRef] [PubMed]

76. Nigam, Y.; Knight, J.; Bhattacharya, S.; Bayer, A. Physiological changes associated with aging and immobility. *J. Aging Res.* **2012**, *2012*. [CrossRef]

77. Navaratnarajah, A.; Jackson, S.H.D. The physiology of aging. *Medicine* **2017**, *45*, 6–10. [CrossRef]

78. Russell, R.M. Factors in aging that effect the bioavailability of nutrients. *J. Nutr.* **2001**, *131*, 1359S–1361S. [CrossRef]

79. Tang, G.W.; Serfaty-Lacrosniere, C.; Camilo, M.E.; Russell, R.M. Gastric acidity influences the blood response to a beta-carotene dose in humans. *Am. J. Clin. Nutr.* **1996**, *64*, 622–626. [CrossRef]

80. Farage, M.A.; Miller, K.W.; Elsner, P.; Maibach, H.I. Functional and physiological characteristics of the aging skin. *Aging Clin. Exp. Res.* **2008**, *20*, 195–200. [CrossRef]

81. Gholamian-Dehkordi, N.; Luther, T.; Asadi-Samani, M.; Mahmoudian-Sani, M.R. An overview on natural antioxidants for oxidative stress reduction in cancers; a systematic review. *Immunopathol. Persa.* **2017**, *3*, e12. [CrossRef]

82. Gaschler, M.M.; Stockwell, B.R. Lipid peroxidation in cell death. *Biochem. Biophys. Res. Commun.* **2017**, *482*, 419–425. [CrossRef]

83. Shen, Y.; Li, J.; Gu, R.; Yue, L.; Wang, H.; Zhan, X.; Xing, B. Carotenoid and superoxide dismutase are the most effective antioxidants participating in ROS scavenging in phenanthrene accumulated wheat leaf. *Chemosphere* **2018**, *197*, 513–525. [CrossRef] [PubMed]

84. Miller, N.J.; Sampson, J.; Candeias, L.P.; Bramley, P.M.; Rice-Evans, C.A. Antioxidant activities of carotenes and xanthophylls. *FEBS Lett.* **1996**, *384*, 240–242. [CrossRef]

85. Krinsky, N.I. The antioxidant and biological properties of the carotenoids. *Ann. N. Y. Acad. Sci.* **1998**, *854*, 443–447. [CrossRef]

86. Eggersdorfer, M.; Wyss, A. Carotenoids in human nutrition and health. *Arch. Biochem. Biophy.* **2018**, *652*, 18–26. [CrossRef]

87. Prasad, K.N.; Wu, M.; Bondy, S.C. Telomere shortening during aging: attenuation by antioxidants and anti-inflammatory agents. *Mech. Ageing Dev.* **2017**, *164*, 61–66. [CrossRef]

88. GBD 2015 DALYs; Hale Collaborators. Global, regional, and national disability-adjusted life-years (DALYs) for 315 diseases and injuries and healthy life expectancy (HALE), 1990–2015: A systematic analysis for the Global Burden of Disease Study 2015. *Lancet* **2016**, *388*, 1603–1658. [CrossRef]

89. Quillen, D.A. Common causes of vision loss in elderly patients. *Am. Fam. Physician* **1999**, *60*, 99–108.

90. Chen, Y.; Bedell, M.; Zhang, K. Age-related macular degeneration: Genetic and environmental factors of disease. *Mol. Interv.* **2010**, *10*, 271–281. [CrossRef]

91. Tosini, G.; Ferguson, I.; Tsubota, K. Effects of blue light on the circadian system and eye physiology. *Mol. Vis.* **2016**, *22*, 61–72.

92. Congdon, N.; O'Colmain, B.; Klaver, C.C.; Klein, R.; Muñoz, B.; Friedman, D.S.; Kempen, J.; Taylor, H.R.; Mitchell, P.; Eye Diseases Prevalence Research Group. Causes and prevalence of visual impairment among adults in the United States. *Arch. Ophthalmol.* **2004**, *122*, 477–485.

93. Resnikoff, S.; Pascolini, D.; Etya'ale, D.; Kocur, I.; Pararajasegaram, R.; Pokharel, G.P.; Mariotti, S.P. Global data on visual impairment in the year 2002. *Bull. World Health Organ.* **2004**, *82*, 844–851.

94. Wong, W.L.; Su, X.; Li, X.; Cheung, C.M.; Klein, R.; Cheng, C.-Y.; Wong, T.Y. Global prevalence of age-related macular degeneration and disease burden projection for 2020 and 2040: A systematic review and meta-analysis. *Lancet Glob. Health* **2014**, *2*, e106–e116. [CrossRef]

95. Eisenhauer, B.; Natoli, S.; Liew, G.; Flood, V.M. Lutein and zeaxanthin-food sources, bioavailability and dietary variety in age-related macular degeneration protection. *Nutrients* **2017**, *9*, 120. [CrossRef]

96. Blasiak, J.; Petrovski, G.; Veréb, Z.; Facskó, A.; Kaarniranta, K. Oxidative stress, hypoxia, and autophagy in the neovascular processes of age-related macular degeneration. *BioMed Res. Int.* **2014**, *2014*. [CrossRef] [PubMed]

97. Liu, X.-H.; Yu, R.B.; Liu, R.; Hao, Z.-X.; Han, C.-C.; Zhu, Z.-H.; Ma, L. Association between lutein and zeaxanthin status and the risk of cataract: A meta-analysis. *Nutrients* **2014**, *6*, 452–465. [CrossRef] [PubMed]

98. Age-Related Eye Disease Study 2 Research Group; Chew, E.Y.; SanGiovanni, J.P.; Ferris, F.L.; Wong, W.T.; Agron, E.; Clemons, T.E.; Sperduto, R.; Danis, R.; Chandra, S.R.; et al. Lutein/zeaxanthin for the treatment of age-related cataract: AREDS2 randomized trial report no. 4. *JAMA Ophthalmol.* **2013**, *131*, 843–850. [CrossRef] [PubMed]

99. Bungau, S.; Abdel-Daim, M.M.; Tit, D.M.; Ghanem, E.; Sato, S.; Maruyama-Inoue, M.; Yamane, S.; Kadonosono, K. Health benefits of polyphenols and carotenoids in age-related eye diseases. *Oxid. Med. Cell. Longev.* **2019**, *2019*. [CrossRef]

100. Sandmann, G. Carotenoids of biotechnological importance. *Adv. Biochem. Eng. Biotechnol.* **2015**, *148*, 449–467. [PubMed]

101. Bernstein, P.S.; Li, B.; Vachali, P.P.; Gorusupudi, A.; Shyam, R.; Henriksen, B.S.; Nolan, J.M. Lutein, zeaxanthin, and meso-zeaxanthin: The basic and clinical science underlying carotenoid-based nutritional interventions against ocular disease. *Prog. Retin. Eye Res.* **2016**, *50*, 34–66. [CrossRef]

102. Gonçalves, A.; Estevinho, B.N.; Rocha, F. Microencapsulation of vitamin A: A review. *Trends Food Sci. Tech.* **2016**, *51*, 76–87.

103. West, K.P. Epidemiology and prevention of vitamin A deficiency disorders. *Retinoids Biol. Biochem. Dis.* **2015**, 505–527.

104. Hammond, B.R.; Fletcher, L.M.; Roos, F.; Wittwer, J.; Schalch, W. A double-blind, placebo-controlled study on the effects of lutein and zeaxanthin on photostress recovery, glare disability, and chromatic contrast. *Investig. Ophthalmol. Vis. Sci.* **2014**, *55*, 8583–8589. [CrossRef] [PubMed]

105. Yao, Y.; Qiu, Q.H.; Wu, X.W.; Cai, Z.Y.; Xu, S.; Liang, X.Q. Lutein supplementation improves visual performance in Chinese drivers: 1-year randomized, double-blind, placebo-controlled study. *Nutrition* **2013**, *29*, 958–964. [CrossRef]

106. Nolan, J.M.; Power, R.; Stringham, J.; Dennison, J.; Stack, J.; Kelly, D.; Moran, R.; Akuffo, K.O.; Corcoran, L.; Beatty, S. Author response: Comments on enrichment of macular pigment enhances contrast sensitivity in subjects free of retinal disease: CREST-Report 1. *Investig. Ophthalmol. Vis. Sci.* **2016**, *57*, 5416. [CrossRef]

107. World Health Organization. Dementia. 2019. Available online: https://www.who.int/news-room/fact-sheets/detail/dementia (accessed on 5 March 2019).

108. Renzi, L.M.; Dengler, M.J.; Puente, A.; Miller, L.S.; Hammond, B.R.Jr. Relationships between macular pigment optical density and cognitive function in unimpaired and mildly cognitively impaired older adults. *Neurobiol. Aging* **2014**, *35*, 1695–1699. [CrossRef]

109. Feeney, J.; Finucane, C.; Savva, G.M.; Cronin, H.; Beatty, S.; Nolan, J.M.; Kenny, R.A. Low macular pigment optical density is associated with lower cognitive performance in a large, population-based sample of older adults. *Neurobiol. Aging* **2013**, *34*, 2449–2456. [CrossRef]

110. Rebecca, P.; Robert, C.; Stephen, B.; Riona, M.; Rachel, M.; Jim, S.; Alan, H.N.; John, N.M. Supplemental retinal carotenoids enhance memory in healthy individuals with low levels of macular pigment in a randomized, double-blind, placebo-controlled clinical trial. *J. Alzheimer's Dis.* **2018**, *61*, 947–961.

111. Rubin, L.P.; Ross, A.C.; Stephensen, C.B.; Bohn, T.; Tanumihardjo, S.A. Metabolic effects of inflammation on vitamin A and carotenoids in humans and animal models. *Adv. Nutr.* **2017**, *8*, 197–212. [CrossRef]

112. Jing, L.; Xiao, M.; Dong, H.; Lin, J.; Chen, G.; Ling, W.; Chen, Y. Serum carotenoids are inversely associated with RBP4 and other inflammatory markers in middle-aged and elderly adults. *Nutrients* **2018**, *10*, 260. [CrossRef]

113. Norseen, J.; Hosooka, T.; Hammarstedt, A.; Yore, M.M.; Kant, S.; Aryal, P.; Kiernan, U.A.; Phillips, D.A.; Maruyama, H.; Kraus, B.J.; et al. Retinol-binding protein 4 inhibits insulin signaling in adipocytes by inducing proinflammatory cytokines in macrophages through c-Jun N-terminal kinase- (JNK) and toll-like receptor 4-dependent and retinol-independent mechanism. *Mol. Cell. Biol.* **2012**, *32*, 2010–2019. [CrossRef]

114. Du, M.; Martin, A.; Hays, F.; Johnson, J.; Farjo, R.A.; Farjo, K.M. Serum retinol-binding protein-induced endothelial inflammation is mediated through the activation of toll-like receptor 4. *Mol. Vis.* **2017**, *23*, 185–197.

115. Moraes-Vieira, P.M.; Yore, M.M.; Dwyer, P.M.; Syed, I.; Aryal, P.; Kahn, B.B. RBP4 activates antigen-presenting cells leading to adipose tissue inflammation and systemic insulin resistance. *Cell MeTable* **2014**, *19*, 512–526. [CrossRef]

116. Christensen, K.; Gleason, C.E.; Mares, J.A. Dietary carotenoids and cognitive function among US adults, NHANES 2011–2014. *Nutr. Neurosci.* **2018**, 1–9. [CrossRef] [PubMed]

117. Hadad, N.; Levy, R. Combination of EPA with carotenoids and polyphenol synergistically attenuated the transformation of microglia to M1 phenotype via inhibition of NF-κB. *Neuromol. Med.* **2017**, *19*, 436–451. [CrossRef]

118. Lin, H.-C.; Lin, M.-H.; Liao, J.-H.; Wu, T.-H.; Lee, T.-H.; Mi, F.-L.; Wu, C.H.; Chen, K.C.; Cheng, C.H.; Lin, C.W. Antroquinonol, a ubiquinone derivative from the mushroom *Antrodia camphorata*, inhibits colon cancer stem cell-like properties: Insights into the molecular mechanism and inhibitory targets. *J. Agric. Food Chem.* **2017**, *65*, 51–59. [CrossRef] [PubMed]

119. Wang, J.; Li, L.; Wang, Z.; Cui, Y.; Tan, X.; Yuan, T.; Liu, Q.; Liu, Z.; Liu, X. Supplementation of lycopene attenuates lipopolysaccharide-induced amyloidogenesis and cognitive impairments via mediating neuroinflammation and oxidative stress. *J. Nutr. Biochem.* **2018**, *56*, 16–25. [CrossRef] [PubMed]

120. Krishnaraj, R.N.; Kumari, S.S.; Mukhopadhyay, S.S. Antagonistic molecular interactions of photosynthetic pigments with molecular disease targets: A new approach to treat AD and ALS. *J. Recept. Signal Transduct.* **2016**, *36*, 67–71. [CrossRef]

121. Xiang, S.; Liu, F.; Lin, J.; Chen, H.; Huang, C.; Chen, L.; Zhou, Y.; Ye, L.; Zhang, K.; Jin, J.; et al. Fucoxanthin inhibits β-amyloid assembly and attenuates β-amyloid oligomer-induced cognitive impairments. *J. Agric. Food Chem.* **2017**, *65*, 4092–4102. [CrossRef] [PubMed]

122. Ono, K.; Yamada, M. Vitamin A and Alzheimer's disease. *Geriatr. Gerontol. Int.* **2012**, *12*, 180–188. [CrossRef] [PubMed]

123. Sachdeva, A.K.; Chopra, K. Lycopene abrogates Aβ (1–42)-mediated neuroinflammatory cascade in an experimental model of Alzheimer's disease. *J. Nutr. Biochem.* **2015**, *26*, 736–744. [CrossRef] [PubMed]

124. Min, J.Y.; Min, K.B. Serum lycopene, lutein and zeaxanthin, and the risk of Alzheimer's disease mortality in older adults. *Dement. Geriatr. Cogn. Disord.* **2014**, *37*, 246–256. [CrossRef]

125. World Health Organization. Cardiovascular Disease. 2019. Available online: https://www.who.int/cardiovascular_diseases/en/ (accessed on 5 March 2019).

126. Leening, M.J.; Ferket, B.S.; Steyerberg, E.W.; Kavousi, M.; Deckers, J.W.; Nieboer, D.; Heeringa, J.; Portegies, M.L.; Hofman, A.; Ikram, M.A.; et al. Sex differences in lifetime risk and first manifestation of cardiovascular disease: Prospective population based cohort study. *BMJ* **2014**, *349*, g5992. [CrossRef] [PubMed]

127. Siti, H.N.; Kamisah, Y.; Kamsiah, J. The role of oxidative stress, antioxidants and vascular inflammation in cardiovascular disease (a review). *Vascul. Pharmacol.* **2015**, *71*, 40–56. [CrossRef]

128. Bugger, H.; Abel, E.D. Molecular mechanisms for myocardial mitochondrial dysfunction in the metabolic syndrome. *Clin. Sci.* **2008**, *114*, 195–210. [CrossRef]

129. Lee, R.; Margaritis, M.; Channon, M.K.; Antoniades, C. Evaluating oxidative stress in human cardiovascular disease: Methodological aspects and considerations. *Curr. Med. Chem.* **2012**, *19*, 2504–2520. [CrossRef] [PubMed]

130. Thies, F.; Mills, L.M.; Moir, S.; Masson, L.F. Cardiovascular benefits of lycopene: Fantasy or reality? *Proc. Nutr. Soc.* **2017**, *76*, 122–129. [CrossRef]

131. Alvi, S.S.; Iqbal, D.; Ahmad, S.; Khan, M.S. Molecular rationale delineating the role of lycopene as a potent HMG-CoA reductase inhibitor: In vitro and in silico study. *Nat. Prod. Res.* **2016**, *30*, 2111–2114. [CrossRef]

132. Sandoval, V.; Rodríguez-Rodríguez, R.; Martínez-Garza, U.; Rosell-Cardona, C.; Lamuela-Raventós, R.M.; Marrero, P.F.; Haro, D.; Relat, J. Mediterranean tomato-based sofrito sauce improves fibroblast growth factor 21 (FGF21) signaling in white adipose tissue of obese ZUCKER rats. *Mol. Nutr. Food Res.* **2018**, *62*, 1700606. [CrossRef]

133. Chang, J.; Zhang, Y.; Li, Y.; Lu, K.; Shen, Y.; Guo, Y.; Qi, Q.; Wang, M.; Zhang, S. NrF2/ARE and NF-κB pathway regulation may be the mechanism for lutein inhibition of human breast cancer cell. *Future Oncol.* **2018**, *14*, 719–726. [CrossRef]

134. Chung, R.W.S.; Leanderson, P.; Lundberg, A.K.; Jonasson, L. Lutein exerts anti-inflammatory effects in patients with coronary artery disease. *Atherosclerosis* **2017**, *262*, 87–93. [CrossRef]

135. Maria, A.G.; Graziano, R.; Nicolantonio, D.O. Carotenoids: Potential allies of cardiovascular health? *Food Nutr. Res.* **2015**, *59*, 26762. [CrossRef]

136. Kishimoto, Y.; Taguchi, C.; Saita, E.; Suzuki-Sugihara, N.; Nishiyama, H.; Wang, W.; Masuda, Y.; Kondo, K. Additional consumption of one egg per day increases serum lutein plus zeaxanthin concentration and lowers oxidized low-density lipoprotein in moderately hypercholesterolemic males. *Food Res. Int.* **2017**, *99*, 944–949. [CrossRef]

137. Leermakers, E.T.; Darweesh, S.K.; Baena, C.P.; Moreira, E.M.; Melo van Lent, D.; Tielemans, M.J.; Muka, T.; Chowdhury, R.; Bramer, W.M.; Kiefte-de Jong, J.C.; et al. The effects of lutein on cardiometabolic health across the life course: A systematic review and meta-analysis. *Am. J. Clin. Nutr.* **2016**, *103*, 481–494. [CrossRef]

138. Costa-Rodrigues, J.; Pinho, O.; Monteiro, P.R.R. Can lycopene be considered an effective protection against cardiovascular disease? *Food Chem.* **2018**, *245*, 1148–1153. [CrossRef]

139. Cheng, H.M.; Koutsidis, G.; Lodge, J.K.; Ashor, A.; Siervo, M.; Lara, J. Tomato and lycopene supplementation and cardiovascular risk factors: A systematic review and meta-analysis. *Atherosclerosis* **2017**, *257*, 100–108. [CrossRef]

140. Greene, C.M.; Waters, D.; Clark, R.M.; Contois, J.H.; Fernandez, M.L. Plasma LDL and HDL characteristics and carotenoid content are positively influenced by egg consumption in an elderly population. *Nutr. MeTable* **2006**, *3*, 6. [CrossRef] [PubMed]

141. Song, B.; Liu, K.; Gao, Y.; Zhao, L.; Fang, H.; Li, Y.; Pei, L.; Xu, Y. Lycopene and risk of cardiovascular diseases: A meta-analysis of observational studies. *Mol. Nutr. Food Res.* **2017**, *61*, 1601009. [CrossRef]

142. Osganian, S.K.; Stampfer, M.J.; Rimm, E.; Spiegelman, D.; Manson, J.E.; Willett, W.C. Dietary carotenoids and risk of coronary artery disease in women. *Am. J. Clin. Nutr.* **2003**, *77*, 1390–1399. [CrossRef] [PubMed]

143. Sesso, H.D.; Liu, S.; Gaziano, J.M.; Buring, J.E. Dietary lycopene, tomato-based food products and cardiovascular disease in women. *J. Nutr.* **2003**, *133*, 2336–2341. [CrossRef]

144. Tavani, A.; Gallus, S.; Negri, E.; Parpinel, M.; La Vecchia, C. Dietary intake of carotenoids and retinol and the risk of acute myocardial infarction in Italy. *Free Radic. Res.* **2006**, *40*, 659–664. [CrossRef] [PubMed]

145. Li, X.; Xu, J. Dietary and circulating lycopene and stroke risk: A meta-analysis of prospective studies. *Sci. Rep.* **2014**, *4*, 5031. [CrossRef]

146. Borel, P.; Desmarchelier, C.; Nowicki, M.; Bott, R. Lycopene bioavailability is associated with a combination of genetic variants. *Free Radic. Biol. Med.* **2015**, *83*, 238–244. [CrossRef]

147. Zubair, N.; Kooperberg, C.; Liu, J.; Di, C.; Peters, U.; Neuhouser, M.L. Genetic variation predicts serum lycopene concentrations in a multiethnic population of postmenopausal women. *J. Nutr.* **2015**, *145*, 187–192. [CrossRef]

148. World Health Organization. Cancer. 2019. Available online: https://www.who.int/cancer/en/ (accessed on 7 March 2019).

149. International Agency for Research on Cancer (IARC). Latest Global Cancer Data: Cancer Burden Rises to 18.1 Million New Cases and 9.6 Million Cancer Deaths in 2018. 2018. Available online: https://www.who.int/cancer/PRGlobocanFinal.pdf?ua=1 (accessed on 7 March 2019).

150. Liu, X.; Song, M.; Gao, Z.; Cai, X.; Dixon, W.; Chen, X.; Cao, Y.; Xiao, H. Stereoisomers of astaxanthin inhibit human colon cancer cell growth by inducing G2/M cell cycle arrest and apoptosis. *J. Agric. Food Chem.* **2016**, *64*, 7750–7759. [CrossRef]

151. Rafi, M.M.; Kanakasabai, S.; Gokarn, S.V.; Krueger, E.G.; Bright, J.J. Dietary lutein modulates growth and survival genes in prostate cancer cells. *J. Med. Food* **2015**, *18*, 173–181. [CrossRef] [PubMed]

152. Shareck, M.; Rousseau, M.C.; Koushik, A.; Siemiatycki, J.; Parent, M.-E. Inverse association between dietary intake of selected carotenoids and vitamin C and risk of lung cancer. *Front. Oncol.* **2017**, *7*, 23. [CrossRef]

153. Tuzcu, M.; Orhan, C.; Muz, O.E.; Sahin, N.; Juturu, V.; Sahin, K. Lutein and zeaxanthin isomers modulates lipid metabolism and the inflammatory state of retina in obesity-induced high-fat diet rodent model. *BMC Ophthalmol.* **2017**, *17*, 129. [CrossRef]

154. Cha, J.H.; Kim, W.K.; Ha, A.W.; Kim, M.H.; Chang, M.J. Anti-inflammatory effect of lycopene in SW480 human colorectal cancer cells. *Nutr. Res. Pract.* **2017**, *11*, 90–96. [CrossRef]

155. De Waart, F.G.; Schouten, E.G.; Stalenhoef, A.F.H.; Kok, F.J. Serum carotenoids, α-tocopherol and mortality risk in a prospective study among Dutch elderly. *Int. J. Epidemiol.* **2001**, *30*, 136–143. [CrossRef]

156. Aizawa, K.; Liu, C.; Tang, S.; Veeramachaneni, S.; Hu, K.Q.; Smith, D.E.; Wang, X.D. Tobacco carcinogen induces both lung cancer and nonalcoholic steatohepatitis and hepatocellular carcinomas in ferrets which can be attenuated by lycopene supplementation. *Int. J. Cancer* **2016**, *139*, 1171–1181. [CrossRef] [PubMed]

157. Middha, P.; Weinstein, S.J.; Männistö, S.; Albanes, D.; Mondul, A.M. β-carotene supplementation and lung cancer incidence in the ATBC study: The role of tar and nicotine. *Nicotine Tob. Res.* **2018**. [CrossRef] [PubMed]

158. Russell, R.M. Beta-carotene and lung cancer. *Pure Appl. Chem.* **2002**, *74*, 1461–1467. [CrossRef]

159. World Health Organization. Diabetes. 2019. Available online: https://www.who.int/news-room/fact-sheets/detail/diabetes (accessed on 7 March 2019).

160. Fowler, M.J. Microvascular and macrovascular complications of diabetes. *Clin. Diabetes* **2011**, *29*, 116–122. [CrossRef]

161. Ullah, A.; Khan, A.; Khan, I. Diabetes mellitus and oxidative stress—A concise review. *Saudi Pharm. J.* **2016**, *24*, 547–553.

162. Wang, J.; Light, K.; Henderson, M.; O'Loughlin, J.; Mathieu, M.E.; Paradis, G.; Gray-Donald, K. Consumption of added sugars from liquid but not solid sources predicts impaired glucose homeostasis and insulin resistance among youth at risk of obesity. *J. Nutr.* **2013**, *144*, 81–86. [CrossRef]

163. Yan, L.-J. Pathogenesis of chronic hyperglycemia: From reductive stress to oxidative stress. *J. Diabetes Res.* **2014**, *2014*. [CrossRef]

164. Wan, T.-T.; Li, X.-F.; Sun, Y.-M.; Li, Y.-B.; Su, Y. Recent advances in understanding the biochemical and molecular mechanism of diabetic retinopathy. *Biomed. Pharmacother.* **2015**, *74*, 145–147. [CrossRef] [PubMed]

165. Newsholme, P.; Cruzat, V.F.; Keane, K.N.; Carlessi, R.; de Bittencourt, P.I.H., Jr. Molecular mechanisms of ROS production and oxidative stress in diabetes. *Biochem. J.* **2016**, *473*, 4527–4550. [CrossRef]

166. Uchiyama, K.; Naito, Y.; Hasegawa, G.; Nakamura, N.; Takahashi, J.; Yoshikawa, T. Astaxanthin protects beta-cells against glucose toxicity in diabetic db/db mice. *Redox Rep.* **2002**, *7*, 290–293. [CrossRef]

167. Sluijs, I.; Cadier, E.; Beulens, J.W.; van der, A.D.; Spijkerman, A.M.; van der Schouw, Y.T. Dietary intake of carotenoids and risk of type 2 diabetes. *Nutr. Metab. Cardiovasc. Dis.* **2015**, *25*, 376–381. [CrossRef] [PubMed]

168. Arnlov, J.; Zethelius, B.; Riserus, U.; Basu, S.; Berne, C.; Vessby, B.; Alfthan, G.; Helmersson, J.; Uppsala Longitudinal Study of Adult Men Study. Serum and dietary beta-carotene and alpha-tocopherol and incidence of type 2 diabetes mellitus in a community-based study of Swedish men: Report from the Uppsala Longitudinal Study of Adult Men (ULSAM) study. *Diabetologia* **2009**, *52*, 97–105. [CrossRef] [PubMed]

169. Maeda, H.; Hosokawa, M.; Sashima, T.; Murakami-Funayama, K.; Miyashita, K. Anti-obesity and anti-diabetic effects of fucoxanthin on diet-induced obesity conditions in a murine model. *Mol. Med. Rep.* **2009**, *2*, 897–902. [CrossRef] [PubMed]

170. Manabe, E.; Handa, O.; Naito, Y.; Mizushima, K.; Akagiri, S.; Adachi, S.; Takagi, T.; Kokura, S.; Maoka, T.; Yoshikawa, T. Astaxanthin protects mesangial cells from hyperglycemia-induced oxidative signaling. *J. Cell. Biochem.* **2008**, *103*, 1925–1937. [CrossRef] [PubMed]

171. Kim, Y.J.; Kim, Y.A.; Yokozawa, T. Protection against oxidative stress, inflammation, and apoptosis of high-glucose-exposed proximal tubular epithelial cells by astaxanthin. *J. Agric. Food Chem.* **2009**, *57*, 8793–8797. [CrossRef]

172. Akbaraly, T.N.; Fontbonne, A.; Favier, A.; Berr, C. Plasma carotenoids and onset of dysglycemia in an elderly population. *Diabetes Care* **2008**, *31*, 1355–1359. [CrossRef]

173. International Osteoporosis Foundation. Facts and Statistics. 2017. Available online: https://www.iofbonehealth.org/facts-statistics (accessed on 8 March 2019).

174. Johnell, O.; Kanis, J.A. An estimate of the worldwide prevalence and disability associated with osteoporotic fractures. *Osteoporos. Int.* **2006**, *17*, 1726–1733. [CrossRef]

175. Melton, L.J., 3rd.; Crowson, C.S.; O'Fallon, W.M. Fracture incidence in Olmsted County, Minnesota: Comparison of urban with rural rates and changes in urban rates over time. *Osteoporos. Int.* **1999**, *9*, 29–37. [CrossRef]

176. Gullberg, B.; Johnell, O.; Kanis, J.A. World-wide projections for hip fracture. *Osteoporos. Int.* **1997**, *7*, 407. [CrossRef] [PubMed]

177. Astley, S.B.; Hughes, D.A.; Wright, A.J.; Elliott, R.M.; Southon, S. DNA damage and susceptibility to oxidative damage in lymphocytes: Effects of carotenoids in vitro and in vivo. *Br. J. Nutr.* **2004**, *91*, 53–61. [CrossRef]

178. Almeida, M.; Han, L.; Martin-Millan, M.; O'Brien, C.A.; Manolagas, S.C. Oxidative stress antagonizes Wnt signaling in osteoblast precursors by diverting beta-catenin from T cell factor- to forkhead box O-mediated transcription. *J. Biol. Chem.* **2007**, *282*, 27298–27305. [CrossRef] [PubMed]

179. Cao, W.T.; Zeng, F.F.; Li, B.L.; Lin, J.S.; Liang, Y.Y.; Chen, Y.M. Higher dietary carotenoid intake associated with lower risk of hip fracture in middle-aged and elderly Chinese: A matched case-control study. *Bone* **2018**, *111*, 116–122. [CrossRef]

180. Dai, Z.; Wang, R.; Ang, L.W.; Low, Y.L.; Yuan, J.M.; Koh, W.P. Protective effects of dietary carotenoids on risk of hip fracture in men: The Singapore Chinese Health Study. *J. Bone Miner. Res.* **2014**, *29*, 408–417. [CrossRef]

181. Zhang, Z.Q.; Cao, W.T.; Liu, J.; Cao, Y.; Su, Y.X.; Chen, Y.M. Greater serum carotenoid concentration associated with higher bone mineral density in Chinese adults. *Osteoporos. Int.* **2016**, *27*, 1593–1601. [CrossRef] [PubMed]

182. Li, H.; Huang, C.; Zhu, J.; Gao, K.; Fang, J.; Li, H. Lutein suppresses oxidative stress and inflammation by Nrf2 activation in an osteoporosis rat model. *Med. Sci. Monit.* **2018**, *24*, 5071–5075. [CrossRef]

183. Tominari, T.; Matsumoto, C.; Watanabe, K.; Hirata, M.; Grundler, F.M.W.; Inada, M.; Miyaura, C. Lutein, a carotenoid, suppresses osteoclastic bone resorption and stimulates bone formation in cultures. *J. Biosci. Biotechnol. Biochem.* **2017**, *81*, 302–306. [CrossRef] [PubMed]

184. Bovier, E.R.; Hammond, B.R. The macular carotenoids lutein and zeaxanthin are related to increased bone density in young healthy adults. *Foods* **2017**, *6*, 78. [CrossRef]

185. Willis, L.M.; Shukitt-Hale, B.; Joseph, J.A. Modulation of cognition and behavior in aged animals: Role for antioxidant- and essential fatty acid-rich plant foods. *Am. J. Clin. Nutr.* **2009**, *89*, 1602–1606. [CrossRef]

186. Zhang, Z.; Han, S.; Wang, H.; Wang, T. Lutein extends the lifespan of *Drosophila melanogaster*. *Arch. Gerontol. Geriatr.* **2014**, *58*, 153–159. [CrossRef]

187. Neena, P.; Thomas, K.; Cynthia, H.; Shannon, H.; Rosemarie, A.; Marvin, T.; Salvador, G. Regulation of the extracellular matrix remodeling by lutein in dermal fibroblasts, melanoma cells, and ultraviolet radiation exposed fibroblasts. *Arch. Dermatol. Res.* **2007**, *299*, 373–379.

188. Bahrami, H.; Melia, M.; Dagnelie, G. Lutein supplementation in retinitis pigmentosa: PC-based vision assessment in a randomized double-masked placebo-controlled clinical trial. *BMC Ophthalmol.* **2006**, *6*, 23. [CrossRef] [PubMed]

189. Yazaki, K.; Yoshikoshi, C.; Oshiro, S.; Yanase, S. Supplemental cellular protection by a carotenoid extends lifespan via Ins/IGF-signaling in *Caenorhabditis elegans*. *Oxid. Med. Cell. Longev.* **2011**, *2011*. [CrossRef]

190. Giannakou, M.E.; Goss, M.; Junger, M.A.; Hafen, E.; Leevers, S.J.; Partridge, L. Long-lived Drosophila with overexpressed dFOXO in adult fat body. *Science* **2004**, *305*, 361. [CrossRef] [PubMed]

191. Lashmanova, E.; Proshkina, E.; Zhikrivetskaya, S.; Shevchenko, O.; Marusich, E.; Leonov, S.; Melerzanov, A.; Zhavoronkov, A.; Moskalev, A. Fucoxanthin increases lifespan of *Drosophila melanogaster* and *Caenorhabditis elegans*. *Pharmacol. Res.* **2015**, *100*, 228–241. [CrossRef]

192. Johnson, E.J. Role of lutein and zeaxanthin in visual and cognitive function throughout the lifespan. *Nutr. Rev.* **2014**, *72*, 605–612. [CrossRef] [PubMed]

193. Ravikrishnan, R.; Rusia, S.; Ilamurugan, G.; Salunkhe, U.; Deshpande, J.; Shankaranarayanan, J.; Shankaranarayana, M.L.; Soni, M.G. Safety assessment of lutein and zeaxanthin (Lutemax 2020): Subchronic toxicity and mutagenicity studies. *Food Chem. Toxicol.* **2011**, *49*, 2841–2848. [CrossRef] [PubMed]

194. Harikumar, K.B.; Nimita, C.V.; Preethi, K.C.; Kuttan, R.; Deshpande, J. Toxicity profile of lutein and lutein ester isolated from marigold flowers (*Tagetes erecta*). *Int. J. Toxicol.* **2008**, *27*, 1–9. [CrossRef]

195. Institute of Medicine (US) Panel on Dietary Antioxidants and Related Compounds. *Dietary Reference Intakes for Vitamin C, Vitamin E, Selenium, and Carotenoids*; National Academies Press (US): Washington, DC, USA, 2000.

196. Joint, F.A.O. *Evaluation of Certain Food Additives: Sixty-Third Report of the Joint FAO/WHO Expert Committee on Food Additives*; World Health Organization: Geneva, Switzerland, June 2004; pp. 23–26.

197. European Food Safety Authority. Scientific opinion on the re-evaluation of lutein [e 161b] as a food additive. *EFSA J.* **2010**, *8*, 1678. [CrossRef]

198. European Food Safety Authority (EFSA). Safety, bioavailability and suitability of lutein for the particular nutritional use by infants and young children—Scientific Opinion of the Panel on Dietetic Products, Nutrition and Allergies. *EFSA J.* **2008**, *823*, 1–24.

199. Zheng, Y.F.; Bae, S.H.; Kwon, M.J.; Park, J.B.; Choi, H.D.; Shin, W.G.; Bae, S.K. Inhibitory effects of astaxanthin, b-cryptoxanthin, canthaxanthin, lutein, and zeaxanthin on cytochrome P450 enzyme activities. *Food Chem. Toxicol.* **2013**, *59*, 78–85. [CrossRef] [PubMed]

200. Amengual, J.; Lobo, G.P.; Golczak, M.; Li, H.N.; Klimova, T.; Hoppel, C.L.; Wyss, A.; Palczewski, K.; von Lintig, J. A mitochondrial enzyme degrades carotenoids and protects against oxidative stress. *FASEB J.* **2011**, *25*, 948–959. [CrossRef]

201. Olmedilla, B.; Granado, F.; Southon, S.; Wright, A.J.; Blanco, I.; Gil-Martinez, E.; van den Berg, H.; Thurnham, D.; Corridan, B.; Chopra, M.; et al. A European multicentre, placebo-controlled supplementation study with alpha-tocopherol, carotene-rich palm oil, lutein or lycopene: Analysis of serum responses. *Clin. Sci.* **2002**, *102*, 447–456. [CrossRef]

202. Satia, J.A.; Littman, A.; Slatore, C.G.; Galanko, J.A.; White, E. Long-term use of beta-carotene, retinol, lycopene, and lutein supplements and lung cancer risk: Results from the Vitamins and Lifestyle (VITAL) study. *Am. J. Epidemiol.* **2009**, *169*, 815–828, Erratum in **2009**, *169*, 1409. [CrossRef] [PubMed]

203. Choi, R.Y.; Chortkoff, S.C.; Gorusupudi, A.; Bernstein, P.S. Crystalline maculopathy associated with high-dose lutein supplementation. *JAMA Ophthalmol.* **2016**, *134*, 1445–1448. [CrossRef]

204. Buscemi, S.; Corleo, D.; Di Pace, F.; Petroni, M.L.; Satriano, A.; Marchesini, G. The effect of lutein on eye and extra-eye health. *Nutrients* **2018**, *10*, 1321. [CrossRef]

205. Gorusupudi, A.; Nelson, K.; Bernstein, P.S. The age-related eye disease 2 study: Micronutrients in the treatment of macular degeneration. *Adv. Nutr.* **2017**, *8*, 40–53. [CrossRef]

15

Insights into Heterologous Biosynthesis of Arteannuin B and Artemisinin in *Physcomitrella patens*

Nur Kusaira Khairul Ikram [1,2], **Arman Beyraghdar Kashkooli** [3,4], **Anantha Peramuna** [5], **Alexander R. van der Krol** [3], **Harro Bouwmeester** [3,6] and **Henrik Toft Simonsen** [5,*]

[1] Institute of Biological Sciences, Faculty of Science, University of Malaya, Kuala Lumpur 50603, Malaysia; nkusaira@um.edu.my
[2] Centre for Research in Biotechnology for Agriculture (CEBAR), University of Malaya, Kuala Lumpur 50603, Malaysia
[3] Laboratory of Plant Physiology, Wageningen University and Research, Droevendaalsesteeg 1, 6708 PB Wageningen, The Netherlands; arman.beyraghdarkashkooli@wur.nl (A.B.K.); sander.vanderkrol@wur.nl (A.R.v.d.K.); h.j.bouwmeester@uva.nl (H.B.)
[4] Bioscience, Wageningen Plant Research, Wageningen University and Research, Droevendaalsesteeg 1, 6708 PB Wageningen, The Netherlands
[5] Department of Biotechnology and Biomedicine, Technical University of Denmark, Søltofts Plads, 2800 Kgs. Lyngby, Denmark; aperamuna@gmail.com
[6] Plant Hormone Biology group, Swammerdam Institute for Life Sciences, University of Amsterdam, 1098 XH Amsterdam, The Netherlands
[*] Correspondence: hets@dtu.dk

Academic Editors: Pinarosa Avato and Thomas J. Schmidt

Abstract: Metabolic engineering is an integrated bioengineering approach, which has made considerable progress in producing terpenoids in plants and fermentable hosts. Here, the full biosynthetic pathway of artemisinin, originating from *Artemisia annua*, was integrated into the moss *Physcomitrella patens*. Different combinations of the five artemisinin biosynthesis genes were ectopically expressed in *P. patens* to study biosynthesis pathway activity, but also to ensure survival of successful transformants. Transformation of the first pathway gene, *ADS*, into *P. patens* resulted in the accumulation of the expected metabolite, amorpha-4,11-diene, and also accumulation of a second product, arteannuin B. This demonstrates the presence of endogenous promiscuous enzyme activity, possibly cytochrome P450s, in *P. patens*. Introduction of three pathway genes, *ADS-CYP71AV1-ADH1* or *ADS-DBR2-ALDH1* both led to the accumulation of artemisinin, hinting at the presence of one or more endogenous enzymes in *P. patens* that can complement the partial pathways to full pathway activity. Transgenic *P. patens* lines containing the different gene combinations produce artemisinin in varying amounts. The pathway gene expression in the transgenic moss lines correlates well with the chemical profile of pathway products. Moreover, expression of the pathway genes resulted in lipid body formation in all transgenic moss lines, suggesting that these may have a function in sequestration of heterologous metabolites. This work thus provides novel insights into the metabolic response of *P. patens* and its complementation potential for *A. annua* artemisinin pathway genes. Identification of the related endogenous *P. patens* genes could contribute to a further successful metabolic engineering of artemisinin biosynthesis, as well as bioengineering of other high-value terpenoids in *P. patens*.

Keywords: artemisinin; *Physcomitrella patens*; sesquiterpenoids; malaria; biotechnology

1. Introduction

Artemisinin is a potent malaria drug that is exclusively produced in the plant *Artemisia annua*. The limited production of artemisinin in glandular trichomes of leaves and flowers has led to an extensive cultivation of *Artemisia* plants to meet the needs of the patients. The complex structure of artemisinin makes the chemical synthesis difficult and expensive. Therefore, various efforts have been performed to improve the production of artemisinin in the plant. As alternative, other hosts for heterologous production have been explored, but currently artemisinin production is still mainly based on the use of cultivated plants.

All genes responsible for the biosynthesis of the direct precursor of artemisinin, dihydroartemisinic acid, have been characterized (Scheme 1) [1]. The final conversion of dihydroartemisinic acid to artemisinin is thought to be a light-induced non-enzymatic spontaneous reaction [2]. The first committed biosynthetic step is the cyclization of endogenous farnesyl diphosphate (FPP) to amorpha-4,11-diene by amorpha-4,11-diene synthase (ADS) [3–6], which is substrate for the next enzyme amorphadiene monooxygenase (CYP71AV1). CYP71AV1 is an important cytochrome P450 enzyme [7] in artemisinin biosynthesis as it catalyses three subsequent oxidations of amorpha-4,11-diene to artemisinic acid, via artemisinic alcohol and artemisinic aldehyde [8]. However, in addition the alcohol dehydrogenase 1 (ADH1, a dehydrogenase/reductase enzyme) has been identified, which specifically produces artemisinic aldehyde from artemisinic alcohol (Scheme 1). This specificity and strong expression in *A. annua* glandular trichomes likely indicates that ADH1 is mainly responsible for biosynthesis of artemisinic aldehyde [9,10]. Artemisinic aldehyde is at a branch point in the bifurcating pathway producing either dihydroartemisinic acid or artemisinic acid [9,10]. In the branch leading to artemisinin, artemisinic aldehyde is reduced to dihydroartemisinic aldehyde by artemisinic aldehyde Δ11(13)-reductase (DBR2) and subsequently is oxidized to dihydroartemisinic acid by an aldehyde dehydrogenase (ALDH1) [11–13]. Besides catalysing the oxidation of dihydroartemisinic aldehyde to dihydroartemisinic acid in one branch, in a second pathway branch ALDH1 also catalyses the oxidation of artemisinic aldehyde to artemisinic acid (a reaction also catalysed by CYP71AV1) [7,12]. Another enzyme, dihydroartemisinic aldehyde reductase (RED1) converts dihydroartemisinic aldehyde into dihydroartemisinic alcohol, a "dead end" product, which negatively affects the yield of artemisinin [11]. The final steps in the two branches of the pathway likely involves photo-oxidation of dihydroartemisinic acid and artemisinic acid to artemisinin and arteannuin B, respectively [2,7].

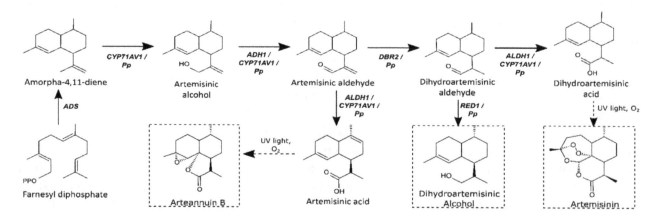

Scheme 1. The biosynthetic pathways of artemisinin and arteannuin B in *Artemisia annua*. *Pp* annotation represents possible native *P. patens* enzyme activity. *ADS*, amorphadiene synthase; *CYP71AV1*, amorphadiene oxidase; *ADH1*, alcohol dehydrogenase; *DBR2*, artemisinic aldehyde double-bond reductase; *ALDH1*, aldehyde dehydrogenase 1. The boxes indicate the products of the pathway.

Taking advantage of the elucidated artemisinin pathway, metabolic engineering has been a popular approach to improve the production of artemisinin or its precursors in heterologous hosts such as *E. coli*, yeast and tobacco. A production of amorpha-4,11-diene at 24 g/L was established through the introduction of the MVA pathway and ADS in *E. coli* along with several other modifications [14]. However, expressing plant P450s (such as CYP71AV1) in *E. coli* is not favourable. Therefore *Saccharomyces cerevisiae* (baker's yeast) was engineered to boost the MVA pathway and ADS through several modifications resulting in a yeast strain producing 153 mg/L amorpha-4,11-diene [8]. Subsequently, CYP71AV1 and a cytochrome P450 reductase (CPR) were introduced resulting in production of up to 100 mg/L of artemisinic acid [8]. The strains were further optimized by adding ADH1, ALDH1 and CYPB5, a native partner of CYP71AV1, that contributed to a significant increase of 25 g/L artemisinic acid via fermentation [9]. Although in these systems complete artemisinin biosynthesis is not accomplished, a 3-step chemical conversion from artemisinic acid to artemisinin has been developed and is currently used in commercial production of artemisinin in combination with yeast fermentation [9,15].

Introducing artemisinin pathway genes in tobacco has also been successful, using both stable and transient expression [16–21]. However, in tobacco pathway intermediates are efficiently glycosylated, resulting in low artemisinin yield [16,19]. Attempts have been made to target pathway enzymes to different compartments such as the chloroplast, and Fuentes et al. were able to produce 120 µg/g dry weight (d.w.) artemisinic acid [20], while Malhotra et al. produced 0.8 mg/g d.w. artemisinin in *Nicotiana benthamiana* [22]. All these attempts involved extensive bioengineering of precursor pathways and pathway localization, which is time consuming and with limited success in increasing final yield. Recent work has shown that *Physcomitrella patens* can be a promising heterologous host for artemisinin production, with a high yield of artemisinin after three days, prior to any production enhancements [21,23].

In the present study, various combinations of the pathway genes are assembled to study the biosynthetic route and the interplay with endogenous metabolism as well as ensuring the survival of successful transformants. We observed biosynthetic routes not previously described in the metabolic network of *P. patens* and demonstrate that some endogenous *P. patens* enzymes have promiscuous substrate recognition, which may substitute for some *A. annua* pathway enzyme activities. This provides new insight into *P. patens* metabolism and offers alternative engineering targets for production of artemisinin in this primitive plant and promising heterologous production platform.

2. Results and Discussion

2.1. Heterologous Expression of Artemisinin Biosynthesis Pathway Genes

The gene encoding the first committed enzyme in the artemisinin biosynthesis pathway (ADS) was introduced into the wild-type (WT) *P. patens*. Integration of the gene was confirmed by PCR on genomic DNA isolated from transformants (Figure S1) and metabolic profiling showed that amorpha-4,11-diene was produced in cultures up to levels up to 200 mg/L [23]. However, localization of the amorpha-4,11-diene remains unclear: is it stored in specific organelles such as lipid bodies or transported out of the cell? Several studies have shown that *P. patens* is able to ectopically produce volatile terpenoids, but the regulation of volatiles production and their potential storage within *P. patens* is yet to be explored [23–25]. Besides amorpha-4,11-diene, the transgenic lines expressing *ADS* also accumulated arteannuin B, which is thought to be derived from artemisinic acid through photo-oxidation. This suggest accumulation of artemisinic acid in the transgenic lines and reveals a promiscuous activity of an endogenous oxidative enzyme (or enzymes) such as the cytochrome P450 in *P. patens*, which can catalyse the triple oxidation of amorpha-4,11-diene via artemisinic alcohol and aldehyde to the acid. In *A. annua* these activities are catalysed by CYP71AV1 and ADH1 [8,26]. Although predominant results indicate that most plant P450s are highly specific in their substrate recognition, increasing evidence shows that some plant P450s can be promiscuous in substrate recognition, similar to mammalian P450s [27–30]. Endogenous *P. patens* oxidative enzymes fully convert amorpha-4,11-diene to artemisinic acid, since the alcohol and aldehyde intermediates were not detected in culture extracts. *P. patens* naturally produces high amounts of *ent*-kaurenoic acid from *ent*-kaurene, which is catalysed by an *ent*-kaurene oxidase (CYP701B1) through three successive oxidations [31,32]. CYP701B1 may therefore be a likely candidate for catalysing the conversion of amorpha-4,11-diene into artemisinic acid in *P. patens*. Other possible candidate enzymes are the numerous cytochrome P450s, ferrodoxin mono-oxygenases, and other oxidoreductases encoded by the *P. patens* genome.

Having established transgenic lines producing a high level of amorpha-4,11-diene, a second transformation introduced the second (*CYP71AV1*) and third (*ADH1*) artemisinin pathway genes. Likewise, the final two artemisinin pathway genes, *DBR2* and *ALDH1* were also introduced into the *ADS* background lines. Having successfully introduced two different sets of 3 artemisinin genes; *ADS-CYP71AV1-ADH1* and *ADS-DBR2-ALDH1* in *P. patens*, the remaining artemisinin pathway genes were introduced into these transgenic lines. This resulted in transgenic lines with all five artemisinin biosynthesis genes in different genomic sequential arrangements. The transgenic lines *ADS-CYP71AV1-ADH1-DBR2-ALDH1* and *ADS-DBR2-ALDH1-CYP71AV1-ADH1* were recovered and genotyping showed the presence of all five artemisinin biosynthesis genes in the genome of *P. patens* (Figure S1).

2.2. Metabolite Profiling of Transgenic P. patens Lines

In total five different transgenic lines were produced (Table 1). Metabolic profiling of these lines showed that artemisinin was produced in all lines, except for the transgenic line solely expressing *ADS*. The *ADS-CYP71AV1-ADH1* line only produced 25% of the artemisinin levels in the *ADS-DBR2-ALDH1* line. This suggests that in the *ADS-DBR2-ALDH1* line the *P. patens* oxidizing enzymes efficiently convert amorpha-4,11-diene to artemisinic aldehyde, which is then converted by DBR2 and ALDH1 to dihydroartemisinic acid (Scheme 1, Table 1). Interestingly, two other metabolites; artemisinic alcohol and dihydroartemisinic alcohol were also detected in the *ADS-DBR2-ALDH1* line. Notably, ADH1 is specific towards artemisinic alcohol [9] and absence of ADH1 in the *ADS-DBR2-ALDH1* lines may explain the accumulation of artemisinic alcohol in this line. The presence of dihydroartemisinic alcohol in the *ADS-DBR2-ALDH1* lines suggests that *P. patens* has an endogenous oxidoreductases similar to *A. annua* RED1 that catalyses the formation of dihydroartemisinic alcohol from dihydroartemisinic aldehyde in *A. annua* [11].

Table 1. Quantification of artemisinin, artemisinin intermediates and arteannuin B produced in transgenic *Physcomitrella patens* and the moss culture liquid media (from 3 weeks moss culture, average of two cultures). The content in the liquid media represents the amount of molecules that have been excreted from the moss cells.

	ADS	ADS-CYP71AV1-ADH1	ADS-CYP71AV1-ADH1-DBR2-ALDH1	ADS-DBR2-ALDH1	ADS-DBR2-ALDH1-CYP71AV1-ADH1
Content in culture liquid media (without moss)	(μg/g FW)	(μg/g FW)	(μg/g FW)	(μg/g FW)	(μg/g FW)
Artemisinic alcohol	ND	ND	ND	ND	ND
Dihydroartemisinic alcohol	ND	ND	ND	0.09	ND
Arteannuin B	1.05	0.04	0.09	1.74	ND
Content in dried moss tissue	(mg/g DW)	(mg/g DW)	(mg/g DW)	(mg/g DW)	(mg/g DW)
Artemisinin	ND	0.01	0.03	0.04	0.01
Artemisinic alcohol	ND	ND	ND	0.13	ND
Dihydroartemisinic alcohol	ND	ND	ND	0.07	ND

ND, not detected.

Arteannuin B is mostly present in the liquid media (see Figure 1, Table 1) indicating transport capacity for artemisinic acid or arteannuin B to the outside of the cells. Alternatively, this could indicate that accumulation of these compounds is toxic to the cells that then die. The artemisinic aldehyde is at the branch point of the biosynthesis pathway, leading to either dihydroartemisinic acid (precursor of artemisinin) or artemisinic acid (precursor of arteannuin B) (Scheme 1). While *DBR2* catalyses the conversion of artemisinic aldehyde toward artemisinin production, *ALDH1* and *CYP71AV1* or *P. patens* hydroxylases catalyse the formation of artemisinic acid.

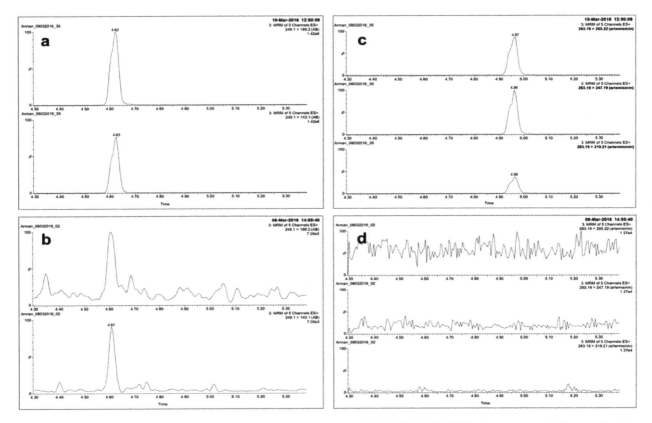

Figure 1. UPLC-MRM-MS analysis of arteannuin B. (**a**) UPLC-MRM-MS of arteannuin B standard fragmented in MRM channels of m/z 249.1 > 189.2; 249.1 > 143.1 (**b**) UPLC-MRM-MS analysis of arteannuin B in transformed *P. patens* with *ADS* (RT = 4.61). (**c**) UPLC-MRM-MS of artemisinin standard fragmented in MRM channels of m/z 283.19 > 219.21; 283.19 > 247.19 and 283.19 > 265.22 (RT = 4.96). (**d**) Demonstration of absence of artemisinin by UPLC-MRM-MS of artemisinin in fragmented in MRM channels of m/z 283.19 > 219.21; 283.19 > 247.19 and 283.19 > 265.22 of extracts from transformed *P. patens* with *ADS*. C+D show that artemisinin is not present in the *ADS* only lines of *P. patens*.

Our transgenic *P. patens* lines were grown under constant (24 h) high light intensity. Thus, all the produced artemisinic acid or dihydroartemisinic acid are presumably photo-chemically converted into arteannuin B and artemisinin, respectively and neither of the two acids were detected in our study.

The accumulation of arteannuin B was correlated with the amount of artemisinin. Transformants with higher levels of arteannuin B, also accumulates higher levels of artemisinin. For instance, *ADS-DBR2-ALDH1* accumulates most artemisinin as well as arteannuin B.

The accumulation of artemisinin in the *ADS-CYP71AV1-ADH1* line shows that *P. patens* has enzymes with similar activities as DBR2 and ALDH1 from *A. annua*. The lower artemisinin accumulation in the *ADS-CYP71AV1-ADH1* line suggests that the affinity of the endogenous *P. patens* enzyme for the pathway intermediates may not be as good as for *A. annua* DBR2 and ALDH1.

Although presence of endogenous enzyme activity might contribute to the accumulation of artemisinin, only arteannuin B was detected in the *ADS* expressing line (see Figure 1). One reason could be that the *P. patens* hydroxylases and oxidoreductases has lower affinity towards the heterologous substrates than the pathway enzymes, CYP71AV1, DBR2 and ALDH1. For example, higher levels of artemisinin was detected when CYP71AV1 was expressed (*ADS-CYP71AV1-ADH1*), which should accumulate artemisinic aldehyde, but this is catalysed into dihydroartemisinic acid by native hydroxylases and oxidoreductases.

Dihydroartemisinic acid spontaneously transform into artemisinin when exposed to light. Meanwhile, in the *ADS*-only line amorpha-4,11-diene accumulates and here the native hydroxylases might favour reactions resulting in a final accumulation of arteannuin B via artemisinic acid (see Scheme 1 for the pathway).

Unlike in other heterologous plants e.g., *Nicotiana benthamiana* [16], no glycosylated and/or glutathione conjugates of the artemisinin biosynthesis intermediate related products were detected in the transgenic *P. patens* lines [23]. The absence of glycosylated products could be due to the much lower number of genes encoding putative glycosyltransferases in *P. patens*, compared to that in higher (vascular) plants [33]. This could be an important feature of *P. patens* to favour full pathway activity toward the accumulation of the two products artemisinin and/or arteannuin B.

2.3. Analysis of Artemisinin Pathway Gene Expression Profiles

Analysis of the artemisinin biosynthetic gene expression profile was performed to investigate the correlation between gene expression and metabolite production in the transgenic lines (Figure 2). The expression of the first committed enzyme, ADS was the highest when it was introduced alone, and decreased with the increasing number of genes introduced; *ADS* > *ADS-CYP71AV1-ADH1* > *ADS-CYP71AV1-ADH1-DBR2-ALDH1*. A similar pattern was observed in the expression of the other constructs with *ADS* > *ADS-DBR2-ALDH1* > *ADS-DBR2-ALDH1-CYP71AV1-ADH1*. For *CYP71AV1*, there was no significant difference in expression between the *ADS-CYP71AV1-ADH1* and *ADS-DBR2-ALDH1-CYP71AV1-ADH1* lines. However, the expression level was 100 fold higher in the *ADS-CYP71AV1-ADH1-DBR2-ALDH1* line showing that higher amount of the enzyme could be present for the higher production of artemisinin. *ADH1* on the other hand exhibited a low expression pattern in all transgenic lines, suggesting its limited contribution to the overall artemisinin pathway in *P. patens*.

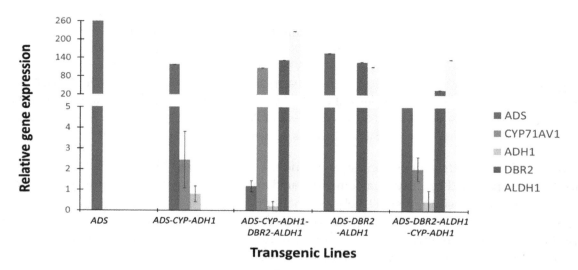

Figure 2. Relative expression of artemisinin pathway genes (*ADS, CYP71AV1, ADH1, DBR2, ALDH1*) in the five transgenic *P. patens* lines. Error bars are shown as SE (n = 3).

Overall, *ADS-DBR2-ALDH1* shows higher gene expressions for all three genes compared to the other transgenic lines and this correlates positively with the product levels. The expression level of the *ADS* gene in *ADS-DBR2-ALDH1* is the second highest, after the *ADS* only expressing line, which may lead to abundant amorpha-4,11-diene to be catalysed by *DBR2* into artemisinic aldehyde and subsequently into dihydroartemisinic acid by *ALDH1*. However, in addition, endogenous *P. patens* hydroxylases and *ALDH1* efficiently catalyse the formation of artemisinic acid, hence contributing to higher accumulation of arteannuin B than artemisinin (Table 1). The transgene expression levels in all the lines expressing *DBR2* and *ALDH1* correlate well with their end product profiles (Figure 2, Table 1). Similarly, lines *ADS-CYP71AV1-ADH1* and *ADS-DBR2-ALDH1-CYP71AV1-ADH1*, which show lower expression of *CYP71AV1*, also show lower levels of artemisinin. Results thus suggest that not only higher affinity for substrates but also abundance of the active *A. annua* enzymes has a positive impact on artemisinin levels. Improving expression and protein levels even further may therefore be targets for future research.

The expression of *DBR2* and *ALDH1* was relatively high and correlates with the amount of metabolite produced. Studies on the artemisinin pathway gene expression in different *A. annua* chemotypes: the high artemisinin producer (HAP) and low artemisinin producer (LAP) as well as the *Nicotiana benthamiana* transiently expressing the artemisinin biosynthetic pathway genes show that the expression of DBR2 is significantly higher in the HAP varieties which is similar to the gene expression pattern found in *P. patens* [16,34]. It is evident that *DBR2* and *ALDH1* appear to be of a great importance in elevating artemisinin production in *P. patens*, *A. annua* and other heterologous plant-based systems [16,20,34,35].

2.4. Lipid Body Formation in Transgenic P. patens

P. patens utilizes lipid bodies (LBs) in its life cycle [36] and because of the hydrophobic nature of artemisinin, we investigated whether ectopic expression of the artemisinin pathway in transgenic *P. patens* favours LB formation by LB staining with BODIPY. Confocal microscopy observations confirmed that abundant and large LBs are present in all transgenic lines (Figure 3). Formation of these LBs in response to production of potentially toxic compounds could indicate an alternative phytotoxic defence mechanism in *P. patens* prior to the development of alternative detoxification strategies through glycosylation as in higher plants. Glycosylation and modification by glutathione of pathway intermediates are the biggest competitor for production of artemisinin and other sesquiterpenes in heterologous plant expression systems. The absence of such detoxification mechanisms and induction of potential sequester structures like LBs in *P. patens* make this organism a potential valuable novel tool for production of artemisinin or other valuable terpenes. To address this, further research on the mechanism of lipid body formation and identification of LB composition in the transgenic *P. patens* will be valuable for an overall understanding on *P. patens* metabolic responses to heterologously produced metabolites.

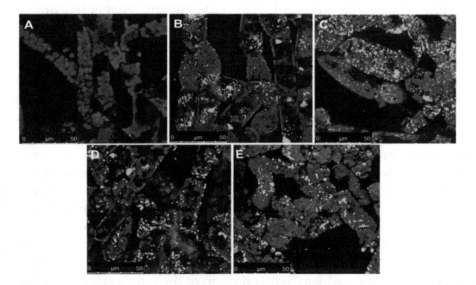

Figure 3. Projections of 8 day old moss obtained by confocal microscopy showing the accumulation of lipid bodies (green spots, stained with BODIPY) in wild type (**A**) and transgenic moss bearing (**B**) *ADS* (**C**) *ADS-CYP71AV1-ADH1* (**D**) *ADS-DBR2-ALDH1* (**E**) *ADS-CYP71AV1-ADH1-DBR2-ALDH1*. Red color represent chlorophyll autofluorescence.

3. Materials and Methods

3.1. Plant Material and Growth Conditions

P. patens (Gransden ecotype, International Moss Stock Center #40001) was grown on solid and liquid PhyB media under sterile conditions, at 25 °C with continuous 20–50 W/m^2 light intensity [37].

3.2. DNA Fragments and Genes

The Pp108 locus homologous recombination flanking regions were amplified from genomic DNA of P. patens. The ADS gene was a kind gift from Assoc. Prof. Dae Kyun Ro, University of Calgary, Calgary, AB, Canada. The synthetic genes of CYP71AV1 (DQ268763), ADH1 (JF910157.1), DBR2 (EU704257.1), and ALDH1 (FJ809784.1) were synthesized by GenScript (city, state abbrev USA) according to the P. paten codon usage. The synthetic genes was linked with a peptide linker LP4/2A from Impatiens balsamina and foot-and-mouth-disease virus (FMDV); CYP71AV1-LP4/2A-ADH1, DBR2-LP4/2A-ALDH1. The Ubiquitin promoter and Ubiquitin terminator from Arabidopsis thaliana (CP002686.1) synthetic genes were also synthesized by GenScript. The Maize Ubiquitin 1 promoter, OCS terminator and G418 selection cassettes was obtained from the pMP1355 vector, a kind gift from Professor Mark Estelle, University of California San Diego, San Diego, CA, USA.

3.3. Transformation Procedures

A detailed description of moss transformation has been previously published [37,38]. Five to seven day old P. patens cultures (from last blending) was harvested and digested with 0.5% DriselaseR enzyme solution in 8.5% mannitol (D9515, Sigma Aldrich) followed by incubation at room temperature for 30 to 60 min. The digested sample was then filtered through a 100 µm pored mesh-filter and the protoplast was collected by centrifugation at 150–200× g for 4 min with slow breaking. The pellet was washed twice with the protoplast wash solution (8.5% mannitol, 10 mM CaCl$_2$) and the protoplast density was measured using a hemocytometer before suspending in MMM solution (9.1% D-mannitol, 10% MES and 15mM MgCl$_2$) to a concentration of 1.6 × 106 protoplasts/mL. 300 µL of the protoplast suspension and 300 µL of PEG solution were added to a 15 mL tube containing 10 µg total DNA and incubated at 45 °C for 5 min and another 5 min at room temperature. 8.5% D-mannitol (300 µL) was then added five times and dilutions with 1 mL of 8.5% D-mannitol another five times. The transformed protoplasts were collected by centrifugation, resuspended in 500 µL of 8.5% D-mannitol and 2.5 mL of protoplast regeneration media (top layer; PRMT). One ml of the mixture was distributed on three plates containing protoplast regeneration media (bottom layer; PRMB) overlaid with cellophane. The plates were incubated in continuous light for 5 to 7 days at 25 °C. The cellophane and regenerating protoplasts was then transferred to PhyB media containing the appropriate selection marker for two weeks, before transferring on PhyB media without antibiotics for another 2 weeks and later transferred back to the final antibiotic selection to confirmed stable transformants.

The first committed precursor of artemisinin biosynthesis pathway, ADS was introduced into wildtype P. patens at the designated neutral locus Pp108. The transformed lines were selected on regeneration medium with geneticin (G418) for two rounds of selection. Next, we transformed the second and third: CYP71AV1-LP4/2A-ADH1 as well as the fourth and fifth; DBR2-LP4/2A-ALDH1 genes respectively into the ADS-expressing transgenic line. Both transformations are targeted to replace the previously transformed G418 selection marker with the new selection of hygromycin. Having successfully introduced three artemisinin genes; ADS-CYP71AV1-ADH1 and ADS-DBR2-ALDH1 in P. patens, we next completed the pathway with addition of the remaining artemisinin genes into both transgenic lines. For this transformation, the previously removed G418 selection marker was used again and hygromycin was targeted for recombination such that this selection marker was removed.

3.4. PCR, DNA Purification and Concentration

All DNA fragments were amplified with PhusionR High-Fidelity DNA Polymerase (New England Biolabs, County Road Ipswich, MA, USA). PCR conditions and annealing temperatures were modified depending on primers and templates used in the reaction. PCR reactions using plasmid DNA as template were digested with DpnI (NEB, County Road Ipswich, MA, USA) for 1 h at 37 °C followed by inactivation at 65 °C for 20 min to lower background after transformation. PCR products were purified using QIAquick PCR Purification Kit (Qiagen GmbH, Strasse 1, Hilden, Germany). The DNA fragments for transformations were concentrated via ethanol precipitation to a final concentration of ~1 µg/µL, determined using NanoDrop2000 (Thermo Fisher Scientific, Waltham, MA, USA). The primers used are listed in Table S1.

3.5. Metabolite Profiling

3.5.1. UPLC-MRM-MS Analysis

Fresh moss samples were harvested, snap-frozen and ground into a fine powder. Samples of 3000 mg were extracted with 3 mL citrate phosphate buffer, pH 5.4, followed by vortexing and sonication for 15 min. One mL of Viscozyme (V2010, Sigma) was added and samples were incubated at 37 °C. The whole mixture was then extracted three times with 3 mL ethyl acetate and concentrated to a volume of 1 mL and stored at −20 °C. For liquid culture extracts, 500 mL of liquid culture was harvested, passed through a filter paper and extracted with 200 mL of ethyl acetate in a separation funnel. Ethyl acetate was concentrated to a volume of 1 mL and stored at −20 °C. Ethyl acetate of both liquid culture and moss sample extracts were then dried under a flow of N_2 and resuspended into 300 µL of 75% MeOH:H_2O (v:v). Extracts were passed through a 0.45 µm membrane filter (Minisart® RC4, Sartorius, Germany) before analysis. Artemisinin and artemisinin biosynthesis pathway intermediates were measured in a targeted approach by using a Waters Xevo tandem quadrupole mass spectrometer equipped with an electrospray ionization source and coupled to an Acuity UPLC system (Waters), essentially as described [16]. For A BEH C18 column (100 × 2.1 mm × 1.7 µm; Waters) was used for chromatographic separation by applying a water:acetonitrile gradient. The gradient started from 5% (v/v) acetonitrile in water with formic acid [1:1000 (v/v)] for 1.25 min, was raised to 50% in 2.35 min and was raised to 90% at 3.65 min. This was kept for 0.75 min before returning to the 5% acetonitrile/water (v/v) with formic acid [1:1000 (v/v)] by using a 0.15 min gradient. The same solvent composition was used to equilibrate the column for 1.85 min. The flow rate was 0.5 mL/min and the column temperature was maintained at 50 °C. Injection volume was set to 10 µL. Desolvation and cone gas flow were set to 1000 and 50 L/h and the mass spectrometer was operated in positive ionization mode. Capillary voltage was set at 3.0 kV. Desolvation and source temperatures were set at 650 and 150 °C, respectively. The cone voltage was optimized for all metabolites using the Waters IntelliStart MS Console. Fragmentation by collision-induced dissociation was done in the ScanWave collision cell using argon. Multiple Reaction Monitoring (MRM) was used for detection and quantification of artemisinin and the other compounds. MRM transitions for artemisinin and pathway intermediates measurement settings were optimized for MRM channels, which are presented in Table S2. Targeted analysis of the fragmentation pattern of authenticated standard was optimized for each of the target compounds. For artemisinin three parent(/daughter) ions (expressed as channels) was obtained and for arteannuin B two channels were identified, as previously described [16,23]. The presence or absence of each compound in samples were checked by comparing the RT of compounds in standard mix with samples. As an additional quality measure the ratio between peak intensity of each compound's channels (e.g., for artemisinin the ratio of 283.19 > 219.21 to 283.19 > 247.19 in samples should be the same as the ratio in what has been measured in artemisinin standard) were checked which was the same in both standards and the identified compounds in samples. Retention time of each compound (positive ionization mode) is presented in Table S3. Artemisinin and dihydroartemisinic acid were gift from Dafra Pharma (Belgium). Other precursors were synthesized from dihydroartemisinic acid by

Chiralix (Nijmegen, the Netherlands) which was checked by NMR (>98% purity). External calibration curves were measured by using reference standards.

3.5.2. LC-QTOF-MS for Analysis of Conjugated Artemisinin Pathway Intermediates

For the artemisinin pathway intermediates glycosides and conjugations, 100 mg of fresh *P. patens* tissue was ground in liquid nitrogen and extracted with 300 μl MeOH:formic acid [1000:1 (*v/v*)]. Samples were briefly vortexed and sonicated for 15 min, followed by 15 min centrifugation at 13,000× g. Extracts were passed through a 0.45 μm membrane filter (Minisart® RC4, Sartorius) before analysis on a Water alliance 2795 HPLC connected to a QTOF Ultima V 4.00.00 mass spectrometer (Waters MS Technologies). The mass spectrometer was operated in negative ionization mode. A precolumn of 2.0 × 4 mm (Phenomenex, Denmark) was connected to the C18 analytical column (Luna 3 μm C18/2 100A; 2.0 × 150 mm; Phenomenex). Degassed eluent A and B were HPLC-grade water:formic acid [1000:1 (*v/v*)] and acetonitrile:formic acid [1000:1 (*v/v*)], respectively. The flow rate was 0.19 mL/min. The HPLC gradient started from 5% eluent B and linearly increased to 75% in 45 min. After that, the column was equilibrated for 15 min with 5% eluent B. 5 μL of each sample was used for injection.

3.6. Lipid Bodies Staining and Microscopy

Equal amount of 14 days old liquid grown cells were suspended in PBS pH 7.4 buffer and stained with a final concentration of 0.5 μg/mL of BIODIPY 505/515 (Invitrogen Molecular Probes, Thermo Fisher). Cells were incubated in the dark for 15 min and visualized with a Leica LAS AF confocal laser microscope. Lipid bodies were visualized with a 488 nm laser excitation line and a 510–530 nm emission window. Chloroplasts were visualized using the same laser line and a 650–700 nm excitation window. Z stacks were performed on each image with a line average of 4 and combined using maximum projection into a single image, and image was visualized with ImageJ [39].

3.7. Expression Profiling in P. patens

100 mg of one week old moss tissue was extracted by RNeasy Plant Mini Kit (Qiagen 74904) according to the protocol provided. The samples were treated with DNase I (Sigma AMPD1) to remove remaining genomic DNA. The RNA quality and concentration was determined by Nanodrop2000 Spectrophotometer (Thermo Fisher Scientific). cDNA synthesis was performed with 500 ng RNA samples using SuperScript III First-Strand Synthesis System for RT-PCR kit (18080-051, Life Technologies, Denmark). Real time quantitative PCR was performed using QuantiFast ® SYBR ® Green PCR (Qiagen, Denmark) according to the protocol provided and run at 95 °C for 5 min, 40 cycles at 95 °C for 10 s followed by 60 °C for 30 s on a CFX Connect Real Time PCR Detection System (BioRad, Denmark). The qPCR was performed with three biological replicates for each sample and three technical replicates for each biological sample. Primers used are listed in (Table S1). Efficiencies of all primers were estimated by generating a standard curve via cDNA serial dilutions using this formula $E = 10^{-1/\text{slope}} - 1$. E values of the primer pairs ranged between 93 to 101% (efficiency between 90 and 110% are acceptable). *P. patens* β-actin was used as the reference gene and the transcripts level was calculated as follows: $\Delta CT = CT(GOI) - CT(Actin)$, $\Delta\Delta CT$ was normalized using ΔCT and the relative change in gene expression is calculated by $2^{-\Delta\Delta CT}$ method [40].

4. Conclusions

Here we show that the anti-malaria drug, artemisinin, can be produced in *P. patens* with either complete or partial introduction and expression of the artemisinin pathway genes. The results demonstrate that *P. patens* expresses endogenous enzymes with similar activity to that of the artemisinin biosynthesis pathway in *A. annua*. This possibly affects the accumulation of artemisinin and arteannuin B. Knocking out the endogenous oxidizing enzyme(s) responsible for the conversion of amorpha-4,11-diene into artemisinic acid could possibly positively affect the yield of artemisinin as it could stimulate the flux towards dihydroartemisinic aldehyde. This work provides novel insights into the metabolic machinery of *P. patens* and shows it has enzymes with activities similar to those that catalyse the artemisinin pathway in *A. annua*. Discovery of these enzymes and the encoding genes may contribute not only to successful metabolic engineering of artemisinin biosynthesis in *P. patens*, but also to the engineering of other high-value terpenes in *P. patens*. Enzymes with promiscuous activity can be of high value for any synthetic biology adventure since they can be used for many purposes. They also shed light on general enzyme activity for the specific classes of enzymes. Work is ongoing to discover these enzymes.

Author Contributions: For this paper the authors contributed as follows: Conceptualization, N.K.K.I., and H.T.S.; Methodology, N.K.K.I., A.B.K., and A.P.; Validation, N.K.K.I. and A.B.K.; Formal analysis, N.K.K.I. and A.B.K.; Investigation, N.K.K.I., A.B.K., and A.P.; Resources, N.K.K.I., A.B.K., and H.T.S.; Data curation, N.K.K.I, A.P. and A.B.K.; Writing—original draft preparation, N.K.K.I.; Writing—review and editing, N.K.K.I., A.B.K., A.P., A.R.v.d.K., H.B., and H.T.S.; Visualization, N.K.K.I., and A.B.K., Supervision, A.R.v.d.K., H.B, and H.T.S.; Project administration, H.T.S; Funding acquisition,, N.K.K.I, A.R.v.d.K., H.B., and H.T.S.

Acknowledgments: The authors would like to thank Mark Estelle, Yuji Hiwatashi and Dae Kyun Ro for kindly providing the pMP1355, and PZAG1 vector and the ADS template.

References

1. Xie, D.-Y.; Ma, D.-M.; Judd, R.; Jones, A.L. Artemisinin biosynthesis in *Artemisia annua* and metabolic engineering: Questions, challenges, and perspectives. *Phytochem. Rev.* **2016**, *15*, 1093–1114. [CrossRef]

2. Sy, L.-K.; Brown, G.D. The mechanism of the spontaneous autoxidation of dihydroartemisinic acid. *Tetrahedron* **2002**, *58*, 897–908. [CrossRef]

3. Bouwmeester, H.J.; Wallaart, T.E.; Janssen, M.H.; van Loo, B.; Jansen, B.J.; Posthumus, M.A.; Schmidt, C.O.; De Kraker, J.-W.; König, W.A.; Franssen, M.C. Amorpha-4, 11-diene synthase catalyses the first probable step in artemisinin biosynthesis. *Phytochemistry* **1999**, *52*, 843–854. [CrossRef]

4. Mercke, P.; Bengtsson, M.; Bouwmeester, H.J.; Posthumus, M.A.; Brodelius, P.E. Molecular cloning, expression, and characterization of amorpha-4, 11-diene synthase, a key enzyme of artemisinin biosynthesis in *Artemisia annua* L. *Arch. Biochem. Biophys.* **2000**, *381*, 173–180. [CrossRef] [PubMed]

5. Picaud, S.; Mercke, P.; He, X.; Sterner, O.; Brodelius, M.; Cane, D.E.; Brodelius, P.E. Amorpha-4,11-diene synthase: Mechanism and stereochemistry of the enzymatic cyclization of farnesyl diphosphate. *Arch. Biochem. Biophys.* **2006**, *448*, 150–155. [CrossRef] [PubMed]

6. Picaud, S.; Olofsson, L.; Brodelius, M.; Brodelius, P.E. Expression, purification, and characterization of recombinant amorpha-4,11-diene synthase from *Artemisia annua* L. *Arch. Biochem. Biophys.* **2005**, *436*, 215–226. [CrossRef]

7. Teoh, K.H.; Polichuk, D.R.; Reed, D.W.; Nowak, G.; Covello, P.S. *Artemisia annua* L. (Asteraceae) trichome-specific cdnas reveal CYP71AV1, a cytochrome p450 with a key role in the biosynthesis of the antimalarial sesquiterpene lactone artemisinin. *FEBS Lett.* **2006**, *580*, 1411–1416. [CrossRef]

8. Ro, D.-K.; Paradise, E.M.; Ouellet, M.; Fisher, K.J.; Newman, K.L.; Ndungu, J.M.; Ho, K.A.; Eachus, R.A.; Ham, T.S.; Kirby, J. Production of the antimalarial drug precursor artemisinic acid in engineered yeast. *Nature* **2006**, *440*, 940. [CrossRef]

9. Paddon, C.J.; Westfall, P.; Pitera, D.; Benjamin, K.; Fisher, K.; McPhee, D.; Leavell, M.; Tai, A.; Main, A.; Eng, D. High-level semi-synthetic production of the potent antimalarial artemisinin. *Nature* **2013**, *496*, 528–532. [CrossRef]

10. Olofsson, L.; Engstrom, A.; Lundgren, A.; Brodelius, P. Relative expression of genes of terpene metabolism in different tissues of *Artemisia annua* L. *BMC Plant Biol.* **2011**, *11*, 45. [CrossRef]

11. Rydén, A.-M.; Ruyter-Spira, C.; Quax, W.J.; Osada, H.; Muranaka, T.; Kayser, O.; Bouwmeester, H. The molecular cloning of dihydroartemisinic aldehyde reductase and its implication in artemisinin biosynthesis in *Artemisia annua*. *Planta Med.* **2010**, *76*, 1778. [CrossRef] [PubMed]

12. Teoh, K.H.; Polichuk, D.R.; Reed, D.W.; Covello, P.S. Molecular cloning of an aldehyde dehydrogenase implicated in artemisinin biosynthesis in *Artemisia annua* this paper is one of a selection of papers published in a special issue from the national research council of canada-plant biotechnology institute. *Botany* **2009**, *87*, 635–642. [CrossRef]

13. Zhang, Y.; Teoh, K.H.; Reed, D.W.; Maes, L.; Goossens, A.; Olson, D.J.; Ross, A.R.; Covello, P.S. The molecular cloning of artemisinic aldehyde δ11 (13) reductase and its role in glandular trichome-dependent biosynthesis of artemisinin in *Artemisia annua*. *J. Biol. Chem.* **2008**, *283*, 21501–21508. [CrossRef] [PubMed]

14. Martin, V.J.J.; Pitera, D.J.; Withers, S.T.; Newman, J.D.; Keasling, J.D. Engineering a mevalonate pathway in *Escherichia coli* for production of terpenoids. *Nat. Biotech.* **2003**, *21*, 796–802. [CrossRef]

15. Paddon, C.J.; Keasling, J.D. Semi-synthetic artemisinin: A model for the use of synthetic biology in pharmaceutical development. *Nat. Rev. Microbiol.* **2014**, *12*, 355. [CrossRef]

16. Ting, H.M.; Wang, B.; Rydén, A.M.; Woittiez, L.; Herpen, T.; Verstappen, F.W.; Ruyter-Spira, C.; Beekwilder, J.; Bouwmeester, H.J.; Krol, A. The metabolite chemotype of *Nicotiana benthamiana* transiently expressing artemisinin biosynthetic pathway genes is a function of CYP71AV1 type and relative gene dosage. *New Phytol.* **2013**, *199*, 352–366. [CrossRef]

17. Farhi, M.; Marhevka, E.; Ben-Ari, J.; Algamas-Dimantov, A.; Liang, Z.; Zeevi, V.; Edelbaum, O.; Spitzer-Rimon, B.; Abeliovich, H.; Schwartz, B. Generation of the potent anti-malarial drug artemisinin in tobacco. *Nat. Biotechnol.* **2011**, *29*, 1072–1074. [CrossRef]

18. Zhang, Y.; Nowak, G.; Reed, D.W.; Covello, P.S. The production of artemisinin precursors in tobacco. *Plant Biotechnol. J.* **2011**, *9*, 445–454. [CrossRef]

19. Wang, B.; Kashkooli, A.B.; Sallets, A.; Ting, H.-M.; de Ruijter, N.C.; Olofsson, L.; Brodelius, P.; Pottier, M.; Boutry, M.; Bouwmeester, H. Transient production of artemisinin in *Nicotiana benthamiana* is boosted by a specific lipid transfer protein from a. Annua. *Metab. Eng.* **2016**, *38*, 159–169. [CrossRef]

20. Fuentes, P.; Zhou, F.; Erban, A.; Karcher, D.; Kopka, J.; Bock, R. A new synthetic biology approach allows transfer of an entire metabolic pathway from a medicinal plant to a biomass crop. *eLife* **2016**, *5*, e13664. [CrossRef]

21. Ikram, N.K.; Simonsen, H.T. A review of biotechnological artemisinin production in plants. *Front. Plant Sci.* **2017**, *8*, 1966. [CrossRef] [PubMed]

22. Malhotra, K.; Subramaniyan, M.; Rawat, K.; Kalamuddin, M.; Qureshi, M.I.; Malhotra, P.; Mohmmed, A.; Cornish, K.; Daniell, H.; Kumar, S. Compartmentalized metabolic engineering for artemisinin biosynthesis and effective malaria treatment by oral delivery of plant cells. *Mol. Plant* **2016**, *9*, 1464–1477. [CrossRef] [PubMed]

23. Ikram, K.; Binti, N.K.; Beyraghdar Kashkooli, A.; Peramuna, A.V.; van der Krol, A.R.; Bouwmeester, H.; Simonsen, H.T. Stable production of the antimalarial drug artemisinin in the moss *Physcomitrella patens*. *Front. Bioeng. Biotechnol.* **2017**, *5*, 47. [CrossRef] [PubMed]

24. Zhan, X.; Han, L.A.; Zhang, Y.; Chen, D.; Simonsen, H.T. Metabolic engineering of the moss *Physcomitrella patens* to produce the sesquiterpenoids patchoulol and α/β-santalene. *Front. Plant Sci.* **2014**, *5*, 636. [CrossRef] [PubMed]

25. Pan, X.-W.; Han, L.; Zhang, Y.-H.; Chen, D.-F.; Simonsen, H.T. Sclareol production in the moss *Physcomitrella patens* and observations on growth and terpenoid biosynthesis. *Plant Biotechnol. Rep.* **2015**, *9*, 149–159. [CrossRef]

26. Brown, G.D.; Sy, L.-K. In vivo transformations of artemisinic acid in *Artemisia annua* plants. *Tetrahedron* **2007**, *63*, 9548–9566. [CrossRef]

27. Hamberger, B.; Bak, S. Plant P450s as versatile drivers for evolution of species-specific chemical diversity. *Philos. Trans. R. Soc. B: Biol. Sci.* **2013**, *368*, 20120426. [CrossRef]

28. Kashkooli, A.B.; van der Krol, A.; Rabe, P.; Dickschat, J.S.; Bouwmeester, H. Substrate promiscuity of enzymes from the sesquiterpene biosynthetic pathways from *Artemisia annua* and *Tanacetum parthenium* allows for novel combinatorial sesquiterpene production. *Metab. Eng.* **2019**.

29. Weitzel, C.; Simonsen, H.T. Cytochrome P450-enzymes involved in the biosynthesis of mono-and sesquiterpenes. *Phytochem. Rev.* **2015**, *14*, 7–24. [CrossRef]

30. Dueholm, B.; Krieger, C.; Drew, D.; Olry, A.; Kamo, T.; Taboureau, O.; Weitzel, C.; Bourgaud, F.; Hehn, A.; Simonsen, H.T. Evolution of substrate recognition sites (srss) in cytochromes P450 from Apiaceae exemplified by the CYP71AJ subfamily. *BMC Evol. Biol.* **2015**, *15*, 122. [CrossRef]

31. Zhan, X.; Bach, S.S.; Hansen, N.L.; Lunde, C.; Simonsen, H.T. Additional diterpenes from *Physcomitrella patens* synthesized by copalyl diphosphate/kaurene synthase (*Pp*CPS/KS). *Plant Physiol. Biochem.* **2015**, *96*, 110–114. [CrossRef] [PubMed]

32. Noguchi, C.; Miyazaki, S.; Kawaide, H.; Gotoh, O.; Yoshida, Y.; Aoyama, Y. Characterization of moss ent-kaurene oxidase (CYP701B1) using a highly purified preparation. *J. Biochem.* **2017**, *163*, 69–76. [CrossRef] [PubMed]

33. Yonekura-Sakakibara, K.; Hanada, K. An evolutionary view of functional diversity in family 1 glycosyltransferases. *Plant J.* **2011**, *66*, 182–193. [CrossRef] [PubMed]

34. Yang, K.; Monafared, R.S.; Wang, H.; Lundgren, A.; Brodelius, P.E. The activity of the artemisinic aldehyde δ11 (13) reductase promoter is important for artemisinin yield in different chemotypes of *Artemisia annua*. *Plant Mol. Biol.* **2015**, *88*, 325–340. [CrossRef] [PubMed]

35. Yuan, Y.; Liu, W.; Zhang, Q.; Xiang, L.; Liu, X.; Chen, M.; Lin, Z.; Wang, Q.; Liao, Z. Overexpression of artemisinic aldehyde δ11 (13) reductase gene–enhanced artemisinin and its relative metabolite biosynthesis in transgenic *Artemisia annua* L. *Biotechnol. Appl. Biochem.* **2015**, *62*, 17–23. [CrossRef] [PubMed]

36. Huang, C.-Y.; Chung, C.-I.; Lin, Y.-C.; Hsing, Y.-I.C.; Huang, A.H.C. Oil bodies and oleosins in *Physcomitrella* possess characteristics representative of early trends in evolution. *Plant Physiol.* **2009**, *150*, 1192–1203. [CrossRef]

37. Bach, S.S.; King, B.C.; Zhan, X.; Simonsen, H.T.; Hamberger, B. Heterologous stable expression of terpenoid biosynthetic genes using the moss *Physcomitrella patens*. In *Plant Isoprenoids. Methods in Molecular Biology (Methods and Protocols), Vol. 1153*; Humana Press: New York, NY, USA, 2014; pp. 257–271.

38. Cove, D.J.; Perroud, P.-F.; Charron, A.J.; McDaniel, S.F.; Khandelwal, A.; Quatrano, R.S. The moss *Physcomitrella patens*: A novel model system for plant development and genomic studies. *Cold Spring Harb. Protoc.* **2009**, *2009*, pdb.emo115. [CrossRef]

39. Schindelin, J.; Rueden, C.T.; Hiner, M.C.; Eliceiri, K.W. The ImageJ ecosystem: An open platform for biomedical image analysis. *Molecular Reproduction and Development* **2015**, *82*, 518–529. [CrossRef]

40. Livak, K.J.; Schmittgen, T.D. Analysis of relative gene expression data using real-time quantitative pcr and the 2− δδct method. *Methods* **2001**, *25*, 402–408. [CrossRef]

Permissions

All chapters in this book were first published by MDPI; hereby published with permission under the Creative Commons Attribution License or equivalent. Every chapter published in this book has been scrutinized by our experts. Their significance has been extensively debated. The topics covered herein carry significant findings which will fuel the growth of the discipline. They may even be implemented as practical applications or may be referred to as a beginning point for another development.

The contributors of this book come from diverse backgrounds, making this book a truly international effort. This book will bring forth new frontiers with its revolutionizing research information and detailed analysis of the nascent developments around the world.

We would like to thank all the contributing authors for lending their expertise to make the book truly unique. They have played a crucial role in the development of this book. Without their invaluable contributions this book wouldn't have been possible. They have made vital efforts to compile up to date information on the varied aspects of this subject to make this book a valuable addition to the collection of many professionals and students.

This book was conceptualized with the vision of imparting up-to-date information and advanced data in this field. To ensure the same, a matchless editorial board was set up. Every individual on the board went through rigorous rounds of assessment to prove their worth. After which they invested a large part of their time researching and compiling the most relevant data for our readers.

The editorial board has been involved in producing this book since its inception. They have spent rigorous hours researching and exploring the diverse topics which have resulted in the successful publishing of this book. They have passed on their knowledge of decades through this book. To expedite this challenging task, the publisher supported the team at every step. A small team of assistant editors was also appointed to further simplify the editing procedure and attain best results for the readers.

Apart from the editorial board, the designing team has also invested a significant amount of their time in understanding the subject and creating the most relevant covers. They scrutinized every image to scout for the most suitable representation of the subject and create an appropriate cover for the book.

The publishing team has been an ardent support to the editorial, designing and production team. Their endless efforts to recruit the best for this project, has resulted in the accomplishment of this book. They are a veteran in the field of academics and their pool of knowledge is as vast as their experience in printing. Their expertise and guidance has proved useful at every step. Their uncompromising quality standards have made this book an exceptional effort. Their encouragement from time to time has been an inspiration for everyone.

The publisher and the editorial board hope that this book will prove to be a valuable piece of knowledge for researchers, students, practitioners and scholars across the globe.

List of Contributors

Seong Soo Moon, Hye Jin Lee, Yu Jin Kim and Jin Woo Min
Department of Oriental Medicinal Biotechnology, College of Life Science, Kyung Hee University, 1 Seocheon-dong, Giheung-gu, Yongin-si, Gyeonggi-do 17104, Korea

Deok Chun Yang
Department of Oriental Medicinal Biotechnology, College of Life Science, Kyung Hee University, 1 Seocheon-dong, Giheung-gu, Yongin-si, Gyeonggi-do 17104, Korea
Graduate School of Biotechnology, College of Life Science, Kyung Hee University, 1 Seocheon-dong, Giheung-gu, Yongin-si, Gyeonggi-do 17104, Korea

Ramya Mathiyalagan and Zuly Jimenez
Graduate School of Biotechnology, College of Life Science, Kyung Hee University, 1 Seocheon-dong, Giheung-gu, Yongin-si, Gyeonggi-do 17104, Korea

Dong Uk Yang
Department of Oriental Medicinal Biotechnology, College of Life Science, Kyung Hee University, 1 Seocheon-dong, Giheung-gu, Yongin-si, Gyeonggi-do 17104, Korea
K-gen (corp), 218, Gajeong-ro, Yuseong-gu, Daejeon 34129, Korea

Dae Young Lee
Department of Herbal Crop Research, National Institute of Horticultural and Herbal Science, RDA, Eumseong 27709, Korea

Stefania Schiavone, Paolo Tucci, Luigia Trabace and Maria Grazia Morgese
Department of Clinical and Experimental Medicine, University of Foggia, Viale Pinto, 1 71122 Foggia, Italy

Huynh Nhu Tuan and Ha Van Oanh
Hanoi University of Pharmacy, 13 Le Thanh Tong Street, Hoan Kiem District, Hanoi 100100, Vietnam

Bui Hoang Minh
Faculty of Pharmacy, Nguyen Tat Thanh University, 300C Nguyen Tat Thanh Street, District 4, Hochiminh City 72820, Vietnam

Phuong Thao Tran and Jeong Hyung Lee
Department of Biochemistry, College of Natural Sciences, Kangwon National University, Chuncheon, Gangwon-Do 24414, Korea

Quynh Mai Thi Ngo
College of Pharmacy, Hai Phong University of Medicine and Pharmacy, 72A Nguyen Binh Khiem, Hai Phong 180000, Vietnam

Yen Nhi Nguyen
Faculty of Biology and Biotechnology, University of Science, Vietnam National University Hochiminh City, 227 Nguyen Van Cu, District 5, Hochiminh City 748000, Vietnam

Pham Thi Kim Lien and Manh Hung Tran
Biomedical Sciences Department, Institute for Research & Executive Education (VNUK), The University of Danang, 158A Le Loi, Hai Chau District, Danang City 551000, Vietnam

Vittoria Graziani, Assunta Esposito, Angela Chambery, Rosita Russo and Nicoletta Potenza
Dipartimento di Scienze e Tecnologie Ambientali Biologiche e Farmaceutiche (DiSTABiF), Università degli Studi della Campania "Luigi Vanvitelli", via Vivaldi 43, I-81100 Caserta, Italy

Monica Scognamiglio
Department of Biochemistry, Max Planck Institute for Chemical Ecology-Beutenberg Campus, Hans-Knöll-Straße, 8 D-07745 Jena, Germany

Fortunato Ciardiello and Teresa Troiani
Dipartimento di Medicina di Precisione, Università degli Studi della Campania "Luigi Vanvitelli" - Via Pansini, 5, 80131 Napoli, Italy

Antonio Fiorentino and Brigida D'Abrosca
Dipartimento di Scienze e Tecnologie Ambientali Biologiche e Farmaceutiche (DiSTABiF), Università degli Studi della Campania "Luigi Vanvitelli", via Vivaldi 43, I-81100 Caserta, Italy
Dipartimento di Biotecnologia Marina, Stazione Zoologica Anton Dohrn, Villa Comunale, 80121 Naples, Italy

Deepika Singh, Yin-Yin Siew, Teck-Ian Chong, Hui-Chuing Yew, Samuel Shan-Wei Ho, Claire Sophie En-Shen Lim, Wei-Xun Tan, Soek-Ying Neo and Hwee-Ling Koh
Department of Pharmacy, Faculty of Science, National University of Singapore, 18 Science Drive 4, Singapore 117543, Singapore

Xuyang Lu
Institute of Mountain Hazards and Environment, Chinese Academy of Sciences, Chengdu 610041, China Key Laboratory of Mountain Surface Processes and Ecological Regulation, Chinese Academy of Sciences, Chengdu 610041, China

Shuqin Ma
College of Tourism, Henan Normal University, Xinxiang 453007, China

Youchao Chen
Wuhan Botanical Garden, Chinese Academy of Sciences, Wuhan 430074, China

Degyi Yangzom
Ecological Monitoring & Research Center, Tibetan Environment Monitoring Station, Lhasa 850000, China

Hongmao Jiang
Institute of Mountain Hazards and Environment, Chinese Academy of Sciences, Chengdu 610041, China University of Chinese Academy of Sciences, Beijing 100049, China

Yinglin Zheng, Yichen Tong, Xinfeng Wang, Jiebin Zhou and Jiyan Pang
School of Chemistry, Sun Yat-Sen University, Guangzhou 510275, China

Tongchai Saesong, Prapapan Temkitthawon and Kornkanok Ingkaninan
Department of Pharmaceutical Chemistry and Pharmacognosy, Faculty of Pharmaceutical Sciences and Center of Excellence for Innovation in Chemistry, Naresuan University, Phitsanulok 65000, Thailand

Pierre-Marie Allard, Emerson Ferreira Queiroz, Laurence Marcourt and Jean-Luc Wolfender
School of Pharmaceutical Sciences, EPGL, University of Geneva, University of Lausanne, CMU Rue Michel Servet 1, 1211 Geneva 4, Switzerland

Nitra Nuengchamnong
Science Lab Center, Faculty of Science, Naresuan University, Phitsanulok 65000, Thailand

Nantaka Khorana
Division of Pharmaceutical Sciences, School of Pharmaceutical Sciences, University of Phayao, Phayao 56000, Thailand

Anja Hartmann, Markus Ganzera and Hermann Stuppner
Institute of Pharmacy, Pharmacognosy, CMBI, University of Innsbruck, Innrain 80-82, 6020 Innsbruck, Austria

Ulf Karsten
Institute of Biological Sciences, Applied Ecology & Phycology, University of Rostock, Albert-Einstein-Str. 3, 18059 Rostock, Germany

Alexsander Skhirtladze
Department of Phytochemistry, Iovel Kutateladze Institute of Pharmacochemistry, Tbilisi State Medical University, 0159 Tbilisi, Georgia

Marco A. Loza-Mejía, Juan Rodrigo Salazar and Juan Francisco Sánchez-Tejeda
Benjamín Franklin 45, Cuauhtémoc, Mexico City 06140, Mexico

Yan Wang, James Zheng Shen, Yuk Wah Chan and Wing Shing Ho
School of Life Sciences, Chinese University of Hong Kong, Shatin, Hong Kong, China

Ya Chen, Conrad Stork and Steffen Hirte
Center for Bioinformatics (ZBH), Department of Informatics, Faculty of Mathematics, Informatics and Natural Sciences, Universität Hamburg, 20146 Hamburg, Germany

Johannes Kirchmair
Center for Bioinformatics (ZBH), Department of Informatics, Faculty of Mathematics, Informatics and Natural Sciences, Universität Hamburg, 20146 Hamburg, Germany
Department of Chemistry, University of Bergen, 5007 Bergen, Norway
Computational Biology Unit (CBU), Department of Informatics, University of Bergen, 5008 Bergen, Norway

Nik Amirah Mahizan, Shun-Kai Yang and Chew-Li Moo
Department of Cell and Molecular Biology, Faculty of Biotechnology and Biomolecular Sciences, Universiti Putra Malaysia, 43400 Serdang, Selangor, Malaysia

Adelene Ai-Lian Song
Department of Microbiology, Faculty of Biotechnology and Biomolecular Sciences, Universiti Putra Malaysia, 43400 Serdang, Selangor, Malaysia

Chou-Min Chong
Department of Aquaculture, Faculty of Agriculture, Universiti Putra Malaysia, 43400 Serdang, Selangor, Malaysia

Chun-Wie Chong
School of Pharmacy, Monash University Malaysia, Jalan Lagoon Selatan, Bandar Sunway 47500, Selangor, Malaysia

Aisha Abushelaibi and Swee-Hua Erin Lim
Health Sciences Division, Abu Dhabi Women's College, Higher Colleges of Technology, 41012 Abu Dhabi, UAE

Kok-Song Lai
Department of Cell and Molecular Biology, Faculty of Biotechnology and Biomolecular Sciences, Universiti Putra Malaysia, 43400 Serdang, Selangor, Malaysia
Health Sciences Division, Abu Dhabi Women's College, Higher Colleges of Technology, 41012 Abu Dhabi, UAE

Bee Ling Tan
Department of Nutrition and Dietetics, Faculty of Medicine and Health Sciences, Universiti Putra Malaysia, Serdang 43400, Selangor, Malaysia

Mohd Esa Norhaizan
Department of Nutrition and Dietetics, Faculty of Medicine and Health Sciences, Universiti Putra Malaysia, Serdang 43400, Selangor, Malaysia
Laboratory of Molecular Biomedicine, Institute of Bioscience, Universiti Putra Malaysia, Serdang 43400, Selangor, Malaysia
Research Centre of Excellent, Nutrition and Non-Communicable Diseases (NNCD), Faculty of Medicine and Health Sciences, Universiti Putra Malaysia, Serdang 43400, Selangor, Malaysia

Arman Beyraghdar Kashkooli
Laboratory of Plant Physiology, Wageningen University and Research, Droevendaalsesteeg 1, 6708 PB Wageningen, The Netherlands
Bioscience, Wageningen Plant Research, Wageningen University and Research, Droevendaalsesteeg 1, 6708 PB Wageningen, The Netherlands

Anantha Peramuna and Henrik Toft Simonsen
Department of Biotechnology and Biomedicine, Technical University of Denmark, Søltofts Plads, 2800 Kgs. Lyngby, Denmark

Harro Bouwmeester
Laboratory of Plant Physiology, Wageningen University and Research, Droevendaalsesteeg 1, 6708 PB Wageningen, The Netherlands
Plant Hormone Biology group, Swammerdam Institute for Life Sciences, University of Amsterdam, 1098 XH Amsterdam, The Netherlands

Nur Kusaira Khairul Ikram
Institute of Biological Sciences, Faculty of Science, University of Malaya, Kuala Lumpur 50603, Malaysia
Centre for Research in Biotechnology for Agriculture (CEBAR), University of Malaya, Kuala Lumpur 50603, Malaysia

Alexander R. van der Krol
Laboratory of Plant Physiology, Wageningen University and Research, Droevendaalsesteeg 1, 6708 PB Wageningen, The Netherlands

Index

Printed in the USA
CPSIA information can be obtained
at www.ICGtesting.com
JSHW051406091023
49903JS00006B/306